Neuropsychological Validation
of Learning Disability Subtypes

Neuropsychological Validation of Learning Disability Subtypes

Edited by

Byron P. Rourke
University of Windsor

THE GUILFORD PRESS
New York   London

© 1991 The Guilford Press
A Division of Guilford Publications, Inc.
72 Spring Street, New York, NY 10012

Printed in the United States of America

This book is printed on acid-free paper.

Last digit is print number: 9 8 7 6 5 4 3 2 1

Library of Congress Cataloging-in-Publication Data

Neuropsychological validation of learning disability subtypes / edited
by Byron P. Rourke.
　　p.　cm.
　　Includes bibliographical references.
　　Includes index.
　　ISBN 0-89862-446-0
　　1. Learning disabilities.　2. Learning disabilities—
Classification.　3. Neuropsychology.　I. Rourke, Byron P. (Byron
Patrick), 1939–
　　[DNLM: 1. Learning Disorders—classification.　2. Learning
Disorders—diagnosis.　3. Neuropsychological Tests.　WS 110 N494]
RC394.L37N48　1991
616.85′889′0012—dc20
DNLM/DLC
for Library of Congress　　　　　　　　　　　　　　　　90-3912
　　　　　　　　　　　　　　　　　　　　　　　　　　　　　CIP

FOR MARILYN

Contributors

Kenneth M. Adams, Ph.D., Psychology Service, V.A. Medical Center, Ann Arbor, Michigan, and Department of Psychiatry, University of Michigan Medical Center, Ann Arbor, Michigan

Dirk J. Bakker, Ph.D., Department of Child Neuropsychology, PPW-Faculty, Free University, Amsterdam, The Netherlands

Linas A. Bieliauskas, Ph.D., Psychology Service, V.A. Medical Center, Ann Arbor, Michigan

Clare F. Brandys, Ph.D., Department of Neuropsychology, St. Michael's Hospital, Toronto, Ontario, Canada

Joseph E. Casey, M.A., Department of Psychology, University of Windsor, Windsor, Ontario, Canada

Jerel E. Del Dotto, Ph.D., Division of Neuropsychology, Henry Ford Hospital, Detroit, Michigan

John W. DeLuca, Ph.D., Psychology Department, Lafayette Clinic, Detroit, Michigan

Kimberly A. Espy, M.A., Department of Psychology, University of Houston, Houston, Texas

Christina A. M. Fiedorowicz, Ph.D., Research and Development, Autoskill Inc., Ottawa, Ontario, Canada

John L. Fisk, Ph.D., Division of Neuropsychology, Henry Ford Hospital, Detroit, Michigan

Jack M. Fletcher, Ph.D., Department of Pediatrics, University of Texas Medical School, Houston, Texas

Jane M. Flynn, Ph.D., Gundersen Foundation Research Center, Gundersen Medical Center, LaCrosse, Wisconsin

David J. Francis, Ph.D., Department of Psychology, University of Houston, Houston, Texas

Darren R. Fuerst, Ph.D., Department of Psychology, University of Windsor, Windsor, Ontario, Canada

Gerald Goldstein, Ph.D., Neuropsychology Research, V.A. Medical Center, Pittsburgh, Pennsylvania, and Departments of Psychiatry and Psychology, University of Pittsburgh, Pittsburgh, Pennsylvania

Robert Licht, Ph.D., Department of Child Neuropsychology, PPW-Faculty, Free University, Amsterdam, The Netherlands

G. Reid Lyon, Ph.D., Department of Education, Johnson State College, Johnson, Vermont

Michael McCue, Ph.D., Behavioral Neuropsychology Associates, Pittsburgh, Pennsylvania

Gerald T. McFadden, Ph.D., Department of Psychology, University of Windsor, Windsor, Ontario, Canada

Robin D. Morris, Ph.D., Department of Psychology, Georgia State University, Atlanta, Georgia

Edite J. Ozols, Ph.D., Department of Psychological Services, Toronto Board of Education, Toronto, Ontario, Canada

Byron P. Rourke, Ph.D., Department of Psychology, University of Windsor, Windsor, Ontario, Canada

Diane L. Russell, Ph.D., Waterman, Russell, Wilkinson & Associates, Nanaimo, British Columbia, Canada

Sara S. Sparrow, Ph.D., Yale University Child Study Center, New Haven, Connecticut

Ronald L. Trites, Ph.D., Faculty of Medicine, University of Ottawa, Ottawa, Ontario, Canada

Harry van der Vlugt, Ph.D., M.D., Department of Neuropsychology, University of Tilburg, Tilburg, The Netherlands

Jan van Strien, Ph.D., Department of Child Neuropsychology, PPW-Faculty, Free University, Amsterdam, The Netherlands

L. Warren Walter, Ph.D., Department of Psychology, Georgia State University, Atlanta, Georgia

Preface

This book is a companion volume to our first effort to deal with the basic scientific and clinical issues involved in learning disability subtypes (Rourke, 1985). Approximately one-half of the contributions to the 1985 volume dealt with considerations regarding the reliability of learning disability subtypes. This is to be expected, since one must first deal with the consistency and stability of psychological phenomena before dealing to any great extent with their validity. Nevertheless, there were a number of contributions to this initial volume that dealt quite explicitly with issues of validation.

The current work expands on these earlier attempts at the validation enterprise, and it continues the tradition of considering these attempts to specify both the reliability and the validity of learning disability subtypes within an explicitly neuropsychological framework. As will become apparent to the reader, the dimensions of reliability take a decidedly second seat to the primary concerns of this volume, namely, the determination of the extent to which various subtyping schemes are valid. A feature that the current work shares in common with its predecessor is the concern for the ecological validity of learning disability subtypes, especially as regards the implications that the subtyping enterprise holds for assessment and intervention for persons who exhibit academic, vocational, and/or socioemotional problems associated with their learning disabilities.

Before launching this endeavor, it would be well to acknowledge the contributions of two persons in particular without whose efforts this book would never have come to fruition. Marilyn Chedour read and commented on all of the chapters; Mary Stewart assiduously edited and critiqued all of the contributions. Both of these persons played crucial roles in the generation of this volume.

In addition to the ordinary duties associated with editing such a volume, I have done my best to arrange and integrate the chapters in a manner that I thought would aid in their understanding. It goes without saying that any and all limitations that remain in the work are my responsibility.

BYRON P. ROURKE

Reference

Rourke, B. P. (Ed.). (1985). *Neuropsychology of learning disabilities: Essentials of subtype analysis.* New York: Guilford Press.

Contents

References, 307

B. Adult Studies

15. *Neuropsychological Aspects of Learning Disability*
    in Adults   311
    Michael McCue and Gerald Goldstein

    Statement of the Problem, 311
    Prototype Neuropsychological Profiles of Learning-Disabled
        Adults, 315
    Neuropsychological Subtypes of Learning-Disabled Adults, 320
    Summary and Implications for Rehabilitation, 326
    References, 327

16. *Subtypes of Arithmetic-Disabled Adults:*
    Validating Childhood Findings   330
    Robin D. Morris and L. Warren Walter

    Deficits in Mathematics-Related Abilities, 331
    SMD in Adults, 333
    Study of SMD in College Students, 334
    Study Results, 335
    Case Illustrations, 338
    Discussion, 339
    References, 343

VI. DIMENSIONS OF CLINICAL VALIDITY

17. *Case Studies of Children with*
    Nonverbal Learning Disabilities   349
    Sara S. Sparrow

    Case Study 1, 349
    Case Study 2, 352

18. *Case Studies of Adolescents with*
    Nonverbal Learning Disabilities   356
    John W. DeLuca

    Introduction
    Case Study 1, 356
    Case Study 2, 363
    Acknowledgments, 369
    Reference, 369

Neuropsychological Validation
of Learning Disability Subtypes

Introduction

CHAPTER 1

Validation of Learning Disability Subtypes: An Overview

Byron P. Rourke

Dimensions of Validity

The notion of validity, in its simplest terms, is the notion of truth. When we ask the question, "What is the validity of a learning disability subtype?" we are, essentially, asking what is true about it. And, just as truth has many facets and dimensions, so too does validity.

Let us, for example, consider *content* validity. This type of validity is usually addressed within the framework of the evaluation of the adequacy of measures such as scholastic tests. Thus, an academic test is valid from a content standpoint insofar as it mirrors the content of the course up to that point, that is, to the extent that it constitutes an adequate sample of what truly went on in it.

At its highest level, of course, we have the notion of *construct* validity. In psychometrics, construct validity involves answers to a rather straightforward question: Does a test actually measure what it purports to measure? In the case of considerations relating to the validity of a learning disability subtype, the question of import is certainly more specific but essentially no different: Do the dimensions of the subtype actually reflect the truth about the way in which the persons so classified within it actually learn?

In both of these first two types of validity considerations we see important dimensions to consider in learning disability subtyping efforts. First, there is the issue of the content of the subtype. In this context we have to ask questions relating to the coverage of the measures used to characterize the subtype. Do these measures actually represent in some truthful fashion the abilities and skills that should have developed in those persons so classified? This leads to a second, intimately related issue: Are these tests sufficient to characterize the dimensions of learning that are being addressed by the subtype exercise? In this way, considera-

3

tions of content validity lead to considerations of construct validity. Consideration of the adequacy of the coverage of the tests and measures on which subtyping is based leads to the crucial question: Do these measures actually reflect in some veridical manner the assets and deficits vis-à-vis learning that the individuals classified in the subtype actually experience?

I stress the interrelatedness of these two types of validity because they are in some senses the purest dimensions of validity, as considered from an epistemological perspective. Of course, the more frequently investigated dimensions of concurrent and predictive validity are also concerned with truth. But the truth that is focused on has a rather more limited spectrum than do considerations of content and construct validity. Let me be specific on this point.

The notion of *concurrent* validity lies at the very heart of psychometrics and every other area of scientific measurement. The question of interest in this context is whether and to what extent the sample of behavior as measured in the test in question mirrors the current status of the organism. Do the results of this blood test truly mirror the presence of health or disease? Does the profile on this psychological test reflect the presence or absence of schizophrenia? Does a score on Test X that falls three standard deviations below the mean reflect the presence of brain damage? Note that these questions relate to a rather limited spectrum of the characteristics of any particular individual so classified; specifically, we may not be interested in how the person in question interacts with other people, how he/she learns to read, or how concepts are formed under various conditions of duress. Rather, we may choose to focus our efforts solely on the determination of the presence or absence of one or more states of being that are relatively superficial as compared to the complex interactions to which I have just alluded.

This does not mean to say that, say, schizophrenia itself, as experienced and lived by the person so afflicted, is a superficial characteristic. Rather, the point to be made here is that the test designed to be truly valid for the diagnosis of schizophrenia has as its aim the relatively superficial aim of designation: it does not aim to specify in detail the complex sets of personal and social interactions that characterize the individual's full existential experience of the disorder.

Of what relevance is this discussion for the determination of the concurrent validity of learning disability subtypes? Just this: The designation of a learning disability subtype as valid from a concurrent standpoint may mean as little (or as much) as the specification of the extent to which this subtype, as compared to other subtypes, is deficient in complex as opposed to simple language skills. Thus, the only truth that is being expressed by this correlation is that being a member of this learning disability subtype implies that one is (concurrently) more or less adept at one of these linguistic dimensions. The establishment of the extent of the concurrent validity in this instance does not explain in any very rich manner how the individual who is in this situation experiences this relationship. Indeed, there is every reason to believe that what is, from the scientist's perspective, a relationship, may, from the individual's perspective, be nothing of the kind. Quite apart from this existential issue is the question that can be answered scientifically: Is there a causal relationship between this subtype of learning disability and relative deficiencies in complex versus simple language skills?

In a similar vein, with a mere change of focus from the present to the future, we have the test of veridicality referred to as *predictive* validity. This type of validity varies from concurrent validity only insofar as the present differs from the future. The task is the same. What do our psychological measures tell us about the true classification into which a limited aspect of the person's attributes fit (e.g., sick or healthy now; sick or healthy 5 years from now)? In the case of learning disability subtypes, we would, for example, be interested in the probability that children classified within a particular subtype on the basis of (say) academic variables are (1) likely to exhibit one or another type or degree of (say) psychopathology now (concurrent validity) or (2) in the future (predictive validity). Note, once again, the fairly restricted scope in terms of human attributes targeted in these cases.

That an aptitude test only predicts outcome in scholastic endeavors at a very high rate may not be very dramatic, but it can be very important. It may not tell us very much about the vicissitudes faced by individual students as they struggle with the learning process. Among other things, however, it does shed some light on issues that are usually very important with respect to (1) student selection for specific courses, (2) the planning of programs of special assistance for those who are likely to need these to cope with academic demands, and (3) the dimensions of performance that, on closer scrutiny, are likely to yield not only better prognostications (predictive validity) but also keener insights into the nature of the skills and abilities that are needed for success—and, presumably, the absence of which lead to failure—in the academic enterprise at a particular time (concurrent validity).

But, once again we must concern ourselves with the individual: What about the multidimensional richness of the individual in all of this? Where are the validity considerations germane to this issue? One way of addressing the issue is to make predictions based on the putative construct validity of a subtype—which is another way of characterizing what is meant by a "model" in the scientific study of subtypes—and then to see if these predictions hold true in the individual case. Thus, one may carry out intensive investigations of individuals to determine if they behave in a manner that would be predicted from the model. The extent to which an individual does, in fact, behave in a fashion predicted from the model designed to explain, say, the neurodevelopmental dimensions of a particular subtype, is the extent to which the construct validity of the subtype and its associated model are "true." On the other hand, if predictions based on the model of the subtype are largely unsupported, then the model must be either modified or abandoned. Here again, the criterion for acceptance of the model (of the subtype) is the extent to which it can be shown to be valid (i.e., a true reflection of what actually transpires in the real world). This reasoning leads to the now-popular notion of "ecological validity," the importance of which in the field of learning disabilities has been commented on extensively (Fisk, Finnell, & Rourke, 1985; Rourke, 1985b, 1989).

With these considerations as background, we now turn to an overview of the chapters that follow. The aim of this exercise is to place these chapters within the context of the considerations of validity outlined above.

Overview of the Book

In Section II, two issues relating to rather basic concerns in the study of learning disability subtypes are addressed. One has to do with definitional issues and the effect of level of psychometric intelligence considerations (Francis et al., Chapter 2); the other is concerned with the stability of the solutions arrived at in subtyping studies (DeLuca et al., Chapter 3). Although these are, in the strict sense, not validity studies, they do involve important "bridging" considerations between earlier work (Rourke, 1985a) devoted largely to issues of reliability, and that contained in the current volume.

The role that "discrepancy" considerations play in the definition of learning disabilities is certainly germane to the truthfulness of the definitions of learning disabilities. Indeed, Francis et al. demonstrate fairly conclusively that different assumptions and starting points will yield different characterizations of who will be designated as learning disabled. Such considerations and the choices that they demand are crucial to the dimensions of learning disability subtypes that are the focus of concern in the other sections of this work.

Another set of choices that must be made in this emerging field is illustrated by DeLuca et al. In this instance, the classificatory system itself is shown to produce differing results depending on the assumptions and starting points that one selects at the beginning of the exercise. Since the stability of subtypes and other considerations relating to reliability are factors that have a crucial impact on validity studies, it was felt that this type of exercise would serve as a salutory reminder of the delicate nature of the subtyping enterprise.

The studies contained within Section III are those that are most easily seen as falling within the framework of traditional considerations of validity. Chapter 4, for example, addresses issues relating to concurrent and predictive validity. The question posed by Russell and Rourke is quite simple: To what extent does the level of phonetic accuracy of the misspellings of disabled learners relate to their current and future neuropsychological status? The astute reader will note that this study constitutes a departure from the subtype endeavor insofar as it deals with the continuous dimension of phonetic accuracy of misspellings rather than with the more usual designation of "phonetically accurate" and "phonetically inaccurate" disabled spellers (Sweeney & Rourke, 1978, 1985). We present this study to demonstrate that there is more than one way to skin the learning disability cat! Our next studies in this series will seek to determine whether or not concurrent and predictive validity are enhanced when disabled spellers are "subtyped" on the basis of this dimension of their spelling performance. More to the point, however, is the rather astounding finding in this study that this rather erstwhile dimension of spelling style relates so strongly to dimensions as diverse as finger-tapping speed and nonverbal concept formation.

Chapter 5 (Brandys & Rourke) has a very different tack. In this instance, children with learning disabilities are subtyped in terms of academic achievement variables, and then their memory capacities are assessed. Note that this is an example of model testing and, as such, is a study that combines concurrent validity with the more extensive dimensions of construct validity. That some of the hypotheses in this study are supported and some are not is a testament to the extent to which the models employed to generate these predictions are bolstered or need modification.

The studies reported in Chapter 6 (Ozols & Rourke) cover a wide gamut of "validity" variables for children subtyped or classified primarily in terms of academic achievement dimensions. Of particular interest are the comparisons made between the patterns of performance of these "younger" (7- to 8-year-old) children with learning disabilities and those "older" (9- to 14-year-old) children with learning disabilities who have been investigated previously (Rourke & Finlayson, 1978; Rourke & Strang, 1978; Strang & Rourke, 1983; see Rourke, 1989, for a summary of these studies). This effort constitutes an example of concurrent validity as well as construct validity: concurrent because of the differences in skills and abilities demonstrated for the three "academic achievement" subtypes; construct because of the testing of specific hypotheses regarding outcomes and because of the developmental similarities and differences noted.

Psychobiological validation of L- and P-type dyslexia is described in Chapter 7. Bakker and his colleagues have produced a large amount of concurrent validity data for this typology. This effort is especially relevant because it involves the testing of predictions based on Bakker's "balance model" within the neurophysiological domain. This is the type of effort that is necessary to expand the construct validity of his model.

In a similar vein, van der Vlugt (Chapter 8) offers descriptions of a series of interrelated studies that run the gamut from cross-cultural validation of the neuropsychological and academic dimensions of learning disability subtypes (a dimension of ecological validity) to the validation of these subtypes on the basis of psychophysiological and neurophysiological measures (concurrent and construct validity). This combination of a variety of types of validation research is the sort of concerted, integrated effort that is likely to lead to advances in model building and hence in our understanding of learning disability subtypes.

Concurrent validity studies that deal with socioemotional dimensions of learning disability subtypes are contained in the next two chapters. In Chapter 9, Fuerst and Rourke present an integrated discussion of a series of studies that have focused on the determination of the relationship between learning disability subtypes and various manifestations of psychosocial disturbance. This effort may be of particular interest to those whose investigative efforts are programmatic in nature, with the conclusions of one study forming the basis for the hypotheses tested in the next. This series of studies also illustrates the relationships that must obtain between the establishment of the reliability of subtypes prior to the determination of their concurrent and predictive validity. Chapter 10 (DeLuca et al.) also illustrates the gamut (some might say gauntlet!) of steps through which one must go in order to establish the reliability and then to test the validity of learning disability subtypes. This chapter also illustrates how one can go about relating neuropsychological and psychosocial dimensions in the investigation of subtypes.

Section IV contains two chapters that address the very important ecological validity considerations relating to the subtype × treatment interaction issue. This has been an abiding concern of those involved in the learning disability subtyping enterprise since its outset. As suggested elsewhere (Fisk et al., 1985; Rourke, 1985b, 1989), this is the issue that lies at the very heart of this area of research for those who seek a rational and productive basis on which to prescribe intervention strategies for different subtypes of learning-disabled youngsters. As the authors of both Chapters 11 and 12 describe and explain very nicely, the process of advancing from subtype identification through reliability tests of the subtypes and finally to various types of validation study is a long and arduous one that is clearly not suited for the faint of heart. The programmatic studies of Lyon and Flynn (Chapter 11) and Fiedorowicz and Trites (Chapter 12), although quite different in focus and scope, provide excellent illustrations of the steps that should be involved in such ventures.

The cross-sectional and longitudinal studies described in Section V, Part A, focus on one learning disability subtype, namely, nonverbal learning disabilities (NLD) (Rourke, 1989). In these offerings by Casey and Rourke (Chapter 13) and Del Dotto et al. (Chapter 14), the aim is to test developmental hypotheses deduced from the NLD model. As such, these efforts would fall under the general rubrics of both predictive validity and construct validity. A close reading of these two chapters will demonstrate the very fine-grained levels of analysis of neuropsychological, behavioral, and psychosocial variables that can be carried out in such validation attempts. It is also easy to see how the results of the studies can lead to modifications in the model.

The investigations in the relatively unexplored area of adult learning disability subtypes in Section V, Part B, are quite different from one another. In Chapter 15, McCue and Goldstein present their integrated attempts to determine the reliability and validity of learning disability subtypes in adults. This presentation mirrors the efforts that have taken place in the study of children over the past few years. Although it is clear that much more needs to be done to develop this classificatory effort, this chapter points the way toward the dimensions of this issue that need to be addressed. Morris and Walter (Chapter 16) present a very explicit attempt to test hypotheses derived from the study of one particular childhood learning disability subtype to adults who manifest the academic achievement patterns in terms of which some arithmetic disability subtypes have been constituted. This is the sort of "cross-validation" within a developmental context that not only illuminates the developmental dimensions of learning disability subtypes but also provides the heuristic bases that are needed for the testing of the neurodevelopmental models that are beginning to appear within this context.

In Section VI, we come to what many might consider to be an example of the "acid test" for learning disability subtype validity considerations, namely, the validation of predictions derived from a model designed to encompass and explain a particular subtype in the individual case. Such investigations fall clearly within the requirements outlined eloquently by Reitan (1974) with respect to the nomothetic/idiographic dilemma, which have been the focus of concern of neuropsychological investigators in the learning disabilities field since the beginning of such efforts (Rourke, 1983). In a word, the validity question within this context is clear: Do individuals who have been identified in terms of the "markers" of the learning disability subtype in question behave in ways that are predictable on the basis of the model proposed for the subtype? The reader can judge for him/herself how adequately these three sets of efforts relating to children (Sparrow, Chapter 17), adolescents (DeLuca, Chapter 18), and adults (Bieliauskas, Chapter 19) answer this question. What may impress the reader is that these very different approaches to neuropsychological assessment of three quite different age groups yield conclusions that are remarkably similar.

A Final Comment

All that remains is for me to welcome the reader to this book. On a personal level, I hope that the enthusiasm and excitement of the authors of these chapters come through to the reader. On a scientific level, I hope that these very remarkable advances in the validation of learning disability subtypes will encourage those with the will, stamina, and resourcefulness to test these interesting waters with their own scientific oars. On a clinical level, I hope that practitioners will find herein the types of insights and suggestions that will enhance their treatment of those afflicted with the academic, vocational, and socioemotional limitations imposed by, and associated with, various subtypes of learning disabilities.

References

Fisk, J. L., Finnell, R., & Rourke, B. P. (1985). Major findings and future directions for learning disability subtype analysis. In B. P. Rourke (Ed.), *Neuropsychology of learning disabilities: Essentials of subtype analysis* (pp. 331-341). New York: Guilford Press.

Reitan, R. M. (1974). Methodological problems in clinical neuropsychology. In R. M. Reitan & L. A. Davison (Eds.), *Clinical neuropsychology: Current status and applications* (pp. 19-46). New York: John Wiley & Sons.

Rourke, B. P. (1983). Outstanding issues in research on learning disabilities. In M. Rutter (Ed.), *Developmental neuropsychiatry* (pp. 564-574). New York: Guilford Press.

Rourke, B. P. (Ed.). (1985a). *Neuropsychology of learning disabilities: Essentials of subtype analysis*. New York: Guilford Press.

Rourke, B. P. (1985b). Overview of learning disability subtypes. In B. P. Rourke (Ed.), *Neuropsychology of learning disabilities: Essentials of subtype analysis* (pp. 3-14). New York: Guilford Press.

Rourke, B. P. (1989). *Nonverbal learning disabilities: The syndrome and the model*. New York: Guilford Press.

Rourke, B. P., & Finlayson, M. A. J. (1978). Neuropsychological significance of variations in patterns of academic performance: Verbal and visual-spatial abilities. *Journal of Abnormal Child Psychology, 6*, 121-133.

Rourke, B. P., & Strang, J. D. (1978). Neuropsychological significance of variations in patterns of academic performance: Motor, psychomotor, and tactile–perceptual abilities. *Journal of Pediatric Psychology, 3,* 62–66.

Strang, J. D., & Rourke, B. P. (1983). Concept-formation/nonverbal reasoning abilities of children who exhibit specific academic problems with arithmetic. *Journal of Clinical Child Psychology, 12,* 33–39.

Sweeney, J. E., & Rourke, B. P. (1978). Neuropsychological significance of phonetically accurate and phonetically inaccurate spelling errors in younger and older retarded spellers. *Brain and Language, 5,* 212–225.

Sweeney, J. E., & Rourke, B. P. (1985). Spelling disability subtypes. In B. P. Rourke (Ed.), *Neuropsychology of learning disabilities: Essentials of subtype analysis* (pp. 147–166). New York: Guilford Press.

Methodology and Measurement

Validity of Intelligence Test Scores in the Definition of Learning Disability: A Critical Analysis

David J. Francis, Kimberly A. Espy, Byron P. Rourke, and Jack M. Fletcher

The relationship of intelligence test performance to learning deficiency is a longstanding issue affecting treatment and research on learning-disabled children. Despite many questions concerning the use of intelligence tests for classifying disabled learners, these tests have become entrenched in every form of work with these children (Kaufman, 1979; Sattler, 1988).

In general, intelligence test scores are used to separate children with generalized impairments of learning (e.g., those who are mentally deficient) from children who have more isolated forms of learning impairment (e.g., those who are learning disabled). Additional distinctions are sometimes made among learning-disabled children in an attempt to separate or classify those children reading at levels appropriate for their measured intellectual potential from those reading below their intellectual potential. Most prominent has been Rutter and Yule's (1975) distinction between "general reading backwardness" and "specific reading retardation."

Although most research involving these types of distinctions concerns children who are deficient in reading, the notion readily generalizes to other academic problems (e.g., arithmetic) and neurobehavioral disorders (e.g., attention deficit–hyperactivity disorder). Virtually any definition of learning disability used for policy (e.g., Kavanaugh & Gray, 1986) employs the concept of intelligence as an index of learning potential. This notion is even more firmly embedded in current definitions used for research on learning disabilities.

The widespread employment of conceptions of intelligence in the definition of disabled learners belies the many problems associated with this practice. Some of these problems are conceptual, whereas others are psychometric/statistical. Unfortunately, well-reasoned argument has been unsuccessful in altering current conceptions, and empirical data have not been adequately employed in addressing these important issues.

Conceptual Problems with the Use of IQ Tests

The conceptual problems underlying the use of IQ test scores with learning-disabled children largely involve the notion that such scores are indices of learning potential. When IQ scores are used as an index of potential, the underlying assumptions revolve around the notion that there is a measurable constant that can be labeled "potential." Historically, this hypothesis is influenced by the idea of a generalized intelligence factor ("*g*") that represents some type of innate, biologically derived factor that sets upper limits on ability attainment (Spearman, 1923). When this limit is not attained, either constitutional or environmental explanations are postulated for the discrepancies. These ideas and their role in definitions of childhood neurobehavioral disorders can be found in Still (1902). Similar notions were the basis of concepts such as "minimal brain injury" (Strauss & Lehtinen, 1947) and were epitomized in policy-based definitions of "minimal brain dysfunction" and "specific learning disability" (Satz & Fletcher, 1980).

As Rutter (1978) suggested, definitions of learning disability that use IQ tests to index potential are vague and poorly operationalized. Taylor, Fletcher, and Satz (1984) summarized many of the problems with the use of IQ tests to measure potential. These problems included the multifactorial nature of composite scores of intellectual functioning. In other words, an IQ score is a summary of several aspects of cognitive functioning. Some aspects are correlated with reading ability (e.g., vocabulary), whereas other aspects have little relationship to reading skill (e.g., puzzle assembly). To the extent that an IQ score is related to reading ability, the IQ score will likely reflect the severity of the reading disorder. Median correlations are approximately .70 (Kaufman, 1979; Sattler, 1988). Lower scores on IQ tests may merely reflect the pervasiveness of cognitive impairment as opposed to an upper limit on cognitive ability. Similarly, some children with lower IQ scores have reading levels in excess of their measured intelligence. All this phenomenon indicates is that the IQ test does not measure some skill that is related to reading proficiency, not that the child is an "overachiever." For example, no intelligence test of which we are aware measures phonological segmentation skills, which are highly related to decoding skills in reading (Rosner & Simon, 1971).

Finally, the use of IQ test scores as an index of learning potential represents a complex causal network in which the joint influences of reading proficiency on IQ and vice versa are difficult to disentangle (Doehring, 1978). It may be that lower IQ scores result from rather than "cause" reading deficiency. These conceptual problems should be considered carefully when IQ scores are used as a primary defining characteristic of learning disability (Fletcher & Morris, 1986).

Psychometric Problems with the Use of IQ Scores

In addition to conceptual problems, the use of IQ test scores to define learning disabilities raises serious psychometric considerations. These problems have been discussed, but they have not seriously been considered in various policy statements and "official" definitions.

What Test?

One obvious problem involves the IQ test score to be used (Morris, 1988). For example, if the Wechsler Intelligence Scale for Children (Wechsler, 1949) is used, should the index of potential be the Verbal IQ, Performance IQ, or Full Scale IQ? What if another IQ test is used (e.g., Stanford–Binet, Fourth Edition, or Kaufman Assessment Battery for Children)? Current implementations of policy at the level of the school lead to unclear arguments among practitioners about various composites and test scores for an individual child. For a child with marked discrepancies in abilities, composite scores that average these discrepancies may mask true potential in the academic area.

What Cut-Off?

A related problem is where to place the cut-off for deciding minimal levels of "average" intelligence. As Morris (1988) suggested, there is little empirical evidence favoring cut-offs of 70, 80, or 90—yet all these scores find their way into empirical studies of disabled learners. Other approaches use some type of discrepancy between achievement and intelligence, but again, the extent of discrepancy necessary to yield a positive diagnosis is vague. Why should a criterion of 1 standard deviation be used as opposed to a criterion of 2 standard deviations?

Age-Based Criteria

When discrepancy-based definitions have been used, the extent of discrepancy has been expressed relative to age and IQ. The problems with age-based criteria are well known (Fletcher & Morris, 1986; Reynolds, 1984). Basically, age-based discrepancies represent unstandardized metrics that vary across age. For example, a child reading 2 years below age level at age 9 is more seriously impaired than is a 16-year-old reading 2 years below age level. Indeed, the level of reading skill representative of most 14-year-olds corresponds with the average literacy level of the United States and Canada. Phillips and Clarizio (1988) recommended this approach because it is possible to compare the academic performance of children who span different grades. In addition, achievement profiles are more easily translatable to educational recommendations. Finally, grade equivalents account for changes in within-grade variability across varying grade levels.

However, Spreen (1976) criticized grade-equivalent discrepancy methodology because dispersion of achievement test scores increases with advancing age (Reynolds, 1984; Salvia & Yesseldyke, 1981). Thus, an older child who performs 2 years below grade level may have a learning disability of similar severity as a younger child whose performance lags by 1 year. Regression between grade and test score is not equivalent across grades or even school subjects (Reynolds, 1984). In addition, Reynolds (1984) illustrated that grade-equivalent difference scores are based on the assumption that a constant rate of learning occurs across the entire school year. Many achievement tests are not administered at each month in the year but rather are extrapolated from both ends of the scale (Salvia & Yesseldyke, 1981). By relying on grade-equivalent discrepancies, small differences in achievement may be exaggerated (Reynolds, 1984).

Discrepancy Scores

IQ-based discrepancies are equally problematic. Two different approaches can be used. One approach simply establishes IQ and achievement cut-offs. If a child has "average" intelligence and reading scores that are below (for example) the 25th percentile, he/she can be considered reading-disabled. Another approach defines discrepancy according to relative levels of IQ and achievement. For example, a child who is reading 1 standard deviation below measured intelligence is considered eligible for special education in Texas and many other states and provinces. Why 1 standard deviation is used, as opposed to 1.5 or 2 standard deviations (comparable with other states and provinces), probably depends on issues involving policy (i.e., funding) and not on clinical characteristics of the child. Equally serious is the failure of these types of definitions to correct for regression artifact (see below).

Phillips and Clarizio (1988) cautioned that standard scores may possess many of the pitfalls associated with grade-equivalent scores. In particular, scaled score differences may not represent equal intervals because of the method of test construction. In fact, the Wide Range Achievement Test (Jastak & Jastak, 1965) derives both standard scores and centiles from grade equivalents converted directly from raw scores. Moreover, the assumption of normality of scores within age or grade groups may not be tenable. By using standard scores, normality may be forced, regardless of the underlying nature of the distribution of scores.

Lastly, Phillips and Clarizio (1988) note that, when differences between standard scores were used to define groups, unusual growth patterns of academic achievement occurred. For example, the Woodcock–Johnson Psycho-Educational Battery (Woodcock & Johnson, 1977) requires an elementary school child to gain 17.7 scaled score points to remain below the 10th centile, 19.2 points to continue to be in the average range (50th centile), and 20.2 points to stay in the superior range (90th centile). However, in high school, the necessary performance pattern changes. An increase of 3.5 scaled score points must have occurred for a student to have remained below average. Students who achieve at least above the 50th centile need to increase their score by at least 2.3 points, and those who had previously demonstrated superior performance had to gain at least 1.7 points to maintain such standing. Moreover, the performance pattern necessary to maintain centile ranking varied as a function of the test employed to assess achievement. Clearly, these findings warrant caution in interpretation of research based on standard score discrepancy definitions. Furthermore, such results necessitate both awareness of and familiarity with the properties of the individual test to be administered.

Regression to the Mean

In addition to objections to appropriate measurement differences, using discrepancy criteria based on comparisons of IQ and achievement scores raises statistical issues involving regression to the mean. If a difference score is formed on the basis of two measures that are neither perfectly correlated nor independent, the resulting distribution differs from the simple subtraction of the two component distributions (Cone & Wilson, 1981). If two measures are moderately correlated and an individual scores above the mean on the first test, on the average, the individual will not be expected to perform at that level or better on the second measure. Because performance on each test is not an independent event, the measures are correlated. Regression toward the mean occurs, in that it is more likely that the score the individual receives on the second test will be closer to the group mean than was the first test score. Correspondingly, the same effect occurs if performance is below the mean. In that case, the second test score is expected to be higher (more toward the mean) than the first score (McLeod, 1979; Yule, 1978).

Reynolds (1984) criticized the use of such discrepancy criteria precisely because regression artifacts are often ignored, especially given the relatively high intercorrelation between IQ and reading achievement. He found that using such comparisons leads to (1) an overidentification of higher-IQ-score children as disabled (in that some difference between IQ and achievement scores is expected) and (2) and underidentification of children with lower IQ scores (because the achievement score is expected to surpass low IQ).

In addition to the misallocation of special education services that accompanies psychometrically imprecise definitions, the use of uncorrected discrepancy criteria may be discriminatory. Often those children who perform more poorly on IQ measures come from educationally deprived environments, may be racially different from traditional reading-disabled samples, or may be of lower socioeconomic status. It is precisely these children who may require appropriate services to achieve successful reading outcomes.

The second approach to the operationalization of standard score discrepancy definitions is the use of regression procedures to predict the actual level of achievement that would be expected on the basis of age or intelligence, hence correcting for regression to the mean. Actual achievement is then compared to the predicted achievement score. If this difference exceeds what would be predicted given normal variation, a designation of reading disabled is indicated.

Rutter and Yule (1975) used regression-based definitional criteria to delineate a group of readers whose achievement was not commensurate with IQ and age (specific reading retardation; SRR). However, Siegel and Heaven (1986) criticized the use of IQ scores to predict reading ability. They argued that by using IQ as an estimate of potential, the same problems occur as when exclusionary definitions are used to define disabled readers (Fletcher & Morris, 1986). Briefly, this argument states that because reading and IQ test scores are positively correlated, the predicted reading score would be biased (in this case depressed) relative to a prediction based on an independent indication of learning potential. Although regression-based approaches do address the problem of regression artifacts that result when using raw score methods, such an approach is in no way a panacea. In general, the issues raised by the use of standard scores and grade-equivalent scores remain, including the comparability of measurement interval over time and the issue of basing assessments of potential on IQ scores.

Specific versus Backward Readers

Even when IQ and achievement scores are corrected for regression, it is not clear that children with discrepancies in IQ and achievement have more specific disabilities than do poor achievers whose IQ scores are not discrepant. Rutter and Yule (1975) defined children with achievement problems according to whether they were "backward readers," who read at IQ-appropriate levels, or "specific reading retarded," who have reading scores below expected levels according to their IQ scores. These designations were based on data derived from children between the ages of 9 and 11 on the Isle of Wight who were then reassessed at the age of 14. Children who scored 2 standard deviations or more below the group mean on nonverbal intelligence and reading attainment measures were subsequently administered a short form of the Wechsler Intelligence Scale for Children and the Neale Analysis of Reading. SRR was defined as an observed difference in reading achievement that was at least 2 standard errors below predicted levels via multiple regression analysis using age and IQ as predictors. "Backward" readers were those children whose reading was deficient on the basis of age alone, regardless of intelligence.

Rutter and Yule (1975) observed that those children identified as SRR differed from the backward readers along a series of measures including educational prognosis. First, there was a greater prevalence of males in the SRR group (76.7%) as compared to the backward readers (54.4%). In addition, the backward readers presented with a greater incidence of overt neurological dysfunction: 11.4% had evidence of "hard" neurological signs such as cerebral palsy, and 25.3% demonstrated evidence of "soft" neurological abnormalities such as developmental delay. None of the SRR children demonstrated "hard" neurological signs, and ony 18.6% showed the possibility of "soft" signs. Moreover, the backward readers were rated as more clumsy, showed more coordinational and constructional difficulties, and were more likely to demonstrate right–left confusion than were SRR children. Motor impersistence and choreiform movements were also more commonly found in the backward reader group. However, both SRR and backward reading groups had a similar incidence of family history of language problems, delayed speech milestones, and poor articulation.

When these children with reading difficulties were assessed as 14-year-olds, educational achievement varied as a function of skill area assessed. The SRR children demonstrated poorer spelling and reading skills than did the backward readers, indicating that they had fallen relatively further behind their age-matched peers. The arithmetic performance of the SRR children improved relative to the backward readers, but it remained significantly below grade levels. Rutter and Yule (1975) concluded that SRR is a relatively distinct disorder that can be summarized as a deficit that is peculiar to language, whereas backward readers demonstrated multiple difficulties in intellectual, neurological, and language areas.

These findings have not been uniformly replicated. Rodgers (1983) did not find evidence for a bimodal distribution of achievement in a large sample of 10-year-olds from Great Britain and Northern Ireland. The actual prevalence of disabled children with a greater than 2 standard deviation difference between actual achievement and that predicted by IQ was 2.29% compared to a predicted prevalence of 2.28%. Rodgers (1983) concluded that the distribution of reading achievement was distributed normally.

Other studies have addressed the original Rutter and Yule (1975) findings. Silva, McGhee, and Williams (1985) assessed 952 children from Dunedin, New Zealand, at 7 and 9 years of age. Children were divided into SRR and backward reader groups in a procedure identical to that used by Rutter and Yule (1975). They found that 74.4% of the backward readers were male, whereas 87.5% of the SRR group were male. Only the backward readers had significantly more neurological abnormalities than either the SRR or normal reader group. Furthermore, backward readers also demonstrated more motor difficulties than did any other group, although the SRR children showed more motor impairment than did normal readers. In contrast to Rutter and Yule (1975), Silva et al. (1985) also found significant differences between the two disabled reading groups on language measures, with the SRR group outperforming the backward readers. The SRR group did, however, achieve below levels of normal readers. The educational attainment was similar for both disabled groups in reading and spelling. Yet, the SRR group performed significantly better on arithmetic measures than did the backward readers, although they continued to achieve below levels of the normal reader group.

Jorm, Share, MacLean, and Matthews (1986) delineated groups of SRR and backward readers among 453 Australian children using the methods described above. They identified 14 retarded readers and 25 backward readers who were subsequently followed during the first three grades. In kindergarten these children were administered a neuropsychological battery consisting of diverse language, motor, and sensory measures. At grade 2 the children were given standardized achievement tests and were classified into diagnostic reading groups using procedures similar to those of Rutter and Yule (1975).

The SRR group differed significantly from backward readers in name writing and reading, letter copying, syntax, receptive vocabulary, sentence memory, and motor impairment. Backward readers differed from normal readers in almost all areas assessed, except motor impersistence, impulsivity, and pseudoword learning. The SRR group differed from normals only on specific language and early literacy skills such as name writing, recognition discrimination, picture and color naming, phoneme segmentation, and finger localization. Jorm et al. (1986) concluded that although the SRR and backward reader groups appeared similar in terms of reading ability, their cognitive competencies differed. SRR children had specific difficulties with language skills, whereas the backward readers had more global difficulties. Finally, they concluded that a common etiology of reading difficulty cannot be assumed for the two groups of disabled readers. It was more likely that the SRR group had academic difficulties because they were prevented from learning because of encoding difficulties (i.e., they were developmentally deviant). Backward readers demonstrated intact, yet reduced, general abilities and thus were considered to learn by a slower, yet normal, process (i.e., they were developmentally delayed).

van der Wissel and Zegers (1985) reviewed the Isle of Wight studies. Observing that there may have been a ceiling effect on the reading test employed, they performed simulation studies that they interpreted as showing that the so-called "hump" in the distribution of achievement test scores is a product of this ceiling effect as well as differences in gender ratios for the groups of backward and SRR children.

Yule (1985) responded to this study by noting that the definition of specific reading retardation used by van der Wissel and Zegers was based solely on a division of IQ scores. The original definitions used by Rutter and Yule (1975) were based across the IQ distribution. Yule also noted that van der Wissel and Zegers (1985) misinterpreted the nature of the reading test and the gender differences. Yule (1985) also disavowed any attempt to link IQ and reading achievement in a casual fashion, stating the "we are not arguing that IQ causes reading disorder, but that the use of our classification identified meaningful subgroups of poor readers" (p. 12).

Fletcher and Morris (1986) noted that the distinction between specific and backward reading is a classification hypothesis that should be subjected to systematic empirical investigation. Finding differences in neurobehavioral characteristics and educational progress supports the viability of the classification. However, there has been little uniformity in such findings.

In an earlier study that did not use regression-based definitions, Taylor, Satz, and Friel (1979) selected children with reading problems (Wide Range Achievement Test Reading below the 30th percentile) according to whether they met exclusionary definitions. They operationally defined the criteria provided by the World Federation of Neurology (Critchley, 1970) by specifying that a diagnosis of dyslexia could only occur in children with a Peabody Picture Vocabulary Test IQ greater than 89, average or above average socioeconomic status as rated by teachers, and an absence of neurological, sensory, or emotional difficulties as noted by teacher or parent. Those children who met the exclusionary criteria and who exhibited deficient reading skills were labeled "dyslexic" disabled readers, and those who did not (i.e., low socioeconomic status or IQ and low reading ability) were labeled "nondyslexic" disabled readers.

These two groups of disabled readers were compared against two groups of normal readers across seven different areas: neuropsychological and academic test performance, severity of reading problems, reversal and/or letter confusion, parental reading proficiency, neurological exam, and personality. Results showed no significant differences in any of the areas assessed between "dyslexic" and "nondyslexic" disabled reading groups of children. The two reading-disabled groups did, however, differ significantly from normal readers on measures in all seven domains. Furthermore, when IQ and socioeconomic variables were controlled, differences continued to be robust between disabled and nondisabled readers.

More recently, Share, McGhee, McKenzie, Williams, and Silva (1987) found no differences in prognosis between generally backward and specific reading-disabled children between 7 and 9 years of age. In addition, they noted that the types of differences found between children in this study and the Isle of Wight study had questionable causal relationships with reading impairment. Share et al. (1987) conlcuded that "on the basis of the data discussed here, there appears to be no firm evidence to support the validity of the distinctions between specific reading retardation and general reading backwardness" (p. 42).

In an investigation based on the Connecticut Longitudinal Study (Shaywitz & Shaywitz, 1988), Shaywitz, Shaywitz, Barnes, and Fletcher (1986) compared the influence of various definitions on the selection of children as learning disabled in an epidemiologic sample of school children in Connecticut. Although variations in the use of IQ indices and definitions resulted in different children being identified as learning disabled, few differences in cognitive ability were apparent among children grouped as learning disabled according to various definitions. There were also few differences among children defined as learning disabled whose scores were discrepant or not discrepant from IQ.

Limitations of Previous Studies

The varying findings of these studies undoubtedly reflect differences in samples and instruments. However, at this point, the major question is not so much whether there is a "hump" in the distribution of IQ-reading scores. Rather, the critical question is whether distinctions are valid between disabled readers whose reading ability is consistent with as opposed to inconsistent with measured intelligence.

The answer to this question appears to depend on how groups are defined, representing a classification problem (Fletcher, Francis, & Morris, 1988). It appears that when a more rigorous definition is used to form groups of disabled readers, group differences often emerge. Specifically, children who meet regression-based discrepancy criteria may be impaired on specific language measures when compared to normal readers (Jorm et al., 1986). Correspondingly, those children whose reading is incompatible with levels estimated by age but is consistent with that predicted by IQ are found to have global difficulties in functioning that span motor, neurological, and language domains.

It is not unexpected that smaller or nonsignificant differences were found by Taylor et al. (1979), because the IQ construct played a less prominent and clearly delineated role in the exclusionary selection criteria employed in that study. When IQ differences between disabled and nondisabled readers were controlled, skill differences between these groups defined by exclusionary criteria remained robust. However, IQ effects were neither considered nor controlled when comparing dyslexic and nondyslexic disabled reading groups, even though the dyslexic disabled childern were clearly of higher IQ. Such IQ differences could potentially mask inferior performance of the dyslexic disabled group. In addition, Taylor et al. (1979) used results from receptive vocabulary level as an estimate of IQ. Consequently, groups defined in this manner may not be comparable to those from research employing a more global measure to estimate intelligence. However, one advantage of the Taylor et al. (1979) study is the large sample size. Other comparisons of backward readers and specifically disabled readers have been hampered by small samples of disabled children derived from large epidemiologic samples.

An alternative approach to these issues is to use a large sample of clinically impaired children. A within-group approach will not address prevalence issues, but it can be used to address the validity of various definitions. In the remainder of this chapter, we discuss a series of three studies addressing the validity of discrepancy-based definitions of reading disability in a large cohort of learning-disabled children.

Comparisons of Various Definitions of Learning Disability

Sample

The children for this study were obtained from a data base of over 2,500 cases representing children referred for evaluation of learning disability in Windsor, Ontario. Each child received a comprehensive neuropsychological evaluation (Rourke, 1981; Rourke, Fisk, & Strang, 1986) along with the Wechsler Intelligence Scale for Children (WISC; Wechsler, 1949), and the Wide Range Achievement Test (WRAT; Jastak & Jastak, 1965). For this study, children were selected who ranged in age from 9 years to 14 years with WISC Full Scale IQ (FSIQ) scores above 70. These children were free of sensory, acquired neurological, and other problems traditionally used as exclusionary criteria. Application of these criteria resulted in a total sample of 1,069 children. The sample, 74% of whom were male, were predominantly white, middle-class children, who averaged 11 years, 4 months in age. The mean WRAT Reading standard score was 89.3 (SD = 14.8) with a mean WISC FSIQ of 98.5 (SD = 10.5).

Definitions

Two different definitions were used to identify children as reading disabled based on the word recognition score from the WRAT and the WISC FSIQ. The first definition employed a cutting-score approach that did not correct for regression artifact. Children were defined as reading disabled if their FSIQ exceeded 79 and their WRAT Reading standard score was below 93. In addition, children were categorized according to whether reading scores were consistent with or inconsistent with FSIQ using a criterion of 15 points: A child was considered "discrepant" if the WRAT score was less than the FSIQ by at least 15 points. This definition corresponds directly with criteria commonly used to define eligibility for special education services as a child with reading disability. Liberal criteria in terms of relative severity of word-recognition deficit and IQ were used in the hope of capturing the largest possible sample unbiased to selection variables.

Joint application of both definitions to all children resulted in four reading groups: normal readers (children not impaired according to either criterion); children impaired under both definitions (low achieving and discrepant); children who were low achievers (below 93) but not discrepant; and children whose reading was discrepant with IQ but exceeded a standard score of 93. In the above definitions, IQ–achievement discrepancy was based on observed standard score differences. Alternatively, this discrepancy can be based on regression formulas as previously discussed, where the discrepancy is between observed and predicted achievement.

Comparison Variables

To address whether differences in ability structure exist among groups formed with different definitional criteria, low-achieving children who were discrepant and not discrepant under the two definitions were compared on a set of tests derived from a modification of the Halstead–Reitan Neuropsychological Battery for Children (HRB; Rourke et al., 1986). These measures constitute a representative sample of neuropsychological skills and abilities and are ordinarily administered in a comprehensive evaluation of children with learning disabilities (Rourke, 1981). The linguistic and auditory–perceptual measures are especially sensitive to the reliable discrimination of children with reading disability from non-disabled children and from children with other types of learning disabilities (Rourke, 1978, 1981; Rourke et al., 1986).

Ten tests from the modified HRB were used. These tests are presented in Table 2.1 along with a summary of the constructs measured by each task. These constructs were defined according to maximum-likelihood factor analyses of the test battery in this sample recently completed by our group. It is apparent that these tests measure a variety of abilities frequently impaired in children with reading disabilities, including language, perceptual, and motor skills.

Comparison of Definitions: Study 1

Fletcher et al. (1989) provided a comparison of children in the sample grouped according to the joint application of the two definitions. Both unadjusted and regression-based approaches to defining IQ–achievement discrepancy were used separately. Joint application of raw score and discrepancy criteria produced four groups: children who scored above or below 92 on WRAT Reading and who had reading scores (regardless of

TABLE 2.1. Modified Halstead–Reitan Neuropsychological Tests
by Factor Structure

Test	Factor
1. Category Test	Executive functions, spatial relations
2. Speech-Sounds Perception Test	General language, acoustic language
3. Auditory Closure Test	General language, acoustic language
4. Sentence Memory Test	General language, acoustic language
5. Verbal Fluency Test	General language, acoustic language
6. Finger-Tapping Test	Simple motor
7. Grooved Pegboard Test	Eye-hand coordination, spatial relations
8. Tactual Performance Test	Spatial relations, executive function, eye–hand
9. Trail Making Test, Parts A and B	Executive function
10. Target Test	Spatial relations, eye–hand

level) that were discrepant or not discrepant with WISC FSIQ. To simplify discussion, unadjusted comparisons of discrepancies between observed IQ and achievement are described as "uncorrected" discrepancies. In contrast, "regression-based" discrepancies (i.e., differences between observed and predicted achievement) are described as "corrected" discrepancies because they adjust for the IQ–achievement correlation.

Tables 2.2 and 2.3 summarize classifications of the 1,069 children for definitions uncorrected (Table 2.2) or corrected for (Table 2.3) the correlation of WRAT Reading and WISC FSIQ. For the uncorrected definition, Table 2.2 shows that there is a small group of children ($n = 36$) with reading standard scores greater than 92 whose reading score is at least 15 points below their FSIQ. The other children are distributed fairly evenly across the 2 × 2 matrix. About 34% have reading standard scores below 90 that are at least 15 points below their FSIQ scores, with 30% regarded as not impaired in reading. Some 32% of the children have poor reading, but, because of their FSIQ, would not qualify for special education services.

Table 2.3 presents the resultant 2 × 2 matrix when regression artifact is accounted for in the definition of an IQ–achievement discrepancy. It is apparent that the distribution of children across the four categories is different from that in Table 2.2. More children are identified as discrepant and fewer as nondiscrepant. In terms of overlap between the two definitions, 70 children (7%) with reading standard scores below 93 become eligible for services using the regression-based definition who were not eligible under the cut-off score definition. In general, these children

TABLE 2.2. Means and Standard Deviations for Full Scale IQ, and Reading Standard Scores of Children Categorized According to Reading Standard Scores and Raw Discrepancies

	Reading standard score	
	≤ 92	> 92
Discrepant	N = 360 (34%)	N = 36 (4%)
	FSIQ[a] = 101.8 (8.7)	FSIQ = 114.9 (5.3)
	RdSS[b] = 78.4 (8.0)	RdSS = 96.1 (5.1)
Not discrepant	N = 347 (32%)	N = 326 (30%)
	FSIQ = 90.6 (6.0)	FSIQ = 101.3 (10.9)
	RdSS = 83.9 (5.7)	RdSS = 106.4 (12.2)

[a]FSIQ, Full Scale IQ on WISC.
[b]RdSS, Reading standard score on WRAT.

scored lower on FSIQ ($M = 87.7$; $SD = 4.5$) and WRAT Reading ($M = 75.5$; $SD = 3.4$) than did the group of discrepant readers identified in the first analysis. However, 22 (2%) children who had reading standard scores below 93 and 15-point discrepancies between IQ and reading were no longer eligible under the regression-based definition. These children had a mean WISC FSIQ of 106.2 ($SD = 3.0$) and mean WRAT Reading standard score of 89.7 ($SD = 3.0$). Of the 36 higher-but-discrepant-achievement children eligible under the uncorrected discrepancy score criterion,

TABLE 2.3. Means and Standard Deviations for Full Scale IQ, and Reading Standard Scores for Children Categorized According to Reading Standard Scores and Regression-Based Discrepancies

	Reading standard score	
	≤ 92	> 92
Discrepant	N = 408 (38%)	N = 5 (1%)
	FSIQ[a] = 99.2 (9.8)	FSIQ = 99.2 (9.8)
	RdSS[b] = 77.3 (7.2)	RdSS = 90.2 (9.1)
Not discrepant	N = 299 (28%)	N = 357 (33%)
	FSIQ = 92.4 (7.1)	FSIQ = 102.5 (11.0)
	RdSS = 86.2 (4.2)	RdSS = 105.6 (12.0)

[a]FSIQ, Full Scale IQ on WISC.
[b]RdSS, Reading standard score on WRAT.

only five remain eligible when the definition takes into account regression effects. Thus, the regression-based criteria make 70 "low-achieving readers" eligible but eliminate eligibility for 22 children with word recognition scores below 93, because these scores are within the range expected given their IQ. These criteria also eliminate eligibility for 31 children who exhibit age-appropriate word recognition scores ($M = 97.1$; $SD = 3.6$) and higher FSIQ ($M = 114.6$; $SD = 4.2$).

Overlap: Study 2

One problem with the Fletcher et al. (1989) study is the failure to account for overlap in the classifications in Tables 2.2 and 2.3. In other words, some children meet (or do not meet) both discrepancy-based definitions, whereas other children meet criteria set forth by only one discrepancy-based definition. To address the issue of overlap, Espy, Francis, Fletcher, and Rourke (1989) compared three groups of children who were "disabled readers" according to various discrepancy-based definitions: (1) both raw score and regression-based discrepancy definitions (IBOTH); (2) only raw score definitions (IRAW); and (3) only regression-based definition (IREG). All of these children met discrepancy-based definitions. Children who did not meet a discrepancy-based definition were placed into a single group regardless of reading level on the assumption that these children describe a continuum of reading impairment.

When the sample was divided in this fashion, 291 children met both definitions (IBOTH), 105 met only uncorrected definitions (IRAW), and 22 met only regression-based definitions (IREG). There were 651 children who met neither discrepancy-based definition of reading disability. Note that of these 651 children, 325 (49.9%) could be considered as low-achieving (WRAT Reading $\leq$ 92) children.

The mean WISC Verbal IQ and Performance IQ scores, and WRAT Reading, Spelling, and Arithmetic scores of these four groups are presented in Table 2.4. Among the more striking findings illustrated in this table are the differences in Full Scale IQ across the four groups. The IRAW group has the highest FSIQ ($M = 106.7$), whereas the IREG group has the lowest FSIQ ($M = 86.0$). In the three disabled groups, achievement and WISC scores fluctuate similarly, reflecting the relationship of IQ scores and WRAT achievement scores. Given this finding and the standard error of measurement associated with the WISC and the WRAT, another implication is that there is substantial skill and ability overlap among the three disabled groups. Such IQ differences among the three groups are a natural consequence of the two definitions and the fact that IQ and achievement are correlated.

TABLE 2.4. Scores on WISC and WRAT Variables for Children Categorized According to Raw and Regression-Based Discrepancies

| | Group[a] | | | | | | | |
| | ND (N = 651) | | IBOTH (N = 291) | | IRAW (N = 105) | | IREG (N = 22) | |
Variable	M	SD	M	SD	M	SD	M	SD
WISC								
Verbal IQ	93.7	10.9	94.1	9.3	99.8	9.3	83.4	5.8
Performance IQ	99.4	11.6	109.8	12.1	113.1	7.9	91.4	5.8
Full Scale IQ	93.1	10.2	101.7	9.7	106.7	7.1	86.0	2.8
WRAT								
Reading	39.0	27.6	8.1	7.4	25.6	13.3	3.8	1.2
Spelling	25.6	22.5	6.4	6.6	16.5	11.7	3.6	1.9
Arithmetic	20.7	15.4	13.6	12.1	23.3	13.4	7.5	4.0

[a]ND, not discrepant; IBOTH, discrepant using raw score and regression-based criteria; IRAW, discrepant using raw score criteria only; IREG, discrepant using regression-based criteria only.

ABILITY PROFILES

Espy et al. (1989) performed a series of analyses to examine the magnitude of group differences and the role of IQ scores as differentiators of the four groups. To facilitate these comparisons, groups were compared on the set of 10 neuropsychological variables used as external validation measures (see Table 2.1). These comparisons were treated as a set of classification hypotheses. If it is valid to classify children as LD or not using either type of discrepancy-based definition, then robust differences on these external variables should emerge. Espy et al. (1989) performed these comparisons using general multivariate analysis of variance (MANOVA). However, an alternative to MANOVA in this situation is profile analysis. In the remainder of this chapter we provide an introduction to profile analysis as an alternative to MANOVA through an extended demonstration involving the four reading groups and the 10 neuropsychological measures referred to earlier.

Profile Analysis: Study 3

The most frequently asked questions in neuropsychological research often involve comparisons of two or more groups on multiple measures of neuropsychological functioning. There are several ways to address such questions in a statistical manner. The least informative approach, and the one most difficult to justify statistically (Huberty & Morris, 1989), is that of isolated multiple univariate comparisons. Yet this approach is chosen more frequently than any other, in part because researchers find multivariate alternatives difficult to carry out and interpret. Profile analysis (PA) represents an attractive multivariate alternative for neuropsychologists because PA directly compares "patterns" of group test performance and is easily performed and interpreted. PA accomplishes this pattern comparison by separating differences among groups and differences among measures into three statistically independent pieces of information. These pieces of information are referred to as the dimensions of (1) shape, (2) elevation, and (3) flatness. The remainder of this chapter describes these three questions addressed in PA, and it compares PA with traditional univariate and multivariate alternatives for examining mean group differences. Finally data from the preceding discussion of reading disability definitions are used to demonstrate PA.

Much of the neuropsychological research focuses on the comparison of performance patterns in two or more groups. Indeed, in the 5 years from 1983 to 1988, no fewer than 83 of the articles in the *Journal of Clinical and Experimental Neuropsychology* (about 50%) involved such a comparison as the primary research question. PA is a conceptually simple procedure that directly examines differences in performance patterns. Surprisingly, PA has not seen widespread application in neuropsychology. In fact, only one of the 83 articles mentioned above formally applied PA, whereas 54 used some form of univariate statistic. Although these points were made previously (Francis, Fletcher, & Davidson, 1988), the potential applications of PA in neuropsychology so greatly outnumber the actual applications in the literature that we feel these points are worth repeating.

THE THREE DIMENSIONS OF PROFILE ANALYSIS

To facilitate the following presentation and discussion of PA, consider the patterns of means displayed in Figure 2.1. Each circle in Figure 2.1 corresponds to the mean T-score for one of four reading groups on 1 of 10 neuropsychological measures. The four reading groups were determined by the adjusted and unadjusted discrepancy-based criteria discussed previously. For each group, adjacent means have been connected by a straight line only to increase the visual impression of an ability "profile"; the lines should not be taken to imply that the horizontal dimension in the figure is continuous.

Roughly speaking, the variables have been ordered along the horizontal axis such that motor measures fall further to the left end, with spatial and verbal measures represented progressively further to the right.

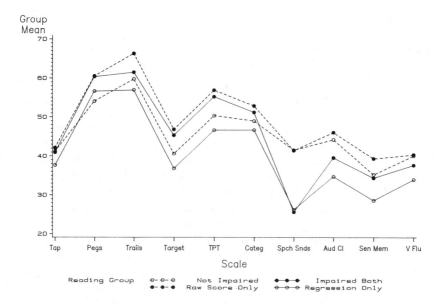

FIGURE 2.1. Mean profiles for four reading groups using 10 measures of neuro-psychological performance. Criteria for forming reading groups are provided in the text. All measures have been transformed to T-scores ($M = 50$) using published norms and scaled such that higher scores indicate better performance. Abbreviations for measures are as follows: Tap, Finger Tapping, average T-score for left and right hands; Pegs, Grooved Pegboard, average T-score for left and right hands; Trails, average T-score for Trail Making A and B; Target, Target Test; TPT, Tactual Performance Test, average T-score for times using left, right, and both hands; Categ, Category Test, total score; Spch Snds, Speech-Sounds Perception; Aud Cl, Auditory Closure; Sen Mem, Sentence Memory; V Flu, Verbal Fluency.

This ordering is strictly arbitrary and was chosen as a matter of convenience to facilitate interpretation of the profiles in Figure 2.1. We return to the issue of variable ordering in due course.

In examining any set of group profiles, such as that of Figure 2.1, three possible questions come to mind. First, we must consider whether the population mean profiles are similarly shaped in the sense that the lines joining adjacent means are parallel for all groups. This is referred to as the "pattern," "shape," or "parallelism" hypothesis. An examination of Figure 2.1 suggests that the hypothesis of parallel profiles is likely to be rejected for these groups on these measures, especially in light of the large sample sizes in three of the four groups.

If one were to conclude that the profiles were parallel, it then becomes reasonable to consider two other hypotheses. First, do the profiles differ in level? This question is commonly referred to as the "levels" or "elevation" hypothesis. As an example of parallel profiles differing in elevation, mean profiles on the four primary verbal scales from the WISC (Wechsler, 1949) are presented in Figure 2.2 for three of the four reading groups. Clearly, in Figure 2.2, the most striking difference among the three profiles is their respective elevation. Second, if one were to conclude that the profiles were parallel, regardless of any possible differences in elevation, it also becomes reasonable to consider whether the population means for the different measures are equal. If the population means for all measures making up the profile were equal, then clearly the average profile (averaging across groups) would be flat. Not surprisingly, this final test is referred to as the "flatness" hypothesis.

From the foregoing discussion, it is clear that PA is quite different from the general MANOVA. MANOVA has been termed an unstructured multivariate analysis (Hand & Taylor, 1987) because MANOVA simply seeks to determine the way in which to combine a set of measures such that group differences on the measures are maximized. PA, in contrast, represents one form of structured multivariate analysis because PA seeks to determine answers to three specific questions concerning differences

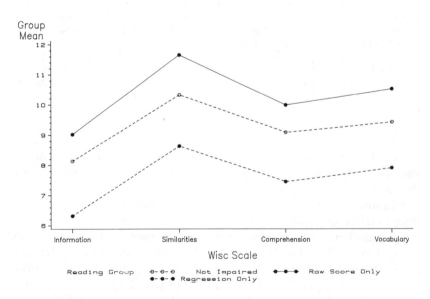

FIGURE 2.2. Mean profiles for three of four reading groups using primary verbal subscales from the WISC. Criteria for forming reading groups are provided in the text. Groups and measures were chosen to demonstrate the appearance of parallel profiles that differ in elevation.

among groups and measures (Hand & Taylor, 1987), each of which can be conceptualized as a specific set of contrasts. Let us consider each question in somewhat greater detail in order to demonstrate how each can be conceptualized as a set of contrasts among groups and measures.

PARALLELISM: THE TEST OF EQUAL SHAPE

The primary question in PA is the question of shape. If profiles do not have the same shape, then questions about elevation and flatness are somewhat meaningless because their answers would depend on which subset of measures or groups was being considered. The precedence of shape over elevation and flatness is analogous to the primary status afforded interactions over main effects in the analysis of variance (ANOVA)—main effects being unambiguous only in the absence of interactions. Actually, PA is directly analogous to the split-plot analysis of variance, representing designs with at least one between- and one within-subjects factor, a point we return to in a moment.

There are two equally legitimate ways to conceptualize the question of shape:

1. Are differences between measures the same for all groups?
2. Are differences between groups the same on all measures?

Consider again the profiles of Figure 2.1. In examining these, the first way of framing the shape question amounts to asking if the line segments joining any adjacent pair of measures have the same slope for all groups. For example, do the four line segments joining the means for Finger Tapping and Grooved Pegboard have equal slope? Similarly, are the slopes of the line segments joining Trails and Grooved Pegboard equal? If the line segments joining a given pair of measures have the same slope in all groups, then, clearly, the group profiles are parallel between those two measures. With p measures it is possible to compute $p - 1$ such linearly independent slopes for each group. For the entire group profiles to be parallel, each of these $p - 1$ slopes would have to be equal for all groups, although it is not necessary for all $p - 1$ slopes to be equal to one another. In the present example, there would be nine such slopes in each group, and it would appear that at least one group differs from the others on all but two of the nine slopes. Of course, we will want to know if these deviations from parallelism are statistically significant or if they could reasonably have resulted from random fluctuations in the data.

In truth, we refer to slopes because it is easy to think of slopes being parallel. However, the line segment slopes referred to are equivalent to differences between the means of adjacent measures. Hence, if we simply compute the difference between adjacent measures for each group, variability between groups in these computed mean differences indicates a lack of parallelism in group profiles. When the number of measures in the profile is three or more, the test of parallelism will involve two or more difference scores, and hence the test will be multivariate in nature.

Using the data presented in Figure 2.1 for the four reading groups, the test of parallelism yields a significant multivariate $F(27,3177) = 10.88$, $p < .0001$. Hence, for these groups we would reject the hypothesis that the profiles are parallel, and we would begin the process of further delineating just how the group profiles differ. Such follow-up questions may involve repeating the profile analysis for a subset of the groups or examining the flatness hypothesis for individual groups. For example, we may desire to know if profiles are parallel for the IQ-adjusted (regression) only and the unadjusted only groups or if the unimpaired group has a flat profile. Alternatively, we may want to know about group differences on specific measures (e.g., do the four groups differ in mean Finger Tapping?). In short, follow-up analyses may entail within-group analyses, between-groups contrasts on individual measures, or interactions between contrasts involving measures and contrasts involving groups, such as repeating the profile analysis for a subset of the groups.

ELEVATION: THE TEST OF EQUAL MEAN PROFILE
HEIGHT AVERAGING OVER MEASURES

The question of equal profile elevation is only addressed if we are willing to conclude that the profiles have the same shape. Clearly, if the profiles do not have the same shape, then it is ambiguous to discuss differences in profile elevation because these differences vary at different points in the profile. The test of equal elevation is the most straightforward of the three tests because it represents a simple between-groups comparison on a single variable. That variable is the group grand mean for the set of measures, that is, the average for each group across the set of p measures. This process of aggregating over the p measures is justified because the existence of parallel profiles implies that differences between groups in profile elevation are the same on all measures. Therefore, averaging across the measures to obtain the group grand means will yield the best estimate of the magnitude of the differences among the groups in profile elevation.

Carrying out a PA on the data in Figure 2.2, we would not reject the parallelism hypothesis, $F(6,1548) = 0.6465$, $p = .69$. However, clear differences exist in mean profile elevation, $F(2,775) = 24.24$, $p < .0001$. At this point we might wish to examine these elevation differences further by performing contrasts between the groups (e.g., pairwise comparisons between the unadjusted only group and the unimpaired group). Regardless of any follow-up tests that might be performed to examine the elevation hypothesis, it is also possible to examine the question of profile flatness.

FLATNESS: THE TEST OF EQUAL MEAN PERFORMANCE
ON ALL MEASURES AVERAGING ACROSS GROUPS

The flatness question is also addressed only in the absence of profile shape differences. Similar to the shape question, flatness is tested by obtaining the mean difference between pairs of adjacent measures. However, in contrast to the shape hypothesis, where slope segments are formed separately for each group, in evaluating the flatness hypothesis, these slope segments are formed by first averaging across groups to obtain the average performance on each measure. Differences are then formed between the grand means for adjacent measures. If the average profile is flat, then the set of $p - 1$ such differences will not be statistically different for 0. As in the test of shape, the test of flatness is a multivariate test whenever p is three or more. Using the data displayed in Figure 2.2 once again, the test of flatness is statistically significant, $F(3,773) = 53.0927$, $p < .0001$, indicating that the average profile among these three groups is *not* flat. This result is not surprising given the large sample sizes in these groups and a visual inspection of Figure 2.2. Having rejected the overall flatness hypothesis, we may wish to perform a more restrictive test of flatness by considering whether the average profile is flat for a subset of the measures (e.g., Information and Vocabulary).

RELATIONS TO MANOVA AND REPEATED-MEASURES ANOVA

As suggested previously, the standard MANOVA represents an unstructured multivariate hypothesis because it fails to distinguish between two types of information about group differences. Specifically, MANOVA combines between-groups differences in profile shape and between groups differences in average profile height into a single effect—group differences on the set of measures. PA separates this information into statistically independent pieces of Elevation and Shape. In addition, PA provides a test of the Flatness of the combined group profile.

The relationship of PA to repeated-measures ANOVA is even more straightforward. Consider a repeated-measures design with one between-subjects factor and one within-subjects factor. Such a design is frequently employed in neuropsychological investigations and is often referred to as a split-plot design. The Elevation hypothesis of PA is exactly the test of the between-subjects main effect in a split-plot design. The Flatness hypothesis of PA equals the test of the main effect of the within-subjects factor. Finally, the Shape hypothesis of PA equals the test of interaction between the within- and between- subjects factors in the split-plot design.

The direct correspondence between PA and the split-plot repeated-measures ANOVA brings up several important considerations. First, readers may or may not be aware that two general approaches exist for analyzing repeated-measures data, regardless of whether the design includes a between-subjects factor. These two general approaches are referred to as the "univariate" and "multivariate" approaches to repeated-measures ANOVA. Given the correspondence between PA and repeated measures, it is not surprising that both univariate and multivariate approaches can also be applied in PA, with the factors governing choice of method being identical in both PA and repeated-measures ANOVA.

We have focused our description on the multivariate approach to PA because we feel this approach is more easily justified statistically in light of the fact that assumptions for the analysis are more likely to be met. We advocate the same approach in analyzing standard repeated-measures designs, and the reader is strongly cautioned that the univariate approach should not be employed in PA or repeated-measures ANOVA unless adjusted for statistical dependence among observations (Maxwell & Arvey, 1982; O'Brien & Kaiser, 1985).

A second point that requires some clarification given the correspondence between PA and repeated-measures ANOVA is the importance of variable ordering in the profiles. The descriptions of the Shape and Flatness hypotheses given above seem to suggest that variable ordering is important. After all, differences are computed between adjacent measures. Obviously, the magnitudes of these differences will depend on which measures are chosen to be adjacent to one another. Yet we have stated that the Shape and Flatness hypotheses of PA correspond to the interaction of the between- and within-subjects factors, and the within-subjects main effect, respectively, in a split-plot design. Furthermore, statistical significance of these latter effects is not altered by reordering the levels of the within-subjects factor at the time of analysis. In fact, the same can be shown to be true for PA—ordering of the measures in the profile will not affect the overall tests of significance, that is, the overall tests of shape and flatness. Clearly, ordering is unimportant for the elevation hypothesis because all measures are averaged to form the grand mean for each group.

In essence, there is a fixed amount of variability attributable to these hypotheses. This total can always be fully explained by a set of $p - 1$ linearly independent single-degree-of-freedom effects (or contrasts). In other words, any set of $p - 1$ linearly independent differences between the p means will completely account for this total effect. Changing the set of single-degree-of-freedom contrasts leaves the total effect unchanged, provided a complete set of $p - 1$ linearly independent contrasts is specified. The set of differences between adjacent measures in a profile is just such a set of $p - 1$ linearly independent contrasts. Put simply, the ordering of variables in a PA is irrelevant to the overall tests of shape, elevation, and flatness.

ASSUMPTIONS

The assumptions underlying the multivariate approach to PA are the same as those for MANOVA: (1) measures must follow a multivariate normal distribution; (2) observations on different subjects must be independent of one another; and (3) variance/covariance matrices must be equal across groups. In addition to these standard MANOVA assumptions, PA requires commensurability of measures. If variables are measured on different metrics (i.e., variables are not commensurable), then shape differences may be an artifact of scale.

This point is most easily understood when one considers the second formulation provided above for the shape hypothesis: namely, parallel profiles imply that differences between groups are equal for all measures. Consider an obvious case where measures are not commensurable. Suppose, for example, that an experimenter has data for two groups on two measures. The measures are high school grade point average (GPA) and junior year Scholastic Aptitude Test (SAT) scores. The range of possible mean differences between groups in GPA is $+4$ to -4, whereas mean differences between groups in SAT scores have a much wider possible range. One would not expect GPA differences between groups to equal SAT differences in magnitude. Consequently, in their original metric, it would make little sense to conduct a PA using GPA and SAT as profile measures because shape differences would reflect artifactual scale differences.

A viable solution when profile measures are not commensurable in their original metrics is to transform the scores to z- or T-scores prior to profile analysis. This yields commensurate scales; however, the metric of the data analysis is changed, and the researcher must determine if the new metric is an acceptable one. We feel that z- or T-score transformation in neuropsychological work is reasonable because most meaures lack a clearly defined metric or one that has more inherent value than the standard deviation metric of T-scores. It is important that any such transformation make use of external information for standardization.

A less obvious example of noncommensurability can be provided by neuropsychological data. Many measures collected by neuropsychologists are scored in a positive direction. Other measures are scored negatively insofar as higher scores indicate poorer performance. The WISC subscales are obvious examples of positively scored scales, whereas the Trail Making Tests, Grooved Pegboard, and time scores of the Tactual Performance Test are examples of negatively scored scales. A PA using both positively and negatively scored scales will almost certainly lead to rejection of the parallelism hypotheses. In this situation, parallel profiles would imply that the best performing group on a positively scored measure is equally the poorest performing group on a negatively scored measure. Obviously, for positively and negatively scored measures to be included in a single PA, one set of measures must be transformed so that the scoring is reversed. For the analyses presented in Figure 2.1, all measures have been scored so that higher scores indicate better performance.

The most important point of the preceding discussion is that PA results are not invariant under transformation of the data. Hence, the choice of metric for analysis must be defensible, and all measures must be scaled similarly. It is our opinion that transformation to normal scores will work well in most neuropsychological applications for reasons just cited and because of the interest in neuropsychological research with distinguishing normative from nonnormative performance.

CONCLUDING COMMENTS ON PROFILE ANALYSIS

The preceding treatment of PA was intentionally nontechnical and relatively narrow in that it dealt only with the primary questions of shape, elevation, and flatness. Interested readers will find more detailed treatment of PA in standard multivariate texts such as Bernstein, Garbin, and Teng (1988), Stevens (1986), Harris (1985), and Morrison (1990), and in the general literature on research methods (e.g., Maxwell & Arvey, 1982). Of the textbooks mentioned, Harris (1985) and Morrison (1990) offer the most complete coverage of PA, but they are also the most mathematically demanding. Stevens (1986) is the most introductory, dealing only with statistical comparison of group profiles as we have done here. Bernstein et al. (1988) is less mathematically demanding than Harris (1985) and Morrison (1990), but it does not deal with statistical inference in the application of PA. Rather, Bernstein et al. presents an overview and discussion of various measures of profile similarity as part of a more general treatment of classification methods. This material is relevant for measuring similarity between group profiles, between an individual's profile and that of a group, or between the profiles of two individuals. The relevance of this latter aspect of PA to research in clinical neuropsychology has been ably discussed and demonstrated by Chelune and his colleagues (Chelune, Heaton, Lehman, & Robinson, 1979; Chelune & Moehle, 1986; Lehman, Chelune, & Heaton, 1979). For that reason, and because this aspect of PA primarily concerns the classification of individuals into known groups, we have chosen to focus on the statistical comparison of mean profiles as an alternative to MANOVA, reflecting the focus on group definition in the preceding section of the chapter.

Conclusions Regarding Discrepancy-Based Definitions of Reading Disability

In the preceding section, we saw that four groups of children meeting different criteria for reading disability differ significantly from one another in their patterns of neuropsychological test performance. When examining the scales from the Halstead–Reitan Battery (Reitan & Davison, 1974) and other measures, clear differences in profile shape emerged. Although visual inspection of profiles suggests that these differences are small in magnitude, it must be kept in mind that these ability profiles are displayed in a standard score metric. With this fact in mind, the most striking characteristic of these profiles is the markedly poor performance of the two regression-based groups on measures heavily influenced by phonological analysis, such as Speech-Sounds Perception and Auditory Closure. As such, these results are reminiscent of Jorm et al. (1986). A second striking characteristic of these profiles is the generally superior performance of the group meeting only the unadjusted discrepancy score criterion. On examination of verbal skill profiles for the regression only, unadjusted score only, and unimpaired groups, clear differences in profile elevation emerged, with the unadjusted score only group showing clearly superior verbal skills. It is not surprising that the unadjusted score only group outperforms the remaining groups on these verbal scales from the WISC (Wechsler, 1949). The very nature of the IQ–achievement discrepancy score criterion dictates that high-IQ children will be identified by this definition when the discrepancy is not adjusted for the correlation between IQ and achievement. It should also be noted that the group showing the poorest performance in these verbal scale profiles is not eligible for special services in many states and provinces because those jurisdictions do not adjust for the correlation between achievement and IQ.

Much work remains to be done in delineating ability differences between and among groups meeting specific criteria for definitions of learning disability. The data presented here suggest that agencies responsible for dealing with the implications of such definitions need to recast their respective nets in establishing diagnostic criteria for determining eligibility for services. There are many reasons that might be put forward for eliminating discrepancy-based criteria for determining eligibility for services. However, it is clear that, if discrepancy-based criteria are to be used, these criteria should adjust for the correlation between IQ and achievement.

Acknowledgments

Supported in part by NICHD Grant HD-21888, Psycholinguistic and Biological Mechanisms in Dyslexia. Portions of this chapter were presented at the 1988 meeting of the American Education Research Association, New Orleans, LA, April 6, 1988.

References

Bernstein, I. H., Garbin, C. P., & Teng, G. K. (1988). *Applied multivariate analysis*. New York: Springer.

Chelune, G. J., Heaton, R. K., Lehman, R. A., & Robinson, A. (1979). Level versus pattern of neuropsychological performance among schizophrenic and diffusely brain-damaged patients. *Journal of Consulting and Clincial Psychology, 47*, 155–163.

Chelune, G. J., & Moehle, K. A. (1986). Neuropsychological assessment and everyday functioning. In D. Wedding, A. M. Horton, Jr., & J. Webster (Eds.), *The neuropsychology handbook: Behavioral and clinical perspectives* (pp. 489–525). New York: Springer.

Cone, T. E., & Wilson, L. R. (1981). Quantifying a severe discrepancy: A critical analysis. *Learning Disability Quarterly, 4*, 359–371.

Critchley, M. (1970). *The dyslexic child*. Springfield, IL: Charles C. Thomas.

Doehring, D. G. (1978). On the tangled web of behavioral research on developmental dyslexia. In A. L. Benton & D. Pearl (Eds.), *Dyslexia: An appraisal of current research* (pp. 125–135). New York: Oxford University Press.

Espy, K. A., Francis, D. J., Fletcher, J. M., & Rourke, B. P. (1989). Implications of raw cut-off score and regression-based definitions of reading disability. *Journal of Clinical and Experimental Neuropsychology, 11*, 31–32.

Fletcher, J. M., Espy, K. A., Francis, D. J., Davidson, K. E., Rourke, B. P., & Shaywitz, S. E. (1989). Comparisons of cut-off and regression-based definitions of reading disabilities. *Journal of Learning Disabilities, 22*, 334–338.

Fletcher, J. M., Francis, D. J., & Morris, R. (1988). Methodological issues in neuropsychology: Classification, measurement, and the comparison of non-equivalent groups. In F. Boller & J. Grafman (Eds.), *Handbook of neuropsychology* (Vol. I, pp. 83–110). Amsterdam: Elsevier.

Fletcher, J. M., & Morris, R. (1986). Classification of disabled learning: Beyond exclusionary definitions. In S. Ceci (Ed.), *Handbook of cognitive, social, and neuropsychological aspects of learning disabilities* (Vol. I, pp. 55–80). New York: Lawrence Erlbaum.

Francis, D. J., Fletcher, J. M., & Davidson, K. C. (1988, February). *Profile analysis and the study of patterns of neuropsychological performance*. Paper presented at the annual meeting of the International Neuropsychological Society, New Orleans, LA.

Hand, D. J., & Taylor, C. C. (1987). *Multivariate analysis of variance and repeated measures: A practical approach for behavioral scientists*. London: Chapman & Hall.

Harris, R. J. (1985). *Multivariate statistics* (2nd ed.). Orlando: Academic Press.

Huberty, C. J., & Morris, J. D. (1989). Multivariate analysis versus multiple univariate analyses. *Psychological Bulletin, 105,* 302–308.

Jastak, J. L., & Jastak, S. R. (1965). *Wide Range Achievement Test.* Wilmington, DE: Guidance Associates.

Jorm, A. F., Share, D. L., MacLean, R., & Matthews, R. (1986). Cognitive factors at school entry predictive of specific reading retardation and general reading backwardness: A research note. *Journal of Child Psychology and Psychiatry, 27,* 45–54.

Kaufman, A. S. (1979). *Intelligent testing with the WISC-R.* New York: Academic Press.

Kavanaugh, D., & Gray, D. (Eds.) (1986). *Biobehavioral measures of dyslexia.* Parkton, MD: York Press.

Lehman, R. A., Chelune, G. J., & Heaton, R. K. (1979). Level and variability of performance on neuropsychological tests. *Journal of Clinical Psychology, 35,* 358–363.

Maxwell, S. E. & Arvey, R. D. (1982). Small sample profile analysis with many variables. *Psychological Bulletin, 92,* 778–785.

McLeod, J. (1979). Educational underachievement: Toward a defensible psychometric definition. *Journal of Learning Disabilities, 12,* 42–50.

Morris, R. D. (1988). Classification of learning disabilities: Old problems and new approaches. *Journal of Consulting and Clinical Psychology, 56,* 789–794.

Morris, R., & Fletcher, J. M. (1988). Classification in neuropsychology: A theoretical framework and research paradigm. *Journal of Clinical and Experimental Neuropsychology, 10,* 640–658.

Morrison, D. F. (1990). *Multivariate statistical methods* (3rd ed.). New York: McGraw-Hill.

O'Brien, R. G., & Kaiser, M. D. (1985). MANOVA method for analyzing repeated measures designs: An extensive primer. *Psychological Bulletin, 97,* 316–333.

Phillips, S. E., & Clarizio, H. F. (1988). Limitations of standard scores in individual achievement testing. *Educational Measurement: Issues and Practice, 7,* 8–15.

Reitan, R. M., & Davison, L. A. (Eds.). (1974). *Clinical neuropsychology: Current status and applications.* New York: John Wiley & Sons.

Reynolds, C. R. (1984). Critical measurement issues in learning disabilities. *Journal of Special Education, 18,* 451–476.

Rodgers, B. (1983). The identification and prevalence of specific reading retardation. *British Journal of Education Psychology, 53,* 369–373.

Rosner, J., & Simon, D. P. (1971). The auditory analysis test: An initial report. *Journal of Learning Disabilities, 4,* 40–48.

Rourke, B. P. (1978). Reading, spelling, arithmetic disabilities: A neuropsychologic perspective. In H. R. Myklebust (Ed.), *Progress in learning disabilities* (Vol. 4, pp. 97–120). New York: Grune & Stratton.

Rourke, B. P. (1981). Neuropsychological assessment of children with learning disabilities. In S. B. Filskov & T. J. Boll (Eds.), *Handbook of clinical neuropsychology* (pp. 453–478). New York: Wiley-Interscience.

Rourke, B. P., Fisk, J. L., & Strang, J. D. (1986). *Neuropsychological assessment of children.* New York: Guilford Press.

Rutter, M. (1978). Prevalence and types of learning disabilities. In A. L. Benton & D. Pearl (Eds.), *Dyslexia: An appraisal of current research* (pp. 3–29). New York: Oxford University Press.

Rutter, M., & Yule, W. (1975). The concept of specific reading retardation. *Journal of Child Psychology and Psychiatry, 16,* 181–197.

Salvia, J., & Ysseldyke, J. (1981). *Assessment in special and remedial education* (2nd ed.). Boston: Houghton Mifflin.

Sattler, J. M. (1988). *Assessment of children's intelligence and special abilities* (2nd ed.). Philadelphia: W. B. Saunders.

Satz, P., & Fletcher, J. M. (1980). Minimal brain dysfunctions: An appraisal of research concepts and methods. In H. E. Rie & E. D. Rie (Eds.), *Handbook of minimal brain dysfunctions: A critical review* (pp. 669-714). New York: John Wiley & Sons.

Share, D. L., McGhee, R., McKenzie, D., Williams, S., & Silva, P. D. (1987). Further evidence relating to the distinction between specific reading retardation and general reading backwardness. *British Journal of Developmental Psychology, 5,* 35-44.

Shaywitz, S. E., & Shaywitz, B. A. (1988). Afftention deficit disorder: Current perspectives. In J. F. Kavanagh & T. J. Truss (Eds.), *Learning disabilities* (pp. 369-523). Parkton, MD: York Press.

Shaywitz, S. E., Shaywitz, B. A., Barnes, M., & Fletcher, J. M. (1986, October). *Prevalence of dyslexia in a epidemiological sample.* Paper presented at the meeting of the Child Neurology Society, Halifax, Nova Scotia, Canada.

Siegel, L. S., & Heaven, R. K. (1986). Categorization of learning disabilities. In S. Ceci (Ed.), *Handbook of cognitive, social and neuropsychological aspects of learning disabilities* (Vol. I, pp. 95-121). Hillsdale, NJ: Lawrence Erlbaum.

Silva, P. A., McGhee, R., & Williams, S. (1985). Some characteristics of nine year old boys with general reading backwardness or specific reading retardation. *Journal of Child Psychology and Psychiatry, 20,* 407-421.

Spearman, C. E. (1923). *The nature of intelligence and the principles of cognition.* London: Macmillan.

Spreen, O. (1976). Neuropsychology of learning disabilities: Post conference review. In R. M. Knights & D. J. Bakker (Eds.), *The neuropsychology of learning disabilities* (pp. 445-468). Baltimore: University Park Press.

Stevens, J. (1986). *Applied multivariate statistics for the social sciences.* Hillsdale, NJ: Lawrence Erlbaum.

Still, G. F. (1902). Some abnormal psychological conditions in children. *Lancet, 1,* 1077-1082.

Strauss, A. A., & Lehtinen, L. E. (1947). *Psychopathology and education of the brain-injured child.* New York: Grune & Stratton.

Taylor, H. G., Fletcher, J. M., & Satz, P. (1984). Neuropsychological assessment of children. In G. Goldstein & M. Hersen (Eds.), *Handbook of psychological assessment* (pp. 211-234). New York: Pergamon Press.

Taylor, H. G., Satz, P., & Friel, J. (1979). Developmental dyslexia in relation to other childhood reading disorders: Significance and clinical utility. *Reading Research Quarterly, 15,* 84-101.

van der Wissel, A., & Zegers, F. E. (1985). Reading retardation revisited. *British Journal of Developmental Psychology, 3,* 3-9.

Wechsler, D. (1949). *Wechsler Intelligence Scale for Children.* New York: Psychological Corporation.

Woodcock, R. W., & Johnson, M. B. (1977). *Woodcock-Johnson Psycho-Educational Battery Achievement Test.* Hingham, MA: Teaching Resources Corporation.

Yule, W. (1978). Diagnosis: Developmental psychological assessment. In A. G. Kalverboer, H. M. van Praag, & J. Mendlewicz (Eds.), *Advances in biological psychiatry: Vol. 1, Minimal brain dysfunction: Fact or fiction* (pp. 1-49). Basel: S. Karger.

Yule, W. (1985). Response to van der Wissel and Zegers. *British Journal of Developmental Psychology, 3,* 11-13.

CHAPTER 3

Methodological and Statistical Issues in Cluster Analysis

John W. DeLuca, Kenneth M. Adams,
and Byron P. Rourke

This chapter raises some important methodological and statistical issues with respect to the use of numerical taxometric methods, in particular cluster analysis. For example, misconceptions regarding cluster methodology, specifically the notion of "internal validity" are noted. Although determination of the reliability and validity of a cluster solution remains a paramount aspect of the classification process, there continues to exist some confusion surrounding definitions. In addition, there are several issues regarding the use of the two-stage cluster procedure that are vague, misleading, or simply in error. Such problems include the following: percentage relocated as a measure of "stability" and an indicator of "internal validity" (reliability); determination of the "best" starting position for the iterative relocation process; and clarification of what constitutes a true two-stage cluster procedure. In this chapter we review these critical issues as they pertain to the use of cluster analysis in classification research.

The role of classification research is growing rapidly within the field of neuropsychology. Nowhere is it more evident than in the application of cluster analytic techniques to the study of learning-disabled children. Several investigators (e.g., Del Dotto & Rourke, 1985; DeLuca, Rourke, & Del Dotto, Chapter 10, this volume; Fletcher & Morris, 1986; Fuerst, Fisk, & Rourke, 1989; Lyon, Stewart, & Freedman, 1982; Morris, Blashfield, & Satz, 1986) have identified various subtypes of children based on either academic, neuropsychological, or personality dimensions. The work of these and other authors has provided some indication of the reliability and validity of the resulting subtypes. However, the emphasis on this phase of the classification process in the general neuropsychological literature had been less than optimal.

Reliability and Validity

One of the major pitfalls associated with the burgeoning use of cluster analysis is that investigators reporting new and varied classification schemes often do so without concern for the actual utility or their product. That is, provisions for establishing reliability and validity of the resulting solutions are often ignored. Morey, Blashfield, and Skinner (1983) contend that, since there are so many cluster methods and no consensus on the "best" cluster method, evaluation of the validity of the resulting cluster solution is critical. Obviously, a classification model has little place in an empirical discipline or, for that matter, in clinical application when it fails to meet these requirements.

However, such haphazard practice is certainly not novel. In fact, many psychologists have been caught in a quagmire of classification models (or at least what is passed off as such) that rely overly much on clinical "insight" or the exalted divinations of various schools of thought and their respective devotees. At the same time, classification schemes based purely on statistical methods, without the benefit of clinical or theoretical insight, prove to be just as erroneous and/or useless. What is required is the formulation of classification models based on the union or interrelationship of clinical insight and empirical method.

One attempt to provide a model for the entire classification process has been promulgated by Skinner (1981). Skinner delineates three major components in classification research: theory formulation, internal validation, and external validation. According to Skinner, theory formulation involves the specification of the typological paradigm including the following: a precise definition of each subtype; a description of the functional relationships among the groups; an elucidation of the development and etiology of the disorders associated with each subgroup; an explication of prognosis; a description of appropriate treatment interventions; and a discussion of the population for which the typological paradigm might apply.

Once such theoretical contructs are formulated, one must decide on the appropriate numerical taxometric methodology. Most common are the use of Q-type (or inverted) factor analysis and cluster analysis. Specific to the use of cluster analysis are decisions regarding choice of cluster method and ordination metric, variable selection, treatment of outliers, determination of the optimal number of clusters, and, in some cases, choice of iterative relocation procedure (see Morris, Blashfield, & Satz, 1981). Decisions with respect to these aspects of the clustering process are best developed in conjuction with one's hypothesized typological paradigm or theoretical model. However, obtaining a cluster solution is not the end of the classification process. Rather, Skinner elucidated the necessary steps involved in the "internal" and external validation of the resulting cluster solutions.

Morris et al. (1981) contend that the *"internal validation"* process is a method to assess the adequacy and stability of a cluster solution. According to Skinner (1981), internal validation involves the operational definition of constructs and the examination of the cluster solution's internal structure. The latter involves an analysis of reliability, coverage, homogeneity, and robustness (replicability) across techniques and sample (Morris & Fletcher, 1988). Coverage is not an issue in cluster analysis *per se* because this technique, with the exception of the number of outliers excluded from the data set, classifies everyone. Homogeneity is also not a problem in cluster analysis because most hierarchical agglomerative clustering methods produce nonoverlapping or distinct clusters. *External validity* involves evidence of prognostic usefulness, descriptive validity, clinical meaningfulness, and generalizability across samples.

For Skinner (1981), *reliability* pertains to the utilization of split-half samples, alternative samples, comparison of multiple clustering methods, data manipulation (i.e., adding additional subjects or using different classification variables), graphic procedures, and Monte Carlo simulation studies. The split-half sample technique involves just that, dividing a sample in half and clustering both samples. Similar subtypes should be generated by both methods. Alternative samples involves replicating the results with different samples. Comparison of different clustering methods may involve a simple comparison of means and standard deviations across classification variables. However, Morris et al. (1986) proposed a novel use for the Rand statistic. Although this statistic is generally used as an external criterion measure (i.e., comparing a cluster solution to some external criterion such as the true cluster structure), these authors employed it to evaluate the similarity of various solutions generated by different clustering methods.

Data manipulation techniques are twofold. In one case, new subjects are added to the sample, and the new cluster solution is compared to the original one. In the second instance, new clustering variables are employed, and the clustering solutions are compared. Graphic procedures involve graphic plots of clusters either in principal component space or in discriminant space (Morris et al., 1981). Monte Carlo simulations typically involve the generation of multivariate normal random samples based on mean vector, standard deviation vector, and covariance matrix from the original or real data sample (Morris et al., 1986).

Milligan (1981) proposed using internal criterion measures (e.g., gamma, *C* index, point-biserial, tau) to assess the "goodness of fit" between the data and the resulting partitions. These procedures use information strictly from within the clustering process.

Another "internal validation" technique specific to the use of two-stage clustering techniques is calculation of the percentage of entities relocated following k-means iterative partitioning. The two-stage cluster process entails using a hierarchical agglomerative method to generate a typology at the first stage. The second stage employs an iterative partitioning cluster method using "seed points" for the cluster variables from the initial cluster solution. Morris et al. (1981) suggest that the number of entities relocated during the second stage of this process is an index of the *stability* of the cluster solution.

Although all of the above methods are legitimate and crucial aspects of classification research, the theoretical terms of internal and external validity employed by Skinner and others are somewhat confusing. Internal validity, in and of itself, begs the question of reliability. More specifically, methods of reliability and other techniques of validity are enmeshed as if they comprised a single construct. This is precisely the point at which confusion is generated.

According to Adams (1985), the concepts of reliability and validity are quite distinct and have unique tasks, neither of which is served by combining the respective contexts of internal consistency and conceptual justification. Adams (1985) contends that speaking of reliability as "internal validity" serves to confuse the pronounced purposes of reliability and validity. More specifically, Kendall and Buckland (1971) state that:

> The *reliability* of a result is conceived of as that part which is due to permanent systematic effects, and therefore persists from sample to sample. (p. 129)

> *Validation* . . . [is] a procedure which provides, by reference to independent sources, evidence that an inquiry is free from bias or otherwise conforms to its declared purpose . . . Validity is to be contrasted with consistency, which is concerned with the internal agreement of data or procedures among themselves. (p. 160, italics added)

These definitions, as well as many other classical statistical definitions of these concepts, should alert researchers to the fact that internal consistency (e.g., split-half samples, adding more subjects to the data set, internal criterion measures) or observational constancy (e.g., alternate samples, multiple-cluster methods) cannot be proclaimed as evidence for validity that is inherently external to the process under scrutiny (Adams, 1985). Thus, when Skinner (1981) and others speak of internal validity and the processes of reliability, coverage, and homogeneity, all are subsumed under the rubric of reliability, *not* validity. The use of split-half samples, alternate samples, comparison of multiple clustering techniques, inclusion of additional subjects, graphic representations, Monte Carlo simulation procedures, internal criterion measures, and the calculation of percentage of relocated entities in two-stage cluster procedures all form the basis of reliability rather than validity. Only the process of replicating clusters using different clustering variables could be considered as a form of validity (in this case, concurrent validity). To classify these concepts otherwise only leads the unwitting researcher into a nebulous realm of muddled thinking.

Two-Stage Cluster Analysis

Not only has there been some confusion regarding the general concepts employed in classification research, there are other methodological issues surrounding the use of two-stage cluster methods. The two-stage cluster method was promulgated in order to circumvent one of the shortcomings in the use of hierarchical agglomerative clustering methods. That is, once an entity is assigned to a particular cluster, it remains in that cluster even though it may better fit into another cluster as the clustering process proceeds. In short, hierarchical clustering methods contain no provision for the *relocation* of entities that may have been poorly classified in earlier stages of the cluster process (Everitt, 1980).

In order to avoid this deficiency, *k*-means iterative partitioning methods are often applied to compensate for any possible misclassification of entities. These methods are thought to reduce within-cluster variance and to maximize between-cluster variance (Morris et al., 1981). However, there remain several problems associated with the use of this procedure: (1) percentage relocated as a measure of stability or internal validity of a cluster solution; (2) the determination of the optimal starting position for the relocation process; and (3) confusion regarding what constitutes a true two-stage cluster method.

Percentage Relocated

Morris et al. (1981) suggested that the percentage of entities relocated (i.e., the number of entities changing cluster membership from the first-stage solution as compared to the second-stage cluster solution) was an "index of stability" of the cluster solution. That is, if many entities change cluster membership during the relocation process, the adequacy of the results must be questioned (Morris et al., 1981). Although this measure of stability appears to be reasonable and logical, it may be neither. For one thing, Morris et al. do not provide any guidelines as to what is an acceptable number of relocated entities. More important, they do not validate percentage relocated as a meaningful measure of cluster stability or "internal validity."

DeLuca, Adams, and Rourke (submitted) employed several relocation techniques as part of a larger investigation of the two-stage cluster methodology. In this study, we utilized two separate data sets, each of known cluster structure. The first was a Monte Carlo data set consisting of 50 entities, four dimensions or variables, and three clusters. This data set was error-free; that is, there were no outliers, overlapping clusters, or other sources of error (see Milligan, 1981). The second was Fisher's (1936) iris data set; it consisted of 150 entities, four variables, and three clusters (two of which overlapped to some degree). Each data set was subjected to the following first-stage cluster methods: Ward's method using squared euclidean distance (SED), average linkage using SED and correlation coefficient (CORR), and centroid using SED and CORR. All first-stage solutions were subjected to several k-means iterative relocation procedures including SED, CORR, and shape (SHP) as ordination metrics (Wishart, 1978).

Several measures were calculated in order to assess the accuracy of the various methods as well as to analyze the measure of percentage relocated. These included calculating the percentage of entities correctly classified (percentage correct), several external criterion measures (Milligan & Cooper, 1986; Milligan & Schilling, 1985), and the number of entities relocated during the second stage of the clustering process. All four external criterion measures correlated very highly with percentage correct. For the Monte Carlo data set, correlations ranged from .9911 to .9998. For the iris data set, correlations ranged from .87 to .99. Thus, in support of Milligan and his co-workers, several of the external criterion measures were found to represent the degree of true cluster recovery in an accurate fashion.

The percentage of relocated entities (percentage relocated) did not fare as well. In fact, the correlations between percentage relocated and percentage correct ranged from −.2173 to −.2183 for the Monte Carlo data set and from −.0700 to −.1192 for the Iris data set. As a result, DeLuca et al. (submitted) concluded that the usefulness measure of percentage relocated as a measure of stability or "internal validity" was nil. Percentage relocated may reflect the degree of similarity between the first-stage cluster algorithm and the second-stage relocation algorithm and nothing more. In any case, the measure has little value in classification research. Given these results, the claim of "internal validity" for typologies based on the percentage of relocated entities may be misleading.

Starting Position

Generally, iterative partitioning methods begin with an initial partition of the data, either a previous cluster solution, estimated seed values, or a random assignment of cases to n clusters (Blashfield & Aldenderfer, 1978; Wishart, 1978). Each entity is assigned to the cluster with the nearest centroid. Once a complete pass is made though all data cases, new centroids are calculated. The latter process is continued until no entities change cluster membership or until a predetermined number of passes are completed (Anderberg, 1973; Blashfield & Aldenderfer, 1978; Wishart, 1978). Blashfield and Aldenderfer (1978) found that different iterative partitioning methods as well as different starting positions affect the solution.

With respect to this data "fix," several methods of using k-means iterative partitioning have been promoted. For example, Wishart (1978) suggested assigning persons to n clusters in a random manner prior to the relocation process. Another option reported by Morey et al. (1983) is inspection of the initial cluster results to determine the optimal number of clusters. One then applies the random relocation process to that number of clusters. A third method (Morris et al., 1981) involves starting with the optimal number of clusters obtained from a previous solution as above, but it uses the actual cluster membership as the "seeds" or starting points for the relocation procedure. However, the iterative relocation procedure providing the "best" retrieval of the true structure of the data is, as yet, unknown.

Blashfield and Aldenderfer (1978) found that different iterative partitioning methods as well as starting positions affect the solution. These authors reported that solutions obtained from CLUSTAN (Wishart, 1978) using random relocation produced higher κ values than did a solution using Ward's method as a starting point (i.e., median κ values of .71 and .64, respectively). In fact, they reported that the random relocation solutions produced the highest median κ values of all eight classification techniques employed. Morris and Aldenderfer concluded that varying the starting position of the second-stage clustering process had a dramatic effect on the results.

In sharp contrast to the above, Milligan (1980) found very good recovery of true cluster structure when "rational" starting positions (e.g., seed values based on the first-stage clustering solution) were employed. Random seeds or starting positions were found to produce the worst recovery rates. In addition, the former method was found to be robust with respect to all types of error examined. Milligan (1980) concluded the following: (1) the starting position must approximate the final solution

for the k-means methods to produce good recovery; and (2) most algorithms were robust and not affected by type of ordination metric. Thus,
Milligan contends that the choice of cluster method is more critical than
is the choice of ordination metric.

The DeLuca et al. (submitted) study outlined above employed several different relocation procedures. Three ordination metrics were
chosen: SED, CORR, and SHP. For each metric, four relocation procedures were employed. Random relocation methods entailed assigning
cluster members to one of n clusters in a random fashion. Initial relocation methods utilized seed values obtained from the first-stage cluster
solution. In addition, both random and initial relocation methods were
calculated using two different starting positions: starting at 10 clusters
and starting at the optimal number of clusters as determined by the first-
stage cluster solution. The results of this study tend to support Milligan's
notion that seed values based on the first-stage clustering solution provide slightly more accurate cluster recovery rates. However, it was also
found that solutions starting at 10 clusters versus three tended to provide
greater recovery rates. The latter may be the result of a greater number of
iterations (or passes through the data to reassign misclassified entities)
having taken place. However, in contrast to the findings presented by
Milligan (1980), we found that choice of ordination metric was more
important than was choice of first-stage cluster method.

Two-Stage versus One-Stage Cluster Methodology

In the analysis of the various aspects of two-stage clustering procedures,
one differentiation must occur. That is, the use of iterative partitioning
methods employing a random assignment of entities to n clusters is not a
two-stage technique. More specifically, by assigning cases randomly to
clusters, one ignores all information from the first-stage cluster solution
save the number of clusters (except for those instances employing a 10-
cluster starting position). By ignoring these initial seed values and replac-
ing them with a random assignment of cases or entities, the resulting
solution is determined solely by the algorithm employed in the second-
stage procedure. That is, the solution reflects clustering by the k-means
iterative relocation method and not an adjustment to the initial hierarchical agglomerative procedure. Hence, this execution of the relocation
process is not at all a two-stage process. The only true two-stage cluster
procedure entails employing estimated seed values (based on some theoretical model or hypothesis) or seed values obtained by stage-one clustering
methods. However, this exposition is not meant to decry the use of random
relocation procedures. Rather, it is only an attempt to clarify definitional

issues. In fact, DeLuca et al. (submitted) found some random relocation methods to be quite accurate in recovering true cluster structure.

Implications

As classification techniques such as cluster analysis play an increasingly important role in neuropsychological research, investigators must become cognizant of the many intricacies and complexities involved in such a task. It goes without saying that valid and reliable techniques are the hallmark of any empirical methodology. The latter becomes even more critical when information about new typologies is disseminated and applied in clinical realms. The application of cluster-analytic techniques places the investigator in the position of making many decisions throughout the classification process. The more such decisions can be made employing objective and empirical criteria, the less likely erroneous or ill-conceived conclusions will occur. This chapter is an attempt to delineate and discuss some of the remaining problems associated with the conceptualization and application of cluster analysis. Although the potential reward of cluster-based research in neuropsychology remains great, prospective investigators must be forewarned of the need for a perspicacious grasp of the labyrinth that awaits them.

References

Adams, K. M. (1985). Theoretical, methodological, and statistical issues. In B. P. Rourke (Ed.), *Neuropsychology of learning disabilities: Essentials of subtype analysis* (pp. 17–39). New York: Guilford Press.

Anderberg, M. R. (1973). *Cluster analysis for applications*. New York: Academic Press.

Blashfield, R. K., & Aldenderfer, M. S. (1978). Computer programs for performing iterative partitioning cluster analysis. *Applied Psychological Measurement, 2,* 533–541.

Del Dotto, J. E., & Rourke, B. P. (1985). Subtypes of left-handed learning-disabled children. In B. P. Rourke (Ed.), *Neuropsychology of learning disabilities: Essentials of subtype analysis* (pp. 89–132). New York: Guilford Press.

DeLuca, J. W., Adams, K. M., & Rourke, B. P. (submitted). *Two stage cluster analysis: Methodological and statistical issues.*

Everitt, B. S. (1980). *Cluster analysis* (2nd ed.). London: Heineman Educational Books.

Fisher, R. A. (1936). The use of multiple measurements in taxonomic problems. *Annals of Eugenics, 7,* 179–188.

Fletcher, J. M., & Morris, R. D. (1986). Classification of disabled learners: Beyond exclusionary definitions. In S. J. Ceci (Ed.), *Handbook of cognitive, social, and neuropsychological aspects of learning disabilities* (pp. 55–80). Hillsdale, NJ: Lawrence Erlbaum.

Fuerst, D. R., Fisk, J. L., & Rourke, B. P. (1989). Psychosocial functioning of learning-disabled children: Replicability of statistically derived subtypes. *Journal of Consulting and Clinical Psychology, 57,* 275–280.

Kendall, M. G., & Buckland, W. P. (1971). *A dictionary of statistical terms.* New York: Hafner.

Lyon, R., Stewart, N., & Freedman, D. (1982). Neuropsychological characteristics of empirically derived subgroups of disabled readers. *Journal of Clinical Neuropsychology, 4,* 343–366.

Milligan, G. W. (1980). An examination of the effect of six types of error perturbation on fifteen clustering algorithms. *Psychometrika, 45,* 325–342.

Milligan, G. W. (1981). A Monte Carlo study of thirty internal criterion measures for cluster analysis. *Psychometrika, 46,* 187–199.

Milligan, G. W., & Cooper, M. C. (1986). A study of the comparability of external criteria for hierarchical cluster analysis. *Multivariate Behavioral Research, 21,* 441–458.

Milligan, G. W., & Schilling, D. A. (1985). Asymptotic and finite sample characteristics of four external criterion measures. *Multivariate Behavioral Research, 20,* 97–109.

Morey, L. C., Blashfield, R. K., & Skinner, H. A. (1983). A comparison of cluster analysis techniques within a sequential validation framework. *Multivariate Behavioral Research, 18,* 309–329.

Morris, R. D., Blashfield, R. K., & Satz, P. (1981). Neuropsychology and cluster analysis. *Journal of Clinical Neuropsychology, 3,* 79–99.

Morris, R. D., Blashfield, R. K., & Satz, P. (1986). Developmental classification of reading-disabled children. *Journal of Clinical and Experimental Neuropsychology, 8,* 371–392.

Morris, R. D., & Fletcher, J. M. (1988). Classification in neuropsychology: A theoretical framework and research paradigm. *Journal of Clinical and Experimental Neuropsychology, 10,* 640–658.

Skinner, H. A. (1981). Toward the integration of classification theory and methods. *Journal of Abnormal Psychology, 90,* 68–87.

Wishart, D. (1978). *CLUSTAN user manual: Version 1C, release 2* (3rd ed.). Edinburgh: Edinburgh University Program Library Unit.

Content Areas

Concurrent and Predictive Validity of Phonetic Accuracy of Misspellings in Normal and Disabled Readers and Spellers

Diane L. Russell and Byron P. Rourke

Neuropsychological investigations of children with reading and spelling disabilities have revealed, among other things, that these children are a heterogeneous group exhibiting various patterns of ability-related deficits (Rourke, 1978). Specific subtypes of learning-disabled children have been identified using empirical strategies, such as the multivariate approach employed by Petrauskas and Rourke (1979). Children can also be divided into groups on the basis of *a priori* considerations. One such approach is that of Boder (1973), who proposed three types of "dyslexia" based on the child's approach to reading and spelling.

According to Boder, "dysphonetic dyslexics" read and spell words by "sight" and produce phonetically inaccurate spelling errors. Their misspellings bear little or no phonetic similarity to the words to be spelled. "Dyseidetic dyslexics" read and spell words in a phonetic manner and their misspellings are usually very accurate from a phonetic standpoint (i.e., they have a striking phonemic resemblance to the target words). Boder also identified a "mixed dysphonetic–dyseidetic dyslexic" group who cannot visualize or phonetically analyze words. Their misspellings are usually phonetically inaccurate. Boder has also developed a standardized way of classifying children into specific groups based on their approach to reading and spelling (Boder & Jarrico, 1982).

Nelson and Warrington (1974) found that children aged 8 to 14 who exhibited a substantial Wechsler Intelligence Scale for Children (WISC; Wechsler, 1949) Verbal IQ–Performance IQ discrepancy (i.e., VIQ < PIQ by at least 15 points) and who had both reading and spelling disabilities also produced phonetically inaccurate spelling errors. These results supported the work of Newcombe (1969) and Kinsbourne and Warrington (1964), who found that phonetically inaccurate spelling errors were associated with aphasia and generalized language impairment in adult patients.

Sweeney and Rourke (1978) compared the performances of normal spellers and two subtypes of disabled spellers at two age levels ($M = 10$ years and 13.5 years). The two subtypes of disabled spellers were equally deficient in their *level* of spelling performance, but differed markedly in their percentages of phonetically accurate misspellings. The phonetically accurate (PA) spellers rendered at least 60% of their misspelled syllables on the Wide Range Achievement Test (WRAT; Jastak & Jastak, 1965) Spelling subtest in a phonetically accurate manner (e.g., "nacher" for "nature"). Disabled spellers who rendered 40% or less of their misspelled syllables on the WRAT Spelling subtest in a phonetically accurate manner were referred to as phonetically inaccurate (PI) spellers (e.g., "diltum" for "nature"). Sweeney and Rourke (1978) found that the PI group performed at levels significantly below those of the normal group on all linguistic tasks except those requiring only very simple auditory discrimination (e.g., Goldman–Fristoe–Woodcock [1970] Test of Auditory Discrimination) and immediate auditory–verbal memory (e.g., WISC Digit Span subtest). On the other hand, the older PA subtype performed at levels indistinguishable from those of the PI subtype only on tasks that involved fairly complex linguistic–cognitive operations (e.g., WISC Information, Comprehension, and Vocabulary subtests). Differences among the three groups were evident primarily at the older age level investigated.

Subsequent studies in this series examined more specific aspects of the ability structure of these disabled spellers. The results of these investigations indicated that disabled spelling ability appears to be related to deficiencies in logical–grammatical skills, particularly for children whose spelling is predominantly phonetically inaccurate (Rourke, 1983; Sweeney & Rourke, 1985). In studies designed to determine the factors operating at the younger age levels, differences were observed among PAs, PIs, and normal spellers. Specifically, the PAs were able to segment words on a phonetic basis and they exhibited adequate visual memory, but they had difficulty in appreciating the visual aspects or the "gestalt" of words. On the other hand, the PIs were deficient in spelling recognition, phonemic segmentation, visual closure, and visual memory, suggesting that a much wider-ranging and debilitating set of problems was operative in the PI group (Sweeney & Rourke, 1985). In reviewing the results of some of the studies in this series, Rourke (1983) suggested the following:

> In general, the PIs at the older age level performed in a fashion very similar to that which would be expected from an impairment in lin-

guistic systems that are thought to be subserved primarily by the temporal (and possibly, adjacent) cortical regions of the left cerebral hemisphere. It is clear that the picture is far different in the case of the PAs. (p. 228)

The later studies (summarized in Sweeney & Rourke, 1985) dealt specifically with younger children and helped to clarify the patterns of abilities and deficits of these two types of disabled spellers. One of the hypotheses generated on the basis of the results of the Sweeney and Rourke (1978) study was that "PIs encounter significant difficulty in carrying out relatively rudimentary operations on language, and that this hampers their capacity to benefit from formal academic instruction in the processing of verbal information" (Sweeney & Rourke, 1985, p. 15).

A study conducted by Sweeney, McCabe, and Rourke (1978) showed that, at the younger age level (9- to 10½-year-olds), PIs were significantly poorer relative to normals (Ns) in comprehending grammatical relationships. The pattern of performance of the three groups on a revised version of the Logico-Grammatical Sentence Comprehension Test (Wiig & Semel, 1974) was consistent (i.e., PI < PA < N) across all five subtests (Comparative, Temporal, Passive, Spatial, and Familial). The performance of the PAs did not differ statistically from that of either the PIs or the Ns on these measures.

Sweeney and Rourke (1978) also hypothesized that PIs experience difficulty in carrying out basic linguistic operations, whereas PAs experience difficulty when a task requires them to go beyond the verbal information provided to them. Coderre, Sweeney, and Rourke (1979) attempted to provide information regarding these two hypotheses in their study of younger Ns, PIs, and PAs (ages 9 to 11 years). The results were as follows:

1. Phonemic Segmentation Test   PA > N > PI
2. Spelling Recognition Test   N > PA > PI
3. Cloze Procedure (Anderson, 1976)   N > PA > PI
4. Visual Memory Test (Vellutino, Steger,
   DeSetto, & Phillips, 1975)   N > PA > PI

Several basic conclusions were arrived at on the basis of these results. In terms of phonemic segmentation, it was hypothesized that PIs had significant difficulty relative to PAs in analyzing phonemic information in a systematic fashion. The PAs, on the other hand, were thought to adhere rigidly to a phonemic system of analysis, whereas the Ns were more flexible in their approach. According to Sweeney and Rourke (1985): "This flexibility may allow for the utilization of other forms of language-related operations (e.g., 'visualizing' the spatial features of the word to be spelled subsequent to phonemic segmentation)" (p. 159).

Results of the Spelling Recognition Test indicated that PAs had considerable difficulty in appreciating the correct graphic representations of words. They tended to overuse phonemic information to compensate for a deficiency in the ability to utilize the visual information in words. PIs were very poor on this test, again confirming their problem in dealing with even basic language operations.

On the Cloze Procedure (a visual–spatial task), the performance of the PAs indicated a difficulty in memory for the visual–spatial features of word configurations. PIs, of course, were even more deficient in this ability. The results of the Visual Memory Test indicated that neither the PAs nor the PIs had significant difficulties with visual memory so long as the visual stimuli had relatively limited symbolic significance. Their difficulties lay mainly with the handling of symbolic information (i.e., words, letters, syllables).

Coderre et al. (1979) found that PAs were significantly deficient in their ability to choose the correct graphic representation of words with a low grapheme–phoneme correspondence. Sweeney and Rourke (1982), in a further analysis of the reading strategies of older and younger PA spellers, found that PAs read significantly more words by phonetic analysis and significantly fewer words by sight than did the Ns at both age levels. The PIs did not utilize a phonetic strategy at the younger age level, but did shift to become more like the PAs in their reading strategy at the older age level.

Other studies have revealed that retarded readers exhibit significantly more phonetically inaccurate spelling errors than do normal readers in grades 2, 4, 5, and 6 (Rourke, 1983). It should also be noted that Sweeney and Rourke (1978) found that the PIs exhibited deficient reading (word recognition) skills, especially at the older age level studied. The persistence of a relationship between reading disability and phonetic inaccuracy in spelling over a 4-year period and the poor reading performance of PIs suggest that phonetic inaccuracy in spelling is a reliable indicator and predictor of potentially serious reading problems. The deficiency of the PIs in performing linguistic operations such as phonemic synthesis and segmentation appears to be a reliable and consistent deficit across time and appears to play a significant role in the reading disability that these children exhibit—a disability that tends not to resolve as the child grows older.

At this point we review two major investigations that have been conducted in our laboratory. The results of these studies have not been reported previously.

Study 1: Russell and Rourke (1984)

Phonetic accuracy has been found to be related to several linguistic-cognitive operations, including reading and spelling. In 1984, we examined the concurrent and predictive validity of level of phonetic accuracy of misspellings in a group of learning-disabled children (Russell & Rourke, 1984). A group of 21 learning-disabled boys, ages 9 to 14, were assessed neuropsychologically five times over a 1-year period (at 3-month intervals). We found that the degree of phonetic accuracy of the subjects' misspellings on the WRAT Spelling subtest was significantly and consistently related to two achievement measures (WRAT Reading and WRAT Spelling subtests), to phoneme/grapheme matching skills (Speech-Sounds Perception Test; Reitan & Davison, 1974), to the ability to repeat a word while omitting a specific phonemic element from that word (Rosner Auditory Analysis Test; Rosner & Simon, 1970), and to fine auditory discrimination/sustained attention (Seashore Rhythm Test; Reitan & Davison, 1974). Performance on two measures of visual–spatial sequencing ability (one utilizing numerical cues alone—Trail Making Test, Part A; and one utilizing both alphabetic and numerical cues—Trail Making Test, Part B; Reitan & Davison, 1974) and on a test measuring phonemically cued verbal fluency skills (Verbal Fluency Test; Strong, 1963) were also related to levels of phonetic accuracy. These results held for relationships between the aforementioned dependent variables and the levels of phonetic accuracy both initially and at each time of testing.

Changes in scores on specific dependent measures over parts of or the entire 12-month period were also related to the initial levels of phonetic accuracy. These included improvements in visual–spatial sequencing and the ability to shift psychological set, in written spelling skills, in complex auditory analysis abilities, and in fine auditory discrimination and sustained attention skills. Initial levels of phonetic accuracy were negatively related to changes on a measure of phoneme–grapheme matching skills, suggesting that greater gains were made in these skills by those children who initially exhibited low levels of phonetic accuracy in their misspellings.

Level of phonetic accuracy was not related at any time of testing to a measure of speeded eye–hand coordination (Grooved Pegboard Test; Kløve, 1963), to the ability to remember and repeat exactly sentences of gradually increasing length (Sentence Memory Test; Benton, 1965), or to a measure of parental perception of academic achievement (the Achievement Scale of the Personality Inventory for Children [PIC]; Wirt, Lachar, Klinedist, & Seat, 1977). Level of phonetic accuracy was less highly and much less consistently related to the three WISC IQ variables (VIQ, PIQ, and FSIQ), to the WRAT Arithmetic subtest, to the Adjustment and Development scales of the Personality Inventory for Children, and to a sound-blending task (the Auditory Closure Test; Kass, 1964). Low variability in scores (e.g., on the IQ measures) and ceiling effects on some of the measures (e.g., the Auditory Closure Test) may have been responsible for the low correlations obtained.

On the basis of these results we concluded that phonetic accuracy was related to several linguistic abilities as well as to academic achievement measures (particularly reading and spelling) and to measures of visual-spatial sequencing ability. These relationships were evident in a learning-disabled population. Correlations between initial levels of phonetic accuracy and abilities measured over a 12-month period, as well an increase in the scores on several measures over the 12-month interval, indicated that phonetic accuracy may well be both an important indicator of current abilities and an important predictor of future ability levels in the learning-disabled child.

Study 2: Russell and Rourke (1989)

On the basis of the results of the Sweeney and Rourke (1978, 1985) and Russell and Rourke (1984) studies, another investigation was undertaken by Russell and Rourke (1989) to evaluate the relationship between level of phonetic accuracy of misspellings and neuropsychological integrity in both normal and disabled readers and spellers. Some of the results of the data analyses of this longitudinal investigation have been reported earlier (Rourke, 1976; Rourke & Orr, 1977). The focus of this most recent study was on the relationship between the average level of phonetic accuracy and various neuropsychological variables.

Forty-two subjects (23 normal readers—NR; 19 disabled readers—DR) were tested four times over a 5-year period. The subjects were selected from a population of grade 1 and grade 2 male students in regular classroom settings. Normal readers (NR) obtained a centile score or 50 or above on the Reading subtest of the Metropolitan Achievement Test (MAT; Durost, Bixler, Hildreth, Lund, & Wrightstone, 1959) and a centile score of 50 or above on either the Word Knowledge or the Word Discrimination subtest of the MAT. Students in the NR group had also been rated by their principal and teacher as being at least "average" students. Subjects in the DR group obtained a centile score of 20 or below on the Reading subtest of the MAT and a centile score of 35 or below on either the Word Knowledge or the Word Discrimination subtest. Students in the DR group had all been rated by their principal and teacher as "poor" students. All subjects included in the study obtained approximately average Full Scale IQ values on the WISC. The two groups (NR and DR) were also age-matched in pairs. At the time of the initial testing, the subjects were screened to insure that they were free of any auditory or visual acuity deficits and any socioemotional disturbances. The subjects were tested each time with a full neuropsychological test battery (Reitan & Davison, 1974) and a number of other supplementary tests. The neuropsychological tests are listed and described in Rourke (1976), Rourke, Bakker, Fisk, and Strang (1983), and Rourke, Fisk, and Strang (1986).

Calculations were made to determine each subject's level of phonetic accuracy of misspellings on the Spelling subtest of the WRAT for each time of testing and also for the average level over all four times of testing. Table 4.1 contains the average level of phonetic accuracy for the NR and DR groups over all four times of testing. Calculations were also made to determine the average percentage of neuropsychological impairment (API) over all four times of testing for each group. Table 4.2 contains the average percentage impairment levels in *each* category of neuropsychological tests for the NR and DR groups across the four times of testing as well as the average percentage impairment levels across *all* categories for the NR and DR groups. Details regarding the aforementioned calculations can be found in Russell and Rourke (1989).

We found that the average level of phonetic accuracy for the NR group (70.70%) was significantly higher than the average level of phonetic accuracy for the DR group (53.04%). These results were comparable to those obtained by Sweeney and Rourke (1978): They found that the average level of phonetic accuracy for the normal spellers (younger and older groups combined) was 70.87% and that the average level of phonetic accuracy for the disabled spellers (younger and older groups combined and PA and PI groups combined) was 51.97%.

The DR group was clearly more impaired from a neuropsychological perspective than was the NR group (API = 18.04% and 7.03% for the DR and NR groups, respectively). In fact, the NR group could be considered to be essentially normal from a neuropsychological perspective if we take the 0.10 or less (i.e., 10% or less) Halstead Impairment Index cut-off value reported by Reitan and Davison (1974) as "normal."

Some interesting observations can be made from the average percentage impairment scores in the various categories. As would be expected, the DR group performed very poorly on both the achievement and the language-related measures. They also obtained impaired scores on higher-order problem-solving and reasoning tests. Many of these tasks can be performed more effectively through the utilization of such language-related skills as verbal mediation (Rourke et al., 1983, 1986). It is possible that the performance of the DR group on higher-order tasks could have been adversely affected by their language-related disabilities.

TABLE 4.1. Average Level of Phonetic Accuracy over Four
Times of Testing

	M	SD
DR group	53.04	15.15
NR group	70.70	9.77
$t = 3.55, p < .001$		

It is interesting to note that the DR group was more impaired on the
tasks classified as "language-related" than on the WISC Verbal measures
(API $= 21.57\%$ and 10.30%, respectively). This is a common finding in
learning-disabled children (Rourke, 1983). It may be the case that many
of the WISC Verbal subtests require merely rote processing of overlearned
information. However, novel (and therefore more cognitively demanding) language-related measures (e.g., Auditory Closure Test, Verbal
Fluency Test, Sentence Memory Test) require much more complex semantic–acoustic processing. Thus, these tasks may better exemplify the
language-related deficits of disabled readers than do the (more prosaic)
Verbal subtests of the WISC.

Figure 4.1 contains a graphic illustration of the relationship between
the average level of phonetic accuracy of misspellings on the WRAT
Spelling subtest and the average level of neuropsychological impairment
for each subject. The correlation between these two variables was -0.661

TABLE 4.2. Average Percentage Impairment across
Four Times of Testing

Category	Percentage impairment	
	DR group	NR group
Achievement	35.62	3.10
Language-related	21.58	9.74
Higher-order	18.42	9.41
Sensory-perceptual	16.33	11.05
Motor and psychomotor	13.96	5.35
WISC Verbal	10.30	3.81
Visual–spatial	8.76	1.82
Mean	18.04	7.03
$t = 7.29, p < .0005$		

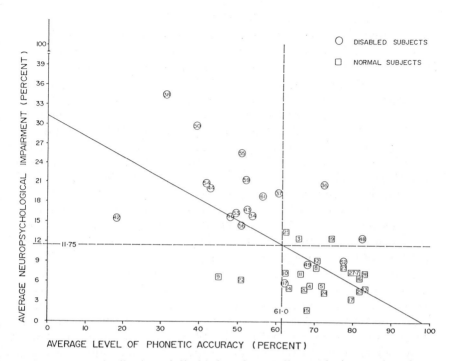

FIGURE 4.1. Distribution of disabled readers/spellers and of normal readers/ spellers based on the average level of phonetic accuracy and the average percentage of neuropsychological impairment.

($p < .0005$), yielding a percentage of variance accounted for by the relationship between these two variables of 44%. This relationship indicates that the higher the average level of phonetic accuracy (i.e., the more phonetically accurate the misspellings), the lower the level of neuropsychological impairment. Conversely, the lower the average level of phonetic accuracy (i.e., the more phonetically inaccurate the misspellings), the higher the level of neuropsychological impairment. As Rourke (1983) pointed out previously, there are some deficiencies that serve to "mark" some subtypes of learning-disabled children and that seem to have particularly debilitating neuropsychological consequences for the children who exhibit them. A preponderance of phonetically inaccurate misspellings in disabled readers and spellers appears to be one such "marker."

In a *post-hoc* analysis of the data presented in Figure 4.1, lines were drawn at the 11.75% level of neuropsychological impairment and the 61.0% average level of phonetic accuracy. The "classification rates" reported by Russell and Rourke (1989) indicate that these two "cut-off" values provide quite high "hit rates" for both the NR and DR groups. A discriminant function analysis and cross-validation study would be valuable in determining the reliability and the validity of these variables and values in discriminating between normal and disabled readers.

It is interesting to note that the 61.0% average level of phonetic accuracy used as a "cut-off" in the Russell and Rourke (1989) study is virtually the same as the 60% phonetic accuracy level used by Sweeney and Rourke (1978) to identify phonetically accurate spellers. In addition, the 11.75% average level of neuropsychological impairment "cut-off" value used in the Russell and Rourke (1989) study is consistent with the 0.10 (10.0%) Halstead Impairment Rating used by Reitan and Davison (1974) to define neuropsychological "normality."

Russell and Rourke (1989) also found that the average level of phonetic accuracy was consistently and highly related to performance on the WRAT Reading subtest (Standard Score and Grade variables) and the MAT Word Knowledge subtest (Standard Score variable). Table 4.3 contains these results. These measures require the child to decode individual words. Therefore, the results seem to indicate that the more phonetically accurate the child's misspellings, the better the performance on decoding measures. These findings are consistent with the results of studies by Nelson and Warrington (1974) and Sweeney and Rourke (1978), who found a relationship between phonetically inaccurate spelling errors and marked reading disability. As suggested by Sweeney and Rourke (1985), phonetic inaccuracy in spelling appears to be a reliable indicator and predictor of serious reading problems. Russell and Rourke (1984) also found that levels of phonetic accuracy were highly and consistently related to reading achievement measures.

Russell and Rourke (1989) found that the average level of phonetic accuracy was significantly related to performance on the Auditory Closure Test at all four times of testing, to the Verbal Fluency Test at three times of testing, to the WISC Information subtest at two times of testing, and to the WISC Vocabulary subtest and the Peabody Picture Vocabulary Test (Dunn, 1965) at one time of testing (see Table 4.4). The average level of phonetic accuracy was not significantly related to the WISC Similarities, Comprehension, and Arithmetic subtests or to the Sentence Memory Test at any of the four times of testing. These results are quite similar to the results of the Russell and Rourke (1984) investigation. In both studies, phonemically cued verbal fluency (i.e., the Verbal Fluency Test) was related to level of phonetic accuracy. The ability to remember and repeat exactly sentences of gradually increasing length (i.e., the Sentence Memory Test) was not related to level of phonetic accuracy in either study.

In the Russell and Rourke (1984) work, the WISC Verbal IQ was related to level of phonetic accuracy at only one time of testing. We felt

TABLE 4.3. Correlations of Achievement Measures with the Average Level of
Phonetic Accuracy (Corrected for Curtailment of Distribution)

Variable	r	Level of significance
Testing 1		
WRAT Reading Standard Score	0.486	$p < .025$
WRAT Reading Grade	0.546	$p < .010$
WRAT Spelling Standard Score	0.531	$p < .010$
MAT Reading Standard Score	0.233	n.s.
MAT Word Knowledge Standard Score	0.623	$p < .005$
Testing 2		
WRAT Reading Standard Score	0.492	$p < .025$
WRAT Reading Grade	0.325	n.s.
WRAT Spelling Standard Score	0.258	n.s.
MAT Reading Standard Score	0.165	n.s.
MAT Word Knowledge Standard Score	0.457	$p < .025$
Testing 3		
WRAT Reading Standard Score	0.427	$p < .050$
WRAT Reading Grade	0.416	$p < .050$
WRAT Spelling Standard Score	0.397	$p < .050$
MAT Reading Standard Score	0.343	n.s.
MAT Word Knowledge Standard Score	0.476	$p < .025$
Testing 4		
WRAT Reading Standard Score	0.432	$p < .050$
WRAT Reading Grade	0.423	$p < .050$
WRAT Spelling Score	0.375	n.s.
MAT Reading Standard Score	0.450	$p < .050$
MAT Word Knowledge Standard Score	0.421	$p < .050$

that low variability in the WISC Verbal IQ could have accounted for this
finding. In the present study, the various WISC Verbal subtests were
much less highly and less consistently related to the average level of
phonetic accuracy than were some of the other neuropsychological variables. Again, low variability on each of the WISC Verbal subtests (i.e.,
$SD < 3.00$) could have accounted for the results obtained.

Russell and Rourke (1989) found that performance on a sound-
blending task (the Auditory Closure Test) and the average level of phonetic accuracy were positively, significantly, and consistently related to

TABLE 4.4. Correlations between the Average Level of Phonetic Accuracy and the Neuropsychological Variables Used in the Sweeney and Rourke (1978) Study

Variable	r	Level of significance
Testing 1		
Auditory Closure Test	0.573	$p < .010$
Verbal Fluency Test	0.542	$p < .010$
PPVT IQ	0.250	n.s.
WISC Vocabulary	0.191	n.s.
WISC Comprehension	0.027	n.s.
Sentence Memory Test	−0.046	n.s.
WISC Arithmetic	−0.076	n.s.
WISC Similarities	−0.091	n.s.
WISC Information	−0.113	n.s.
Testing 2		
Auditory Closure Test	0.591	$p < .005$
WISC Information	0.499	$p < .025$
Verbal Fluency Test	0.472	$p < .025$
PPVT IQ	0.326	n.s.
WISC Vocabulary	0.319	n.s.
WISC Arithmetic	0.280	n.s.
WISC Comprehension	0.103	n.s.
WISC Similarities	0.079	n.s.
Sentence Memory Test	−0.180	n.s.
Testing 3		
WISC Vocabulary	0.676	$p < .005$
Auditory Closure Test	0.620	$p < .005$
Verbal Fluency Test	0.596	$p < .005$
PPVT IQ	0.333	n.s.
WISC Similarities	0.271	n.s.
WISC Information	0.193	n.s.
WISC Comprehension	0.064	n.s.
Sentence Memory Test	0.004	n.s.
WISC Arithmetic	−0.262	n.s.
Testing 4		
Auditory Closure Test	0.674	$p < .005$
PPVT IQ	0.559	$p < .010$
WISC Information	0.456	$p < .025$
WISC Vocabulary	0.388	n.s.
Verbal Fluency Test	0.378	n.s.
WISC Similarities	0.252	n.s.
WISC Arithmetic	0.135	n.s.
WISC Comprehension	−0.022	n.s.
Sentence Memory Test	−0.349	n.s.

each other. This is in sharp contrast to the results of the Russell and Rourke (1984) study, in which performance on the Auditory Closure Test was not related to the level of phonetic accuracy. Russell and Rourke (1984) suggested that a ceiling effect for this measure may have accounted for the lack of relationship between these two variables. This ceiling effect was not observed in the Russell and Rourke (1989) study, since the subjects were tested only once per year instead of five times in 1 year, as in the Russell and Rourke (1984) study.

The results reported by Russell and Rourke (1984, 1989) are consistent with those of Boder (1973). She found that children with reading/spelling disabilities often have difficulties with tasks requiring auditory perception, auditory discrimination, auditory sequencing, and word analysis/synthesis. These skills appear to be quite necessary to perform such tasks as phonemically cued verbal fluency and sound blending (as on the Verbal Fluency Test and the Auditory Closure Test, respectively).

The results of the Russell and Rourke (1989) investigation indicated that the average level of phonetic accuracy of misspellings was highly related to the level of neuropsychological impairment. The average level of phonetic accuracy was also highly, positively, and consistently related to achievement measures (particularly oral word decoding) and language-related tasks (particularly sound blending, the rapid production of words on the basis of phonemic cues, and the ability to access one's long-term store of general information). These results provide further evidence of the need to examine not only the child's *level* of spelling achievement, but also the *quality* of the spelling errors that the child makes. The case could certainly be made for inclusion of some indicator of phonetic accuracy of misspellings in all studies with reading/spelling-disabled children. It would certainly be informative to include this variable in studies examining various predictors of future reading/spelling performance.

Implications for Remediation

Although most of the research reported in this chapter was not specifically designed to address the issue of remediation for reading/spelling-disabled children, several implications for remedial assistance can be suggested on the basis of the information presented. Sweeney and Rourke (1985) discussed several remedial strategies that may be helpful for PA and PI spellers. Specifically, they suggested the following:

1. PIs should be provided with as many opportunities as possible to deal with words through phonetic analysis. This could include both segmenting words into their phonemic elements and blending together

individual segments to form words. Sight-word strategies could be introduced as an additional approach to words once phonemic analysis has been mastered. However, it may be necessary to rely solely on sight-word strategies if phonetic approaches prove to be fruitless.

2. Since PAs tend to overutilize phonetic analysis in their approaches to reading and spelling, it may be of more benefit to use remedial strategies that are more visual in nature. These could include sight-word strategies, "visualizing" the graphic features of words, using "flashcard" exercises and/or tachistoscopic presentations, trying multisensory methods such as VAKT, and other techniques that focus on the visual–spatial aspects of words.

The results of the Russell and Rourke (1989) study suggest that different remedial strategies may be appropriate for different "subtypes" of learning-disabled children. Clearly, this is the implication from past research in the field (Lyon, 1985; Rourke et al., 1983; Sweeney & Rourke, 1985). One particular aspect of the Russell and Rourke (1989) research may be especially relevant to a discussion of remedial strategies. In this connection, we offer the following suggestions:

1. A child with a high average level of phonetic accuracy *and* a low average level of neuropsychological impairment may benefit from an instructional method such as a "synthetic phonics" approach. The high level of PA suggests that the child is capable of understanding and utilizing phonetic information. The low level of impairment suggests that the child would not be as likely to "overutilize" phonics, thus preventing the problems associated with fluent oral reading and accompanying comprehension deficits.

2. On the other hand, it would be advisable to decrease the emphasis on phonetic approaches with children who have lower average levels of phonetic accuracy and/or who have higher average levels of neuropsychological impairment. It would be important to determine the child's level on each of these two variables and then structure his/her remedial program accordingly. The lower the level of PA and the higher the level of impairment, the more the remedial approach should be tailored to utilize multisensory methods.

In all cases, however, it is important to consider not only the degree of neuropsychological impairment, but also the type of impairment(s). Each child's individual strengths and weaknesses should be carefully delineated and considered when a remedial program is designed. However, it would still be instructive to consider these two variables (i.e., level of phonetic accuracy of misspellings and level of neuropsychological impairment) in the initial planning stages of remedial programming.

Obviously much more research of the type reported by Lyon (1985; Lyon & Flynn, Chapter 11, this volume) is necessary in order to provide evidence regarding the efficacy of different remedial strategies for various subtypes of learning-disabled children. The results of this type of research will be invaluable for those professionals involved in the habilitation/ rehabilitation of children with learning disabilities.

References

Benton, A. L. (1965). *Sentence Memory Test*. Iowa City, IA: Author.

Boder, E. (1973). Developmental dyslexia: A diagnostic approach based on three atypical reading-spelling patterns. *Developmental Medicine and Child Neurology, 15*, 663-687.

Boder, E., & Jarrico, S. (1982). *The Boder Test of Reading-Spelling Patterns*. New York: Grune & Stratton.

Coderre, D. J., Sweeney, J. E., & Rourke, B. P. (1979). *Spelling recognition, word analysis and visual memory in children with qualitatively distinct types of spelling errors*. Unpublished manuscript, University of Windsor and Windsor Western Hospital Centre.

Dunn, L. M. (1965). *Expanded manual for the Peabody Picture Vocabulary Test*. Minneapolis: American Guidance Services.

Durost, W. N., Bixler, H. H., Hildreth, G. H., Lund, K. W., & Wrightstone, J. W. (1959). *Metropolitan Achievement Tests*. New York: Harcourt, Brace & World.

Goldman, R., Fristoe, M., & Woodcock, R. W. (1970). *Goldman-Fristoe-Woodcock Test of Auditory Discrimination*. Circle Pines, MN: American Guidance Service.

Jastak, J. F., & Jastak, S. R. (1965). *The Wide Range Achievement Test*. Wilmington, DE: Guidance Associates.

Kass, C. E. (1964). Auditory Closure Test. In J. J. Olson & J. L. Olson (Eds.), *Validity studies on the Illinois Test of Psycholinguistic Abilities*. Madison, WI: Photo Press.

Kinsbourne, M., & Warrington, E. K. (1964). Disorders of spelling. *Journal of Neurology, Neurosurgery, and Psychiatry, 27*, 224-228.

Kløve, H. (1963). Clinical neuropsychology. In F. M. Forster (Ed.), *The medical clinics of North America*. New York: Saunders.

Lyon, G. R. (1985). Educational validation studies of learning disability subtypes. In B. P. Rourke (Ed.), *Neuropsychology of learning disabilities: Essentials of subtype analysis* (pp. 228-253). New York: Guilford Press.

Nelson, H. E., & Warrington, E. K. (1974). Developmental spelling retardation and its relation to other cognitive abilities. *British Journal of Psychology, 65*, 265-274.

Newcombe, F. (1969). *Missile wounds to the brain*. London: Oxford University Press.

Petrauskas, R. J., & Rourke, B. P. (1979). Identification of subtypes of retarded readers: A neuropsychology, multivariate approach. *Journal of Clinical Neuropsychology, 1*, 17-37.

Reitan, R. M., & Davison, L. A. (Eds.). (1974). *Clinical neuropsychology: Current status and applications*. New York: John Wiley & Sons.

Rosner, J., & Simon, D. P. (1970). *The Auditory Analysis Test*. Pittsburgh: Authors.

Rourke, B. P. (1976). Reading retardation in children: Developmental lag or deficit? In R. M. Knights & D. J. Bakker (Eds.), *Neuropsychology of learning disorders: Theoretical approaches*. Baltimore: University Park Press.

Rourke, B. P. (1978). Neuropsychological research in reading retardation: A review. In A. L. Benton & D. Pearl (Eds.), *Dyslexia: An appraisal of current knowledge* (pp. 139-171). New York: Oxford University Press.

Rourke, B. P. (1983). Reading and spelling disabilities: A developmental neuropsychological perspective. In U. Kirk (Ed.), *Neuropsychology of language, reading, and spelling* (pp. 209–234). New York: Academic Press.

Rourke, B. P., Bakker, D. J., Fisk, J. L., & Strang, J. D. (1983). *Child neuropsychology*. New York: Guilford Press.

Rourke, B. P., Fisk, J. L., & Strang, J. D. (1986). *Neuropsychological assessment of children: A treatment-oriented approach*. New York: Guilford Press.

Rourke, B. P., & Orr, R. R. (1977). Prediction of the reading and spelling performances of normal and retarded readers: A 4-year follow-up. *Journal of Abnormal Child Psychology, 5*, 9–20.

Russell, D. L., & Rourke, B. P. (1984). *Concurrent and predictive validity of level of phonetic accuracy of misspellings for learning-disabled children*. Unpublished manuscript, University of Windsor.

Russell, D. L., & Rourke, B. P. (1989). *Phonetic accuracy of misspellings: Neuropsychological significance for normal and disabled readers and spellers*. Unpublished manuscript, University of Windsor.

Strong, R. T., Jr. (1963). *Intellectual deficits associated with minimal brain disorders in primary school children*. Unpublished manuscript, Columbus State School, Columbus, OH.

Sweeney, J. E., McCabe, A. E., & Rourke, B. P. (1978). *Logical–grammatical abilities of retarded spellers*. Unpublished manuscript, Windsor Western Hospital Centre and University of Windsor.

Sweeney, J. E., & Rourke, B. P. (1978). Neuropsychological significance of phonetically accurate and phonetically inaccurate spelling errors in younger and older retarded spellers. *Brain and Language, 6*, 212–225.

Sweeney, J. E., & Rourke, B. P. (1982). *Reading strategies of qualitatively distinct disabled spellers*. Unpublished manuscript, District of Parry Sound Child and Family Centre and Windsor Western Hospital Centre.

Sweeney, J. E., & Rourke, B. P. (1985). Subtypes of spelling disabilities. In B. P. Rourke (Ed.), *Neuropsychology of learning disabilities: Essentials of subtype analysis* (pp. 147–166). New York: Guilford Press.

Vellutino, F. R., Steger, J. A., DeSetto, L., & Phillips, F. (1975). Immediate and delayed recognition of visual stimuli in poor and normal readers. *Journal of Experimental Child Psychology, 19*, 223–232.

Wechsler, D. (1949). *Wechsler Intelligence Scale for Children*. New York: Psychological Corporation.

Wiig, E. H., & Semel, E. M. (1974). Development of comprehension of logico-grammatical sentences by grade school children. *Perceptual and Motor Skills, 38*, 171–176.

Wirt, R. D., Lachar, D., Klinedist, J. K., & Seat, P. D. (1977). *The Personality Inventory for Children*. Los Angeles: Western Psychological Services.

CHAPTER 5

Differential Memory Abilities in Reading- and Arithmetic-Disabled Children

Clare F. Brandys and Byron P. Rourke

As a result of research over the last 15 years, it has become increasingly clearer that recognizable subtypes of learning disability exist. These are distinguishable not only on the basis of academic achievement scores and patterns but also on the basis of neuropsychological test performance configurations. Neuropsychologists interested in studying the brain–behavior relationships of learning-disabled (LD) children have carried out extensive investigations in this area, showing that specific LD groups can be distinguished on the basis of auditory–verbal, psycholinguistic, visual–perceptual, problem-solving, and tactile–perceptual abilities. This provides external validation for the notion that various patterns of academic performance are a function of unique underlying neuropsychological deficits/strengths.

For example, Q-type factor analysis and cluster analysis research have shown that children with reading disabilities frequently exhibit deficits in auditory–verbal and psycholinguistic skill areas, including depressed Wechsler Intelligence Scale for Children (WISC) Verbal subtest scores (Doehring, Trites, Patel, & Fiedorowicz, 1981), impairments on tests of sound–symbol association (Doehring et al., 1981; Rourke & Finlayson, 1978), letter and temporal sequencing tasks (Denckla, 1979; Doehring et al., 1981; studies reviewed by Rourke, 1978), naming tasks (Denckla, 1979; Mattis, 1978), and phonemic segmentation tasks (Shankweiler & Liberman, 1976), These deficits are usually found in the context of relatively intact visual–perceptual skills, particularly on tasks involving nonverbal material (Rourke & Finlayson, 1978), adequate nonverbal problem-solving skills (Strang & Rourke, 1983), and well-developed psychomotor skills (Rourke & Strang, 1978). Nonetheless, there is some evidence to suggest that one or more subtypes may exist that display deficiencies on certain visual–perceptual tasks as well (Boder, 1973; Mattis, 1978).

In contrast to children with disabilities in reading and spelling, children with relatively poor mechanical arithmetic skills yet good reading and spelling achievement have been the subject of much less research. Nonetheless, several fairly consistent results can be summarized in regard to these "specific" arithmetic-disabled youngsters. In direct contrast to reading-disabled children, arithmetic-disabled children frequently exhibit well-developed auditory–perceptual and verbal-related skills but deficient visual–perceptual–organizational skills (Rourke & Finlayson, 1978). Rourke and Strang (1978) have demonstrated bilateral impairments on tests of psychomotor and tactile–perceptual skill as well. These were found to be somewhat more marked on the left side of the body. Furthermore, on a test of complex nonverbal reasoning skills, arithmetic-disabled children have been found to perform in a below-average fashion (Strang & Rourke, 1983). These findings are generally interpreted as suggestive of dysfunctional right hemisphere processes (Rourke, 1982) in the context of well-developed left hemisphere (language-related) functions (see DeLuca, Rourke, & Del Dotto, Chapter 10, this volume, for more extensive investigations of various subtypes of arithmetic-disabled children).

In the quest for external validation of these "academic" subtypes, one facet of higher-order neuropsychological skills that has been largely overlooked is short-term memory ability. Although literally hundreds of studies have been undertaken in the last several years exploring the relationship between memory skills in general and reading disabilities, very little work has focused on the interrelationships between specific academic subtypes (e.g., reading, arithmetic disabilities) and memory skills. In keeping with the requirement that external validation research begin with *a priori* hypotheses based on a theoretical framework for the subtypes to be studied (Fletcher, 1985a), the unique configurations of other neuropsychological strengths and weaknesses associated with specific reading and arithmetic learning disabilities suggest that such children may be expected to display unique differences in the realm of mnestic functions. Within this neuropsychological framework, these differences may be expected to obtain on the basis of the symbolic nature of the material (i.e., verbal versus nonverbal) and the modality of material input (i.e., visual, auditory) as well as other task variables.

Among the pertinent information-processing theories of memory is the notion of separate memory systems—one visual, one auditory—or one semantic memory system with multiple access routes (Paivio, 1971). Baddeley (1978) has conceptualized verbal short-term memory as involving an articulatory loop that processes short-term information. A second larger component of memory is considered to be a central executive that controls the articulatory loop. In accordance with Paivio's (1971) dual-code theory of memory, a corresponding "visual spatial scratch pad" (Baddeley & Hitch, 1974) has been proposed to account for visual nonverbal memory representations; this is also believed to be controlled by the central executive. Researchers interested in exploring the memory skills of LD children have used this explanatory model frequently; however, relatively little research has investigated different LD subtypes simultaneously in an effort to understand both their memory difficulties and differences.

Unique Memory Performances in LD Subtypes

An important validation study investigating these questions was carried out by Fletcher (1985b). In this study, various groups of LD youngsters, classified on the basis of their performance on the Wide Range Achievement Test (Jastak & Jastak, 1978), were compared on verbal and nonverbal memory tasks. The results of this study suggest a between-groups dissociation of auditory–verbal and visual–nonverbal memory skills. As Fletcher predicted, reading- and spelling-disabled children performed poorly when learning lists of words through a selective reminding technique, whereas they performed in a manner similar to normals in learning nonverbal dot-matrix patterns. Arithmetic-disabled children performed in an opposite fashion on both tasks. Furthermore, the pattern of academic achievement appeared to affect group performance in a manner compatible with other neuropsychological test findings: Children uniformly deficient in reading, spelling, and arithmetic performed poorly on both verbal and nonverbal memory tasks. Another group, not previously studied, who were deficient in spelling and arithmetic resembled the arithmetic-disabled (only) group. In a general discussion of LD-subtyping research, Fletcher (1985a) has discussed the important research potential of such studies in providing external validation of already-derived LD subtypes.

A similar study comparing academically based LD groups involved specific aspects of verbal memory skills. In this study, Siegel and Linder (1984) compared normally achieving youngsters, a group of reading/spelling-disabled children, and a group of arithmetic-disabled children on visually and auditorially presented verbal memory tasks. To explore further the relationships among phonemic coding processes, short-term memory skills in general, and various types of learning disability, they included in the lists of words in the memory tasks phonetically confusable items. Results showed that both the reading/spelling- and arithmetic-disabled groups were insensitive to the effects of phonetic confusability at younger ages. However, whereas reading/spelling-disabled children were poor on both auditory and visual memory conditions, arithmetic-disabled children were only deficient in the visual condition. This interesting result is similar to the findings cited by Strang and Rourke (1985a). (See the latter study for an extensive discussion of visual-organizational impairments found in arithmetic-disabled [their "Group 3"] children.) Although they give short shrift to the complexity of their findings, Siegel and Linder (1984) conclude more generally, "Short-term memory abilities are related to functions other than learning to read. Short-term memory may have a significant role in a variety of cognitive functions of which reading is only one" (p. 206).

The results of the Fletcher (1985b) and Siegel and Linder (1984) studies are consistent with the findings of research that has investigated the separate LD populations. Specifically, the large number of memory studies undertaken with children exhibiting reading deficiencies has shown quite consistently that these children, relative to their nondisabled same-age peers, have difficulty with short-term verbal memory tasks. Verbatim, sequential memory appears to be one area of primary deficit. Reading-disabled children exhibit difficulties on a large number of short-term memory tasks that require recall of letters, digits, words, or phrases in exact sequence (Corkin, 1974; Lindgren & Richman, 1984; McKeever & VanDeventer, 1975; Ritchie & Aten, 1976). Impaired naming and phonemic encoding skills are believed to underlie these difficulties, as suggested by the poor performances of reading-disabled children on tasks involving visual material with an intermediary naming stage (Done & Miles, 1978; Ellis & Miles, 1978; MacKinnon & McCarthy, 1973) and by their relative insensitivity to phonetic distractor items on various memory tasks (Brady, Shankweiler, & Mann, 1983; Liberman & Mann, 1981; Liberman, Mann, Shankweiler, & Werfelman, 1982; Shankweiler & Liberman, 1976).

In contrast to the verbal memory deficits of reading-disabled children, other studies have demonstrated that these children perform similarly to normals on specific controlled nonverbal memory tasks. Visual memory for nonverbal material such as pictures (Kastner & Rickards, 1974), designs (Bauserman & Obrzut, 1981), and abstract figures (Vellutino, Steger, Kaman, & DeSetto, 1975) appears to be free of deficit in reading-disabled children on such tasks that do not require, or are not facilitated by, naming strategies.

Very little research has examined the performances of "specific" arithmetic-disabled children on memory tasks. What little has been done suggests that these children may have difficulties on certain visual–verbal memory tasks (Siegel & Feldman, 1983). In contrast, the results of other research suggest better performances in the aural than in the visual modality in a severely arithmetic-disabled group, whereas a mildly impaired group performed in a fashion similar to normals (Webster, 1979).

A Recent Study in the Windsor Laboratory

To address the issues of memory in relation to these academic subtypes, a study was conducted by the present authors. Various experimental memory tasks were compared to investigate the questions of the importance to the various LD subtypes of content (verbal versus nonverbal), modality (visual versus auditory), and format (recall versus recognition) variables of memory tasks. As Fletcher (1985a, 1985b) has discussed, such an external validation study allows one to understand better the importance of subtype differences and aids in the determination of reliable typologies to which new members can be assigned. Should clear-cut between-group differences obtain on measures not used in the original subtyping analysis, one can infer with greater confidence that these skill groups represent actual unique clinical populations. In turn, remediation techniques based on each group's cognitive and behavioral needs can be designed and applied with greater precision for each group. Examples of this type of remediation technique, based on clinical-statistical findings, are presented by Strang and Rourke (1985a) in relation to a neuropsychological subtype characterized by outstanding and specific arithmetic deficiencies and deficient socioemotional coping skills.

Comparisons for the present study were made between normals (Group C) and two groups of age-matched LD youngsters placed in learning disability classrooms, one exhibiting significant deficiencies in reading (Group RD) and another exhibiting significant deficiencies in mechanical arithmetic (Group AD). In contrast to previous validation studies comparing memory abilities, the present study employed a somewhat older population of disabled children (aged 10–14) to investigate the generalizability of the findings of the more commonly studied younger group.

In this study, 54 children were administered the Wide Range Achievement Test (WRAT; Jastak & Jastak, 1978) and a series of experimental memory measures. According to preestablished criteria, 11 subjects were classed as RD, 12 subjects as AD, and 31 as controls. In addition, subjects were administered four subtests of a psychometric intelligence test (Wechsler Intelligence Scale for Children—Revised [WISC-R; Wechsler, 1974], Information, Vocabulary, Picture Arrangement, and Block Design subtests), and the scores were prorated to obtain an estimate of Full Scale IQ (FSIQ) according to the method described by

Tellegen and Briggs (1967, cited in Sattler, 1982). This prorated FSIQ measure was administered in order to limit the length of the testing session, thereby reducing the chances of subject fatigue as an interference. Normal intelligence was established as a prerequisite for the definition of learning disability used in this study (Rourke, 1975). Table 5.1 presents descriptive characteristics of the three achievement groups.

Among the experimental memory tasks were four lists of words, two presented visually and two presented through the auditory modality. In each sensory modality, memory was tested under each of two conditions: one list was presented and then followed by a free-recall format; one list was presented and then followed by a forced-choice recognition format in which the child chose among three words. This latter recognition condition also included phonetically similar distractor words among the choices in order to study the disabled and normal groups with respect to the phonetic confusability hypothesis (Liberman & Mann, 1981; Siegel & Linder, 1984), which relates to an individual's sensitivity to phonetic characteristics of words. A rhyme fluency task (Doehring, 1968; Ridgley, 1970) was also administered to each child to investigate long-term phonetic memory and word-production skills.

To study nonverbal memory, the Rey–Osterrieth Complex Figure task (Osterrieth, 1944) was administered to each child. This task was

TABLE 5.1. Descriptive Characteristics of Achievement Groups Used in This Study

	RD	AD	C
N	11	12	31
Males	10	10	23
Females	1	2	8
Right hand dominant	10	9	27
Left hand dominant	1	3	4
Mean age (mo)	141.73	147.50	147.35
Mean FSIQ	98.09	97.92	101.84
Mean Verbal IQ index	82.41	92.54	96.61
Mean Performance IQ index	112.73	100.00	109.19
WRAT Reading* (grade-equivalent)	4.57	7.49	8.01
WRAT Reading* (percentile)	19.91	64.88	75.68
WRAT Arithmetic** (grade-equivalent)	5.88	4.12	6.81
WRAT Arithmetic** (percentile)	40.64	9.17	53.87

*$p < .0005$; RD < AD,C.
**$p < .0005$; AD < RD < C.

administered and scored according to the method described by Waber and Holmes (1985), with minor modifications to allow for separate scoring of "gestalt" and "internal" feature elements. Raw scores and percentage of features retained from copy to recall phases of the task were compared; an overall "organization" score was also generated.

Several hypotheses were proposed, as follows:

1. Reading-disabled Group RD was expected to perform in an inferior manner, relative to arithmetic-disabled Group AD and control Group C, on the various verbal memory tasks. Specifically, it was expected that Group RD would have difficulty in the recall conditions under both visual and auditory presentation conditions.

2. Phonetic distractor words in the verbal recognition tasks were expected to result in less phonetic confusability for Group RD as a result of difficulties with phonetic encoding. Furthermore, Group RD was expected to obtain poorer scores on the long-term measure of phonetic ability, the rhyme fluency task.

3. Group AD was expected to obtain poorer scores, relative to Groups RD and C, on the nonverbal memory task in both copy and recall phases, with particularly poor recall for gestalt elements and poor organization scores overall.

Group means for the various memory tasks are presented in Table 5.2, as well as *T*-score comparisons based on the mean and standard deviation of control Group C to illustrate meaningful relationships across groups and measures. A series of analysis of variance tests resulted in the expected dissociation between verbal and nonverbal memory measures across groups. In general, the results of this study appear to be consistent with the two-tiered working memory model proposed by Baddeley and Hitch (1974). That is, verbal material is processed through an "articulatory loop" before reaching long-term semantic stores, whereas nonverbal material is processed through a nonverbal memory corollary, the "visual scratch pad." What follows, as suggested by the results of this and similar research (e.g., Fletcher, 1985b), is that an individual may have difficulty with one of these systems while the other system continues to process information of its respective mode with relative ease.

However, it is interesting to note that the Group RD children obtained only slightly poorer scores than did control Group C subjects on the various measures of verbal memory, a less robust effect than what might be expected on the basis of previous investigations into verbal memory functions of reading-disabled children (e.g., Brady et al., 1983; Cohen, Netley, & Clark, 1984) and other verbal processing skills of such children (e.g., Doehring, 1985; Petrauskas & Rourke, 1979; Rourke & Finlayson, 1978). A major difference between this study and many of the previous memory studies is the older age of the subject groups employed

TABLE 5.2. Means (Standard Deviations) and *T*-Scores for Various Dependent Measures, Contrasted by Group Membership

Measure	RD	AD	C
	Means (standard deviations)		
Verbal list A: aud, recall[a]	5.36(0.67)	4.83(1.47)	6.03(1.14)
Verbal list B: vis, recall[b]	3.73(1.62)	5.33(1.61)	5.71(1.74)
Verbal list C: aud, recog	7.36(1.50)	8.08(1.62)	7.68(1.33)
Verbal list D: vis, recog	8.27(1.62)	7.67(1.92)	7.84(1.86)
Percentage phonetic errors[c]	71.27(32.25)	55.27(33.34)	76.13(20.81)
Rhyme fluency task[d]	20.27(5.24)	26.08(6.42)	26.19(7.12)
Rey–Osterrieth nonverbal task			
Total copy accuracy[e]	61.18(5.46)	56.92(7.43)	63.42(1.75)
Total recall accuracy[f]	39.55(9.71)	30.25(9.16)	38.84(9.03)
Percentage retained copy (recall)	64.45(14.25)	53.75(16.41)	61.19(13.92)
Organization score (recall)	3.23(1.13)	2.79(1.05)	3.05(1.16)
Percentage gestalt retained	73.00(14.91)	61.75(20.79)	66.87(16.19)
Percentage internal retained	50.82(20.78)	39.50(18.68)	52.74(20.43)
	T-Scores ($M = 50$, $SD = 10$)		
Verbal list A: aud, recall	44.1	39.5	50
Verbal list B: vis, recall	38.6	47.8	50
Verbal list C: aud, recog	47.6	53.1	50
Verbal list D: vis, recog	52.6	49.1	50
Percentage phonetic errors	47.7	40.1	50
Rhyme fluency task	41.7	49.8	50
Rey–Osterrieth nonverbal task			
Total copy accuracy	37.2	12.8	50
Total recall accuracy	50.8	40.5	50
Percentage retained copy (recall)	52.3	44.7	50
Organization score (recall)	51.6	47.8	50
Percentage gestalt retained	53.8	46.8	50
Percentage internal retained	49.1	43.5	50

[a]AD < C, $p < .01$; [b]RD < AD,C, $p < .01$; [c]AD < C, $p < .10$; [d]RD < AD,C, $p < .05$; [e]AD < RD,C, $p < .005$; [f]AD < RD,C, $p < .05$.

in the present research. Reading-disabled children in the primary grades (the age group most frequently studied) appear to be quite different from their normal counterparts on verbal processing and verbal memory tasks (Ozols & Rourke, 1988; Chapter 6, this volume). In contrast, the present study found that Group AD children were particularly poor in the encoding and recall of nonverbal material; this is clearly consistent with the limited body of previous research into this subtype of disabled learners (Fletcher, 1985b).

In exploring the verbal memory skills of both Group RD and Group AD children in more detail, the distinction of modality of presentation (and response) did not produce the expected result, namely, that Group AD children would have modality-specific difficulties with visual–verbal material (as reported by Siegel & Feldman, 1983; Siegel & Linder, 1984) and that Group RD children would have difficulties with verbal material in either visual (Corkin, 1974; Gerber & White, 1983) or auditory modalities (Cohen et al., 1984; Farnham-Diggory & Gregg, 1975; Holmes & McKeever, 1979; Koppitz, 1975; McKeever & VanDeventer, 1975; Ritchie & Aten, 1976). It appears that the present verbal memory tasks, which utilized words (with their inherent semantic aspects) and somewhat long intervals between stimulus and response, placed fewer demands on limited-capacity modality channels. It is possible that this state of affairs thereby enabled the children to process the words past modality-dependent immediate memory stores into semantic memory (Lindsay & Norman, 1977), thus effectively obscuring any modality-specific strengths or weaknesses between groups. These results suggest that modality of presentation is a presemantic variable primarily relevant only at the initial sensory input/immediate memory stage (Stanley & Hall, 1973).

Another aspect of verbal memory task performance investigated in the present study related to phonetic coding ability. This was assessed by comparing Groups RD, AD, and C on their percentage of phonetic errors using a forced-choice recognition task with phonetically similar foil words as some of the distractor items. Whereas previous research comparing reading-disabled with normal subjects strongly suggests a lower phonetic error rate or less confusability with phonetically similar stimuli (Brady et al., 1983; Mann, Liberman, & Shankweiler, 1980; Mark, Shankweiler, Liberman, & Fowler, 1977), the present findings did not reflect similar tendencies. Age differences among studies may account for this difference, as some research suggests a tendency toward "more precise phonetic codes" in older reading-disabled children (Olson, Davidson, Kliegl, & Davies, 1984). It is also important to remember that the Group RD subjects assessed in the present study had all enjoyed the benefits of one or more years of intensive remedial education, one focus of which is drill work in phonetic decoding skills. The results of the present analysis may therefore reflect recent learning in the RD group.

In contrast, Group AD showed an unexpected low percentage of phonetic errors. Although one study showed young arithmetic-disabled children to be similar to reading-disabled children obtaining low phonetic error rates (Siegel & Linder, 1984), this was not expected because of the older age group studied in the present research. This latter assertion was based on the research and clinical reports suggesting that older arithmetic-disabled children have extremely well-developed phonetic coding skills (Strang & Rourke, 1985b). Nonetheless, the finding of a low percentage of phonetic errors in Group AD children may reflect similar tendencies to those reported by Rourke and Finlayson (1978). Despite the strong verbal nature of certain neuropsychological tasks, arithmetic-disabled children often fare poorly as a function of task novelty (e.g., low average scores obtained on the Auditory Closure Test). A further arithmetic-disabled group phenomenon is suggested by Rourke and Finlayson's results with the Benton Sentence Memory Test: Low average scores obtained by arithmetic-disabled children may be suggestive of difficulties with the semantic requirements of the test. This possibility is consistent with the present results, as the novel forced-choice nature of the tasks may have resulted in semantic confusions for these children. Semantic limitations may be suggested by the lower Verbal IQs (VIQs) found in the present AD group (in contrast to high-average VIQs in Rourke and Finlayson's [1978] "Group 3" subtype).

To clarify this matter, it is also important to consider the results of the rhyme fluency task analysis. In this instance, the predicted Group RD inferiority obtained, and Group AD children performed as well as did controls. This suggests, as reported by other LD-subtyping studies (Boder, 1973; Petrauskas & Rourke, 1979), that reading-disabled children have especial difficulty appreciating or producing phonologically related words, whereas arithmetic-disabled children exhibit well-developed skills on *rote* phonological tasks. The memory task results with respect to phonological codes may therefore point to two separate processes: phonological competence (poor in Group RD children) versus the ability to deploy this competence on a novel, semantically confusing memory task (poor in Group AD children). Perhaps, as other research and descriptions of this subtype of children suggest (Rourke, 1982, 1987, 1988, 1989; Strang & Rourke, 1985b; Tellier, 1986), generating a new strategy in an unfamiliar learning situation poses considerable difficulty for the arithmetic-disabled child. (The present results suggest *dramatically* better memory under recognition as opposed to recall conditions for both LD groups.) To explore this possibility in somewhat more detail, it would be interesting to compare the two disability and control groups using specific training of learning strategies (Pressley, Johnson, & Symons, 1987; Torgeson, Murphy, & Ivey, 1979). The present results suggest that, given a concrete strategy as in the rhyme fluency task, the adverse effects of task novelty and semantic confusion may abate for arithmetic-disabled children as well.

In relation to nonverbal memory abilities, the use of the Rey–Osterrieth Complex Figure memory task allows one to compare not only the oft-studied recall/retrieval measure of mnestic function but also the important aspect of memory encoding (copy phase). The hypotheses made in relation to Group AD were, for the most part, supported. As predicted, Group AD was far inferior to both RD and C groups in both copy and delayed recall aspects of the complex figure. However, when the performances of all three groups are "normalized" by using "percentage retained" as the memory measure, a different result obtains. That is, when the memory bias against "poor copiers/encoders" (particularly subjects in Group AD) is removed, no group is significantly different from the others. Haith (1971) has suggested that increases in children's normal memory capacity can be attributed primarily to *encoding* strategies that improve naturally in the development of the child. (He further states that such strategies are not necessarily verbally based). The present results thus imply a marked deficiency in arithmetic-disabled children's information-processing abilities, as they appear to have difficulty with encoding strategies—*the* definitive skill of developing mnestic function in children.

A surprising result was that comparison of the organization scores failed to show any between-group differences. In terms of more discrete nonverbal memory elements (the gestalt and internal features of the figure), analysis of the raw recall scores revealed inferior scores of both types in Group AD. The hypothesized lower internal feature scores for Group RD (believed to be a function of their impaired verbal mediational skills) did not obtain. Similarly, after correcting for the amount of information encoded (using "percentage retained" scores), the predicted gestalt/internal dissociation did not obtain. Rather, all subjects performed significantly better in recalling gestalt than internal elements, a finding consistent with the reports of Waber and Holmes's (1986) normative sample on the Rey–Osterrieth recall productions. As these authors report in relation to their nonclinical sample, it appears that older children require organizing structures for recall; perhaps this is the form in which material is directly encoded and, thus, later retrieved from storage. The AD, RD, and C groups did not differ in the recall of internal elements. It is possible that a "floor effect" occurs in children's ability to recall detailed elements in an incidental memory task, as only a limited amount of such specific features can be recalled by the average child in this age group.

While not reaching commonly accepted levels of statistical signifi-cance, Group AD obtained the poorest retention scores overall on both gestalt and internal elements. This provides further evidence of their marked difficulties with both encoding and retrieval of nonverbal input (Fletcher, 1985b). It is also important to note the possible difficulties inherent in the dichotomizing of gestalt and internal elements (derived from Waber & Holmes's [1985, 1986] scoring methods). This difficulty is briefly illustrated in Figure 5.1 with characteristic Group AD and RD children's recall reproductions of the Rey–Osterrieth figure. As is evident, although the differences in gestalt and internal *quantitative* scores are sometimes slight, the *quality* of memories may be quite marked in the "configuration-oriented" or "internal detail-oriented" directions sug-gested by Waber and Holmes (1985, 1986) in their clinical ratings scheme. To characterize fully these reproductions, it may be necessary to devise a "weighted" quantitative scoring method that also accounts for severity of difficulty (e.g., more points subtracted for distorted or misplaced line segments).

The finding that Group RD equaled and even surpassed control subjects on the various measures of nonverbal encoding and recall is noteworthy. This has been reflected clearly in other studies that have compared reading-disabled and normal children in their abilities to recall purely nonverbal memory material such as spatial configurations (Bauser-man & Obrzut, 1981; Fletcher, 1985b), faces and abstract designs (Holmes & McKeever, 1979; Liberman et al., 1982; Swanson, 1978). Reading-disabled children have also been shown to be quite adept at making mnemonic associations between auditory and visual nonverbal stimuli (Vellutino, Pruzek, Steger, & Meshoulam, 1973). In fact, the nonverbal abilities of Group RD approaching the superior level of performance in the present study suggest a *superior* skill in this area, perhaps developed to this extent as a compensation for below-average verbal skills and stronger day-to-day reliance on this form of mnestic encoding and processing (Aaron, 1981). An alternative explanation is that their above-average Performance IQs (PIQs) reflect their true superior "learning potential" and that their lowered Verbal IQs (VIQs) represent a drop in skills: "the commonly encountered situation in which a child's general learning potential is not fully realized in the academic situation because of a specific psycholinguistic deficit" (Rourke, Bakker, Fisk, & Strang, 1983, p. 350).

Neuropsychological Implications

As a whole, these test results are quite consistent with previous research conducted on the distinct LD subtypes of children, lending validity to the

Reproduction A

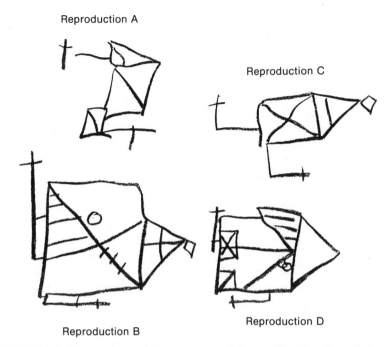

Reproduction C

Reproduction D

Reproduction B

FIGURE 5.1. Illustrations of Group AD and Group RD Rey–Osterrieth recall performances. Reproductions A and B completed by Group AD children. These reflect varying degrees of difficulty with "gestalt" aspects. According to quantitative criteria, Reproduction A scored gestalt = 18, internal = 1; Reproduction B scored gestalt = 25, internal = 6. Reproductions C and D completed by Group RD children. These reflect varying degrees of difficulty with "internal" aspects. Reproduction C scored gestalt = 20, internal = 5; Reproduction D scored gestalt = 20, internal = 14.

separateness of the academic subclassifications. For the purposes of this discussion, the RD and AD groups studied are compared, respectively, to the "Group 2" and "Group 3" subtypes isolated by Rourke and his associates (Rourke & Finlayson, 1978; Rourke & Strang, 1978) and discussed in other research (Fletcher, 1985b). Although the specific identification criteria used here were somewhat different (e.g., Rourke and his colleagues also included cut-off scores on the WRAT Spelling subtest), the general similarities in WRAT Reading and Arithmetic subtest performances suggest that adequate comparisons can be made. In addition, for Group RD, the present IQ-related Verbal and Performance indices are in keeping with those of the "Group 2" subtypes. However, the Verbal and Performance indices (each based on only two WISC-R subtests) suggest discrepant results when comparing Group AD (low-average Verbal, average Performance) to the low-Performance, average-Verbal "Group 3" type (Rourke & Finlayson, 1978). Thus, it appears that generalization of these results to the larger reading disability subtype can be made with greater confidence than can the generalization of these results to the larger subtype of arithmetic-disabled children. The present Group AD may, in fact, not be representative of the larger clinical subtype previously studied, although the consistency in deficient nonverbal abilities is certainly noteworthy.

Generally, these test results are consistent with previous clinical descriptions of children with reading disability and relative strengths in mechanical arithmetic. On "nonmemory" tasks they frequently exhibit mild to moderate impairments in the analysis and synthesis of verbal symbolic and phonological material (Doehring, 1885; Petrauskas & Rourke, 1979), with average or better abilities in the processing of nonverbal, particularly visual–spatial information (Lyon, Watson, Reitta, Porch, & Rhodes, 1981; Petrauskas & Rourke, 1979; Rourke & Finlayson, 1978). The present memory test results combined with reports of neuropsychological performances in previous studies provide support for Orton's early notion of cortical dysfunction of verbal-oriented systems of the left cerebral hemisphere (1937, as discussed in Holmes & McKeever, 1979). Later researchers have also implicated dysfunction in verbal-linguistic–analytic left hemispheric systems (Obrzut, 1979; Rourke, 1982). Specifically, Jorm (1979) has hypothesized that dysfunction in the inferior parietal lobule of the left cerebral hemisphere accounts for both short-term verbal memory impairment and difficulties with decoding the printed letter and word for reading. Byrne (1981) favors an explanatory model in which limited "linguistic access" results in both memory (mostly serialized) deficits and reading problems; the neurological determinants *per se* are not specifically addressed in Byrne's formulation.

The complex neuropsychological correlates of "specific" arithmetic disorders, on the other hand, include a number of nonverbal deficits such as difficulties with processing and analyzing pictorial (Ozols & Rourke, 1985) and visual–constructional materials (Rourke & Finlayson, 1978). The results of the present study, which reflect clear and significant deficits relative to both normal and reading-disabled children on various aspects of nonverbal mnestic tasks, are consistent with previous reports on this subtype. This is a particularly interesting finding, as it obtained with the present sample in spite of their average Performance index on the WISC-R.

Furthermore, the present findings suggest that arithmetic-disabled children may encounter mild difficulties on certain verbal memory tasks, particularly when novel; such findings are consistent with the mild deficits reported on other complex, novel verbal tasks (Rourke & Finlayson, 1978; Webster, 1979). Generalized difficulties in the generation and application of novel concepts and strategies have also been reported in the literature on the arithmetic disability subtype (Rourke, 1989; Strang & Rourke, 1983). In contrast are these children's well-developed skills on rote verbal tasks (Rourke & Finlayson, 1978). This tendency was confirmed in the results of the phonological production task used in the present study. Whereas the present test results are consistent with a generally held theory (Rourke, 1982) concerning dysfunctional systems of the right hemisphere believed to subserve visual–spatial, novel analytic, and "holistic processing" (Reynolds, 1981) functions, a more recent formulation proposed by Rourke (1987, 1988, 1989) concerning dysfunction in connective and integrative white-matter systems of the brain may well provide a more comprehensive explanatory model.

The present results were far less robust with respect to the Group RD verbal impairments predicted. Since many of the comparisons are made with studies of younger disabled learners, these results may be suggestive of a *lag* in certain verbal attentional (Tarver, Hallahan, Kauffman, & Ball, 1976) and/or phonemic and linguistic processing (Beech & Harding, 1984; Ozols & Rourke, 1988) skills among reading-disabled children. These may improve gradually over time as neural systems mature (Satz & Van Nostrand, 1973). However, data exist to suggest that this is not the case (Rourke, 1976). The data of the present study suggest that arithmetic-disabled children exhibit more pervasive difficulties with the encoding of various types of nonverbal information; this seems to indicate rather serious learning impairments in this subtype. Recent reports suggest that these learning impairments may extend throughout the life span (Rourke, Young, Strang, & Russell, 1985). Further developmental studies, comparing reading and arithmetic disability subtypes across various age groups and more closely mimicking "real-life" memory demands are clearly warranted.

Educational/Remedial Implications

The practical ramifications that these findings have for the present educational system can be hypothesized. In recent years, the extension of the neuropsychological model beyond assessment into remedial strategy planning and predictive outcome has become widely recognized (Rourke et al., 1983; Torgeson, 1986). The clarification of specific remedial techniques is especially pertinent for both the specific learning disability teacher as well as regular classroom teachers who are likely to encounter both reading-disabled and arithmetic-disabled children in their classrooms. Although these children sometimes perform at similar levels on the memory tasks administered to them, their differential performances shown in this study and in previous research suggest that they may sometimes do so for entirely different reasons. This was particularly evident on the various verbal tasks. Whereas both Group RD and, to a lesser extent, AD children exhibited mild weaknesses relative to controls, the pattern of Group RD performances suggests that they have particular difficulty with normal verbal mnemonic organization (Dallago & Moely, 1980) or elaborative encoding through a speech code (Alegria & Pignot, 1984). Group AD children, in contrast, appear to have difficulty with the encoding of novel information in spite of good phonemic coding.

Therefore, the following approaches are proposed for subtypes of LD children with respect to mnestic functions. These approaches are specifically focused at the educational setting. Of course, the implications of specific memory deficits for the everyday life of the LD child (both academic and nonacademic) are considerable. Many of the following suggestions may be adapted for use when giving an LD child instructions in the home, when the child is following complex directions in playing games, assembling toys, and the like, and in the learning of adaptive behaviors such as interpersonal relating skills, activities of daily living and self-care, community awareness, and new forms of sport and recreation.

For reading-disabled children:

1. Specific training in "short-cuts" for the encoding of linguistic information (Bauer, 1977; Torgeson, 1979) appear to be fruitful. Techniques such as "chunking" (Dallago & Moely, 1980), elaborative semantic rehearsal (Torgeson et al., 1979), and distinguishing relevant from irrelevant facts (Oakhill, Shaw, & Folkard, 1983) have been shown to produce positive results and are consistent with the evidence relating to the intact semantic stores of reading-disabled children (Wiig & Roach, 1975) and other adaptive abilities of these children (e.g., conceptual grouping skills). In light of their specific difficulties with the retention of letter strings for encoding/decoding purposes, it seems useful to emphasize the encoding of letter chunks such as vowel digraphs (e.g., oo, oi) and word affixes (e.g., ment, ing) to promote "holistic" learning and reduce the processing demands of the visual memory–phonemic memory system (Samuels, 1987).

2. Whenever possible, the results presented here suggest that it would be useful to train such reading-disabled children to exploit their relative strengths in nonverbal areas. This might involve encouraging them to draw pictures or diagrams to illustrate complex verbal concepts and material (thereby recoding the information via the "visual scratch pad"). The increased use of microcomputers in the school system also provides an excellent alternative to teachers and students for designing

visual presentations of material and lessons. Training reading-disabled students in the use of visual imagery mnemonics as an alternative to verbal encoding with specific types of material may also be helpful (Lorayne, 1985; Pressley et al., 1987; Seamon & Gazzaniga, 1973). The results of a study by Bayliss and Livesey (1985) underscore this need to teach children to utilize their "preferred" cognitive strategies in order to maximize individual performance.

For arithmetic-disabled children, the similar lowered performances of arithmetic-disabled children on certain verbal recall tasks suggest that elaborative encoding mechanisms may be faulty and that specific training in these skills, as with reading-disabled children, would be useful. As with the reading-disabled group, perceptual training, favoring one modality over another, does not appear to be a useful aid to memory in the 10- to 14-year age group. In contrast, arithmetic-disabled children's performances on other memory tasks implies that their verbal "memory" problems are not linguistically or phonetically based, but rather, the problems appear to stem from the poor application of test strategies and in dealing with novel information efficiently. Their memory task performances suggest a deficiency in a normal developmental trend, that of relating "learning strategies to changing recall task demands" (Belmont & Butterfield, 1971). Thus, more specific remedial approaches (apparently not needed by many reading-disabled or normal children) appear to be required by this LD subtype. These approaches should emphasize their well-developed rote verbal and phonological processing skills.

1. Arithmetic-disabled children would likely benefit from practice and training in a careful, step-by-step, verbally mediated approach in which they review available test strategies and choose the best alternative. Pressley et al. (1987) have discussed extensively the LD child's need for learning new strategies, as well as learning how and when to utilize each strategy effectively; they refer to this latter area as "metastrategic knowledge." These authors further compare the training methods of "direct explanation," a teacher-directed presentation of the strategies, versus "dyadic instruction," a method dependent on direct interaction of the students and teacher in experimenting with new strategies. This latter type of active, experiential approach, although it may pose initial difficulties for the arithmetic-disabled child who is accustomed to a more withdrawn, noninteractive role (suggested in Strang & Rourke, 1983, 1985a), would likely lead to greater learning of strategies and metastrategic information.

2. The difficulties that these children exhibit in encoding, particularly of novel and nonverbal information, suggest that they would benefit from more time to encode information, carefully recoding it through verbally mediated strategies (as suggested in Strang & Rourke, 1985a, in

reference to remediation of socioemotional coping difficulties). In the learning of new verbal material, an information-processing technique known as "semantic mapping," in which words are related to superordinate and subordinate examples within the child's lexicon, would likely be a beneficial aid to this subtype of verbally competent learners.

3. Because novel information appears to pose specific difficulty for this group of children, behavioral methods of gradual stimulus desensitization may also be of use. This might be facilitated by presenting smaller units of novel material, drawing parallels to already-learned/encoded facts and concepts. A secondary benefit of anxiety reduction may also result.

4. When dealing with largely nonverbal (e.g., pictorial) information, these children would likely profit from training in talking their way through such tasks and through labeling and listing information in highly redundant, sequential steps. This should aid in circumventing general difficulties with organization of material to be encoded (Farnham-Diggory, 1978; Rourke & Strang, 1983). Hicks (1980) has demonstrated the utility of such training in improving visual recall scores for both disabled and normal readers. Verbal mnemonic strategies, such as first-letter cuing (Lorayne, 1985), may also be helpful as a means of exploiting their rote phonological and verbal symbolic abilities. As many younger arithmetic-disabled children appear to exhibit writing as well as arithmetic deficits (Strang & Rourke, 1985b), arithmetic-disabled children who persist in having such difficulties may benefit from additional time to complete written assignments and use of multiple-choice or orally administered examination methods. Older children in this group might profit from reliance on tape recorders to supplement verbal memory while circumventing writing difficulties (Siegel & Feldman, 1983). Because many arithmetic-disabled children encounter difficulty when required to align or visually organize written material for study purposes, they may also benefit from recoding it into its oral form (Strang & Rourke, 1985b). (For a more general approach to the treatment of children with specific arithmetic disabilities, see Rourke, 1989).

The future directions for research on these subtypes of LD children clearly should include testing of these and other remedial recommendations through specific, controlled studies. The next task for researchers is to compare these disability groups on teaching methods to show a differential response to treatment, as suggested by validation experts (Fletcher, 1985b; Lyon, 1985; Lyon & Flynn, Chapter 11, this volume). An example of such an approach is suggested in the work of Condus, Marshall, and Miller (1986) and others. In such research, it has been suggested that the "keyword mnemonic" system, a combined verbal–visual imagery mnemonic approach, can be an extremely helpful and effective strategy for reading-disabled children to use in learning various types of academic material, including vocabulary–definition associations (Condus et al., 1986) and scientific facts (Mastropieri, Scruggs, & Levin, 1985). Long-term retention using this strategy appears to be quite good. Furthermore, unlike other recommended strategies, the practical benefits in an applied (classroom) setting have been demonstrated directly (Condus et al., 1986). A developmental framework for future remedial research along these lines would also be most useful, as many test results, including the present, suggest changing patterns of ability throughout the school years.

Summary

1. Research suggests that children with "specific" learning disabilities in reading and arithmetic exhibit impairments in short-term memory. Individual studies suggest a preponderance of difficulties in the verbal realm for reading-disabled children, whereas arithmetic-disabled children display memory deficits in the nonverbal realm as well as in some aspects of verbal memory. Little research has investigated both LD groups simultaneously.

2. A recent investigation in the Windsor laboratory compared these two subgroups of LD children to each other and to age-matched controls. A similar dissociation in memory skills was found between the two groups, with only minimal verbal memory deficits in the reading-disabled group yet marked nonverbal deficits in the arithmetic-disabled group. The arithmetic-disabled children's performances also suggested difficulties on novel memory tasks.

3. Separate underlying neuropsychological mechanisms were proposed. Specifically, the pattern of mild reading-disabled verbal memory deficits suggested difficulties in phonemic codes, in the context of superior nonverbal memory encoding and recall and good use of novel strategies. The more marked nonverbal memory deficits in arithmetic-disabled children suggested poor visual–spatial recall and what appear to be difficulties in novel strategy generation. Other neuropsychological research supports this hypothesis, implicating the existence of unique LD subtypes. Dysfunction in left hemisphere systems is suggested by the reading-disabled children's deficits; a more serious dysfunction in right hemisphere and connective systems of the brain is suggested by the arithmetic-disabled children's deficits.

4. On the basis of this study and other research into the two subtypes, practical educational approaches were suggested to circumvent areas of deficit while exploiting strengths. In reading-disabled children, nonverbal visual–spatial strategies were suggested, whereas rote verbal strategies were suggested for arithmetic-disabled children.

5. Directions for future validation research in this area include comparisons of verbally and nonverbally based, rote and novel, teaching and mnemonic strategies for each LD subgroup to confirm or disconfirm differential effects.

References

Aaron, P. G. (1981). Diagnosis and remediation of learning disabilities in children—A neuropsychological key approach. In G. W. Hynd & J. E. Obrzut (Eds.), *Neuropsychological assessment and the school-aged child* (pp. 303–334). New York: Grune & Stratton.

Alegria, J., & Pignot, E. (1984). Lexical information in reading and memory. *Reading Research Quarterly, 19,* 173–183.

Baddeley, A. D. (1978). The trouble with levels: A reexamination of Craik and Lockhart's framework for memory research. *Psychology Review, 85,* 139–152.

Baddeley, A. D., & Hitch, G. (1974). Working memory. In G. A. Bower (Ed.), *The psychology of learning and motivation* (Vol. 8, pp. 47–90). New York: Academic Press.

Bauer, R. H. (1977). Memory processes in children with learning disabilities: Evidence for deficient rehearsal. *Journal of Experimental Child Psychology, 24,* 415–430.

Bauserman, D. N., & Obrzut, J. E. (1981). Spatial and temporal matching ability among subgroups of disabled readers. *Contemporary Educational Psychology, 6,* 306–313.

Bayliss, J., & Livesey, P. J. (1985). Cognitive strategies of children with reading disability and normal readers in visual sequential memory. *Journal of Learning Disabilities, 18,* 326–333.

Beech, J. R., & Harding, L. M. (1984). Phonemic processing and the poor reader from a developmental lag viewpoint. *Reading Research Quarterly, 19,* 357–366.

Belmont, J. M., & Butterfield, E. C. (1971). What the development of short-term memory is. *Human Development, 14,* 236–248.

Boder, E. (1973). Developmental dyslexia: A diagnostic approach based on three atypical reading–spelling patterns. *Developmental Medicine and Child Neurology, 15,* 663–687.

Brady, S., Shankweiler, D., & Mann, V. (1983). Speech perception and memory coding in relation to reading ability. *Journal of Experimental Child Psychology, 35,* 345–367.

Byrne, B. (1981). Reading disability, linguistic access and short-term memory: Comments prompted by Jorm's review of developmental dyslexia. *Australian Journal of Psychology, 33,* 83–95.

Cohen, R. I., Netley, C., & Clark, M. A. (1984). On the generality of the short term memory/reading ability relationship. *Journal of Learning Disabilities, 17,* 218–221.

Condus, M. M., Marshall, K. J., & Miller, S. R. (1986). Effects of the keyword mnemonic strategy on vocabulary acquisition and maintenance by learning disabled children. *Journal of Learning Disabilities, 19,* 609–613.

Corkin, S. (1974). Serial-ordering deficits in inferior readers. *Neuropsychologia, 12,* 347–354.

Dallago, M. L. L., & Moely, B. E. (1980). Free recall in boys of normal and poor reading levels as a function of task manipulations. *Journal of Experimental Child Psychology, 30,* 62–78.

Denckla, M. B. (1979). Childhood learning disabilities. In K. M. Heilman & E. Valenstein (Eds.), *Clinical neuropsychology* (pp. 535–573). New York: Oxford University Press.

Doehring, D. G. (1968). *Patterns of impairment in specific reading disability.* Bloomington: Indiana University Press.

Doehring, D. G. (1985). Reading disability subtypes: Interaction of reading and nonreading deficits. In B. P. Rourke (Ed.), *Neuropsychology of learning disabilities: Essentials of subtype analysis* (pp. 133-146). New York: Guilford Press.

Doehring, D. G., Trites, R. L., Patel, P. G., & Fiedorowicz, C. A. (1981). *Reading disabilities: The interaction of reading, language, and neuropsychological deficits.* New York: Academic Press.

Done, D. J., & Miles, T. R. (1978). Learning, memory and dyslexia. In M. M. Gruneberg & N. R. Stratton (Eds.), *Practical aspects of memory* (pp. 553-560). London: Academic Press.

Ellis, N. C., & Miles, T. R. (1978). Visual information processing in dyslexic children. In M. M. Gruneberg & R. N. Stratton (Eds.), *Practical aspects of memory* (pp. 561-569). London: Academic Press.

Farnham-Diggory, S. (1978). *Learning disabilities: A psychological perspective.* Cambridge, MA: Harvard University Press.

Farnham-Diggory, S., & Gregg, L. W. (1975). Short-term memory function in young readers. *Journal of Experimental Child Psychology, 19,* 279-298.

Fletcher, J. M. (1985a). External validation of learning disability typologies. In B. P. Rourke (Ed.), *Neuropsychology of learning disabilities: Essentials of subtype analysis* (pp. 187-211). New York: Guilford Press.

Fletcher, J. M. (1985b). Memory for verbal and nonverbal stimuli in learning disability subgroups: Analysis by selective reminding. *Journal of Experimental Child Psychology, 40,* 244-259.

Gerber, M. J. P., & White, D. R. (1983). Verbal factors in visual recognition memory for poor readers. *Perceptual and Motor Skills, 57,* 851-857.

Haith, M. M. (1971). Developmental changes in visual information processing and short-term visual memory. *Human Development, 14,* 249-261.

Hicks, C. (1980). The ITPA visual sequential memory task: An alternative interpretation and the implications for good and poor readers. *British Journal of Educational Psychology, 30,* 16-25.

Holmes, D. R., & McKeever, W. F. (1979). Material specific serial memory deficit in adolescent dyslexia. *Cortex, 15,* 51-62.

Jastak, J., & Jastak, S. (1978). *Wide Range Achievement Test.* Wilmington, DE: Guidance Associates.

Jorm, A. F. (1979). The cognitive and neurological basis of developmental dyslexia: A theoretical framework and review. *Cognition, 7,* 19-33.

Kastner, S. B., & Rickards, C. (1974). Mediated memory with novel and familiar stimuli in good and poor readers. *Journal of Genetic Psychology, 124,* 105-113.

Koppitz, E. M. (1975). Bender Gestalt Test, Visual Aural Digit Span Test and reading achievement. *Journal of Learning Disabilities, 8,* 32-35.

Liberman, I. Y., & Mann, V. A. (1981). *Should reading instruction and remediation vary with the sex of the child?* New Haven: Haskins Laboratory.

Liberman, I. Y., Mann, V. A., Shankweiler, D., & Werfelman, M. (1982). Children's memory for recurring linguistic and nonlinguistic material in relation to reading ability. *Cortex, 18,* 367-375.

Lindgren, S. D., & Richman, L. C. (1984). Immediate memory functions of verbally deficient reading disabled children. *Journal of Learning Disabilities, 17,* 222-225.

Lindsay, P. H., & Norman, D. A. (1977). *Human information processing* (2nd ed.). New York: Academic Press.

Lorayne, H. (1985). *Page-a-minute memory book.* New York: Rinehart & Winston.

Lyon, R. (1985). Educational validation studies of learning disability subtypes. In B. P. Rourke (Ed.), *Neuropsychology of learning disabilities: Essentials of subtype analysis* (pp. 228–256). New York: Guilford Press.

Lyon, R., Watson, B., Reitta, S., Porch, B., & Rhodes, J. (1981). Selected linguistic and perceptual abilities of empirically derived subgroups of learning disabled readers. *Journal of School Psychology, 19,* 152–166.

MacKinnon, G. E., & McCarthy, N. A. (1973). Verbal labelling, auditory–visual integration, and reading ability. *Canadian Journal of Behavioural Science, 5,* 124–132.

Mann, V. A., Liberman, I. Y., & Shankweiler, D. (1980). Children's memory for sentences and word strings in relation to reading ability. *Memory and Cognition, 8,* 329–335.

Mark, L. S., Shankweiler, D., Liberman, I. Y., & Fowler, C. A. (1977). Phonetic recoding and reading difficulty in beginning readers. *Memory and Cognition, 5,* 623–629.

Mastropieri, M. A., Scruggs, T. E., & Levin, J. R. (1985). Mnemonic strategy instruction with learning disabled adolescents. *Journal of Learning Disabilities, 18,* 94–100.

Mattis, S. (1978). Dyslexia syndromes: A working hypothesis that works. In A. L. Benton & D. Pearl (Eds.), *Dyslexia: An appraisal of current knowledge* (pp. 43–60). New York: Oxford University Press.

McKeever, W. F., & VanDeventer, A. D. (1975). Dyslexic adolescents: Evidence of impaired visual and auditory language processing associated with normal lateralization and visual responsivity. *Cortex, 11,* 361–378.

Oakhill, J., Shaw, D., & Folkard, S. (1983). Selective impairment of educationally subnormal children's delayed memory for text. *Nature, 303,* 800–801.

Obrzut, J. G. (1979). Dichotic listening and bisensory memory skills in qualitatively diverse dyslexic readers. *Journal of Learning Disabilities, 12,* 304–314.

Olson, R. K., Davidson, B. J., & Kliegl, R., & Davies, S. E. (1984). Development of phonetic memory in disabled and normal readers. *Journal of Experimental Child Psychology, 37,* 187–206.

Osterrieth, P. A. (1944). Le test de copie d'une figure complexe. *Archives de Psychologie, 30,* 206–356.

Ozols, E. J., & Rourke, B. P. (1985). Dimensions of social sensitivity in two types of learning-disabled children. In B. P. Rourke (Ed.), *Neuropsychology of learning disabilities: Essentials of subtype analysis* (pp. 281–301). New York: Guilford Press.

Ozols, E. J., & Rourke, B. P. (1988). Characteristics of young learning-disabled children classified according to patterns of academic achievement: Auditory–perceptual and visual–perceptual abilities. *Journal of Child Clinical Psychology, 17,* 44–52.

Paivio, A. (1971). *Imagery and verbal processes.* New York: Holt, Rinehart & Winston.

Petrauskas, R. J., & Rourke, B. P. (1979). Identification of subtypes of retarded readers: A neuropsychological, multivariate approach. *Journal of Clinical Neuropsychology, 1,* 17–37.

Pressley, M., Johnson, C. J., & Symons, S. (1987). Elaborating to learn and learning to elaborate. *Journal of Learning Disabilities, 20,* 76–91.

Reynolds, C. R. (1981). The neuropsychological basis of intelligence. In G. W. Hynd & J. E. Obrzut (Eds.), *Neuropsychological assessment and the school-age child* (pp. 87–124). New York: Grune & Stratton.

Ridgley, B. A. (1970). *The neuropsychological abilities of young normal and retarded readers.* Unpublished doctoral dissertation, University of Windsor.

Ritchie, D. J., & Aten, J. L. (1976). Auditory retention of nonverbal and verbal sequential stimuli in children with reading disabilities. *Journal of Learning Disabilities, 9,* 312–318.

Rourke, B. P. (1975). Brain-behavior relationships in children with learning disabilities. *American Psychologist, 30,* 911–920.

Rourke, B. P. (1976). Reading retardation in children: Developmental lag or deficit? In R. M Knights & D. J. Bakker (Eds.), *Neuropsychology of learning disorders: Theoretical approaches* (pp. 125-137). Baltimore: University Park Press.

Rourke, B. P. (1978). Neuropsychological research in reading retardation: A review. In A. L. Benton & D. Pearl (Eds.), *Dyslexia: An appraisal of current knowledge* (pp. 141-171). New York: Oxford University Press.

Rourke, B. P. (1982). Central processing deficiencies in children: Toward a developmental neuropsychological model. *Journal of Clinical Neuropsychology, 4,* 1-18.

Rourke, B. P. (1987). Syndrome of nonverbal learning disabilities: The final common pathway of white-matter disease/dysfunction? *The Clinical Neuropsychologist, 1,* 209-234.

Rourke, B. P. (1988). The syndrome of nonverbal learning disabilities: Developmental manifestations in neurological disease, disorder, and dysfunction. *The Clinical Neuropsychologist, 2,* 293-330.

Rourke, B. P. (1989). *Nonverbal learning disabilities: The syndrome and the model.* New York: Guilford Press.

Rourke, B. P., Bakker, D. J., Fisk, J. L., & Strang, J. D. (1983). *Child neuropsychology: An introduction to theory, research, and clinical practice.* New York: Guilford Press.

Rourke, B. P., & Finlayson, M. A. J. (1978). Neuropsychological significance of variations in patterns of academic performance: Verbal and visual–spatial abilities. *Journal of Abnormal Child Psychology, 6,* 121-133.

Rourke, B. P., & Strang, J. D. (1978). Neuropsychological significance of variations in patterns of academic performance: Motor, psychomotor, and tactile-perceptual abilities. *Journal of Pediatric Psychology, 2,* 62-66.

Rourke, B. P., & Strang, J. D. (1983). Subtypes of reading and arithmetical disabilities: A neuropsychological analysis. In M. Rutter (Ed.), *Developmental neuropsychiatry* (pp. 473-488). New York: Guilford Press.

Rourke, B. P., Young, G. C., Strang, J. D., & Russell, D. L. (1985). Adult outcomes of central processing deficiencies in childhood. In I. Grant & K. M. Adams (Eds.), *Neuropsychological assessment in neuropsychiatric disorders: Clinical methods and empirical findings* (pp. 244-267). New York: Oxford University Press.

Samuels, S. J. (1987). Information processing abilities and reading. *Journal of Learning Disabilities, 20,* 18-22.

Sattler, J. M. (1982). *Assessment of children's intelligence and special abilities* (2nd ed.). Boston: Allyn & Bacon.

Satz, P., & Van Nostrand, G. K. (1973). Developmental dyslexia: An evaluation of a theory. In P. S. Ross & J. Ross (Eds.), *The disabled learner: Early detection and intervention* (pp. 45-62). Rotterdam: Rotterdam University Press.

Seamon, J. G., & Gazzaniga, M. S. (1973). Coding strategies and cerebral laterality effects. *Cognitive Psychology, 5,* 249-256.

Shankweiler, D., & Liberman, I. Y. (1976). Exploring the relations between reading and speech. In R. M. Knights & D. K. Bakker (Eds.), *Neuropsychology of learning disorders* (pp. 297-313). Baltimore: University Park Press.

Siegel, L. S., & Feldman, W. (1983). Nondyslexic children with combined writing and arithmetic learning disabilities. *Clinical Pediatrics, 22,* 241-244.

Siegel, L. S., & Linder, B. A. (1984). Short-term memory processes in children with reading and arithmetic learning disabilities. *Developmental Psychology, 20,* 200-207.

Stanley, G., & Hall, R. (1973). Short-term visual information processing in dyslexics. *Child Development, 44,* 841-844.

Strang, J. D., & Rourke, B. P. (1983). Concept-formation/nonverbal reasoning abilities of children who exhibit specific academic problems with arithmetic. *Journal of Clinical Child Psychology, 12,* 33-39.

Strang, J. D., & Rourke, B. P. (1985a). Adaptive behavior of children who exhibit specific arithmetic disabilities and associated neuropsychological abilities and deficits. In B. P. Rourke (Ed.), *Neuropsychology of learning disabilities: Essentials of subtype analysis* (pp. 302–330). New York: Guilford Press.

Strang, J. D., & Rourke, B. P. (1985b). Arithmetic disability subtypes: The neuropsychological significance of specific arithmetical impairment in childhood. In B. P. Rourke (Ed.), *Neuropsychology of learning disabilities: Essentials of subtype analysis* (pp. 167–186). New York: Guilford Press.

Swanson, L. (1978). Verbal encoding effects on the visual short term memory of learning disabled and normal readers. *Journal of Educational Psychology, 70*, 539–544.

Tarver, S. G., Hallahan, D. P., Kauffman, J. M., & Ball, D. W. (1976). Verbal rehearsal and selective attention in children with learning disabilities: A developmental lag. *Journal of Experimental Child Psychology, 22*, 375–385.

Tellier, A. (1986). *Memory functions of learning-disabled children with different neuropsychological profiles.* Unpublished manuscript, University of Windsor.

Torgeson, J. K. (1979). Performance of reading-disabled children on serial memory tasks: A selective review of recent research. *Reading Research Quarterly, 14*, 57–87.

Torgeson, J. K. (1986). Learning disabilities theory: Its current state and future prospects. *Journal of Learning Disabilities, 19*, 399–407.

Torgeson, J. K., Murphy, H. A., & Ivey, C. (1979). The influence of an orienting task on the memory performance of children with reading problems. *Journal of Learning Disabilities, 12*, 43–48.

Vellutino, F. R., Pruzek, R. M., Steger, J. A., & Meshoulam, U. (1973). Immediate visual recall in poor and normal readers as a function of orthographic-linguistic familiarity. *Cortex, 9*, 368–384.

Vellutino, F. R., Steger, J. A., Kaman, M., & DeSetto, L. (1975). Visual form perception in deficient and normal readers as a function of age and orthographic–linguistic familiarity. *Cortex, 11*, 22–30.

Waber, D. P., & Holmes, J. M. (1985). Assessing children's copy productions of the Rey-Osterrieth Complex Figure. *Journal of Clinical and Experimental Neuropsychology, 7*, 264–280.

Waber, D. P., & Holmes, J. M. (1986). Assessing children's memory productions of the Rey-Osterrieth Complex Figure. *Journal of Clinical and Experimental Neuropsychology, 8*, 563–580.

Webster, R. E. (1979). Visual and aural short-term memory capacity deficits in mathematics disabled students. *Journal of Educational Research, 72*, 277–283.

Wechsler, D. (1974). *Manual for the Wechsler Intelligence Scale for Children—Revised.* New York: Psychological Corporation.

Wiig, E. H., & Roach, M. A. (1975). Immediate recall of semantically varied "sentences" by learning-disabled adolescents. *Perceptual and Motor Skills, 40*, 119–125.

CHAPTER 6

Classification of Young Learning-Disabled Children According to Patterns of Academic Achievement: Validity Studies

Edite J. Ozols and Byron P. Rourke

Many typologies for the classification of learning disabilities have been introduced in recent years, and many of the studies addressing classification issues have used a clinical–inferential approach to achieve this aim. In this approach, subjects are classified into groups on an *a priori* basis, and the groups are then compared statistically on their performance on a variety of measures presumed to be related to their learning disabilities. For the most part, subtypes have been proposed on the basis of etiological variables, neuropsychological variables, spelling-error types, and patterns of academic achievement.

In this chapter, we discuss studies that have used the classification approach that is based on patterns of academic achievement. This method has proved to be quite successful in revealing differences between groups of older (9- to 14-year-old) learning-disabled children. In some recent investigations, we applied this method of classification to a group of younger (7- and 8-year-old) learning-disabled children, examining their performance on the same or similar variables as those explored in the studies with older children. The primary purpose of this chapter is to present and discuss the results of our recent studies with young learning-disabled children, examining their performance on five sets of variables: auditory–linguistic skills; visual–spatial–organizational skills; motor, psychomotor, and tactile–perceptual abilities; a test of concept formation; and social behavior.

Classification of Older Learning-Disabled Children According to Patterns of Academic Achievement

The Principal Groups of Interest

Three groups of 9- to 14-year-old learning-disabled children, classified according to their patterns of performance on the Wide Range Achievement Test (WRAT; Jastak & Jastak, 1965), have been compared in a series of investigations alluded to in several chapters of this book. Children in Group 1 were uniformly deficient in reading, spelling, and arithmetic; Group 2 children were relatively adept, although still impaired, at arithmetic as compared to their performance in reading and spelling; and Group 3 children exhibited average or above-average reading and spelling skills but were relatively deficient in arithmetic. All three groups were deficient relative to age-based norms in arithmetic.

When the performances of the three groups were compared on a number of auditory–perceptual and visual–perceptual measures, it was found that Group 3 children performed in a superior manner to Groups 1 and 2 on verbal and auditory–perceptual measures, whereas Groups 1 and 2 performed at significantly superior levels to Group 3 on visual–perceptual measures (Rourke & Finlayson, 1978). Subsequent studies demonstrated that Group 3 children also exhibited marked deficiencies relative to Groups 1 and 2 on certain psychomotor and tactile–perceptual skills (Rourke & Strang, 1978) and that the performance of Group 3 was inferior to that of Group 2 on a test designed as a measure of complex concept formation (Strang & Rourke, 1983). These three studies form the basis on which the groups in our investigations of 7- and 8-year-old learning-disabled children were formed; these studies are discussed in more detail in subsequent sections of this chapter.

Investigative Efforts in Other Laboratories

Although negative results have also been reported (Nolan, Hammeke, & Barkley, 1983), at least two other studies using this classification approach have reported significant group differences. Children classified according to their patterns of academic achievement were found to differ in their performance on memory tasks according to whether the task was verbal or spatial in nature (Fletcher, 1983). Significant group differences were also reported in a study assessing recall of rhyming and nonrhyming letters that were presented in visual and auditory modalities (Siegel & Linder, 1984). In particular, the relationship between reading/arithmetic achievement patterns and tasks emphasizing verbal/nonverbal processing has been demonstrated repeatedly (Badian, 1983; Fletcher, 1985).

Furthermore, the relative independence of arithmetic and reading disabilities was suggested by the results of an early study that involved the factor analysis of test data of children who were identified as severe underachievers in mathematics and/or reading (Goodstein & Kahn, 1974). These investigators report that stable and independent factors for arithmetic computation, reading achievement, and measured intelligence were found when they analyzed children's scores on the Wechsler Intelligence Scale for Children (WISC; Wechsler, 1949), Gates–MacGinitie Reading Test, and the SRA Achievement Series in Arithmetic. Similar groups to those studied in the series of investigations by Rourke and Finlayson (1978), Rourke and Strang (1978), and Strang and Rourke (1983) have also been isolated using cluster-analytic techniques (Satz & Morris, 1981).

Children in Group 3 have been the focus of considerable concern, as their problems in adaptive functioning appear to be pervasive. In conjunction with their arithmetic disability, they exhibit outstanding problems in visual–spatial organization and synthesis, bilateral psychomotor and tactile–perceptual deficiencies, and impaired nonverbal concept formation and reasoning (Rourke, 1988, 1989). Because these children appear to be at considerable risk for the development of socioemotional disturbance, it is vital that clinical methods be developed to identify them at young ages. It is also clear that such specification of subtypes would be of potential use in the development of academic intervention programs for the children so classified.

Subtype Research with Younger Learning-Disabled Children

Previous studies of younger learning-disabled children have generally been unsuccessful in demonstrating reliable differences between subtypes of children who were classified on the basis of the WISC (Rourke, Dietrich, & Young, 1973). When groups of 5- to 8-year-old children were formed on the basis of Verbal IQ–Performance IQ (VIQ–PIQ) differences on the WISC, the clear-cut differences that had been found for older children (Rourke & Telegdy, 1971; Rourke, Young, & Flewelling, 1971) were not evident at this young age. This classification method has also been shown to be quite unsuccessful in predicting reading achievement for 6-year-olds, although this was the case for older children (Reed, 1967). It is possible that the absence of significant group differences for young children is related to the relative unreliability of the psychological tests at these ages and/or the relatively undifferentiated ability structures of young children. The variability seen in the test performances of young children has also often been attributed to an attentional deficit that masks basic information-processing deficiencies at young ages (Rourke, 1983).

Alternatively, it could be that group differences *can* be demonstrated in the young learning-disabled population when a different method of classification is used. In the following sections, we describe a series of studies that were designed to address whether 7- and 8-year-old learning-disabled children differ in their patterns of functioning when they are classified according to patterns of academic achievement. Full descriptions of the variables used in this study may be found in Rourke, Fisk, and Strang (1986). Norms for the neuropsychological tests have been provided by Knights and Norwood (1980); norms for the WISC, the WRAT, and the Peabody Picture Vocabulary Test (PPVT; Dunn, 1965) are provided by the authors of these tests.

Investigations of the Neuropsychological and Behavioral Characteristics of 7- and 8-Year-Old Learning-Disabled Children Classified According to Patterns of Academic Achievement

Participants in All Studies

The 45 participants in this study were selected from a population of over 1,500 children of this age who had been assessed at the neuropsychology service of a large urban children's mental health center. These children were referred for neuropsychological assessment because of a learning or "perceptual" handicap to which it was thought that cerebral dysfunction might be a contributing factor. Each child had received an extensive battery of neuropsychological tests administered in a standardized manner by technicians trained specifically for that purpose. Participants ranged in age from 84 to 107 months. The selected children, who met our usual (exclusionary) criteria for "learning disability" (Rourke, 1983), exhibited average levels of psychometric intelligence as defined by obtaining a WISC Full Scale IQ (FSIQ) score between 85 and 115. Only right-handed children were used in this study, and parents of all children selected indicated that English was spoken in the home. On the basis of information derived from a parent questionnaire, school records, and a hearing test administered as part of the neuropsychological test battery, none of the children showed evidence of the following: inadequate visual or auditory acuity; neurological disease; severe cultural, educational, or environmental deprivation; significant emotional disturbance.

Group 1 children (*n* = 15) exhibited uniformly deficient performances on the Reading, Spelling, and Arithmetic subtests of the WRAT. Specifically, their centile scores on all three subtests were less than or equal to 16, and there was no more than a 7-centile-point difference or a one-half grade-level difference between any two of the three WRAT subtests. Group 2 children (*n* = 15) presented with a pattern of deficient Reading and Spelling scores in conjunction with higher Arithmetic scores. The Group 2 children obtained WRAT Reading and Spelling centile scores less than or equal to 16 and obtained WRAT Arithmetic centile scores less than or equal to 34 (range = 16 to 34). Their Arithmetic scores were at least 10 centile points or one-half of a grade level higher than their Reading and Spelling scores. Group 3 children (*n* = 15) exhibited average or above-average performances on the Reading and Spelling subtests but performed in an inferior manner on the Arithmetic subtest. Specifically, Group 3 children obtained WRAT Reading and Spelling scores greater than or equal to 45 (range = 47 to 93) and WRAT Arithmetic centile scores less than or equal to 34 (range = 12 to 34). Their Arithmetic scores were at least 25 centile points and 1 grade level lower than their Reading and Spelling scores.

The exact criteria for child and group selection that were used in the parallel studies with older children could not be employed in the present study because of factors related to the young age of the children. The large grade-level differences on the WRAT seen at the older ages cannot be obtained at ages 7 and 8 because appropriate grade levels for younger children are close to the basal level of the test. Therefore, a slightly modified combination of centile score differences and grade-level differences was used to form the groups in the present study.

Results of one-way analyses of variance (ANOVAs) indicated that Groups 1, 2, and 3 did not differ significantly from one another in age or FSIQ. As expected, one-way ANOVAs indicated that there were highly significant differences in group performance on the three WRAT subtests: In Reading and Spelling, Group 3 performed better than Groups 1 and 2; in Arithmetic, Groups 2 and 3 performed better than Group 1; there was no significant difference between Groups 2 and 3 on the Arithmetic subtest. Group performances on the selection variables are seen in Table 6.1.

Study 1: Auditory–Linguistic Variables

The first study in the series of investigations with older children examined group performance on auditory–linguistic variables (Rourke & Finlayson, 1978). The three groups of 9- to 14-year-old learning-disabled children were compared in their performance on 10 auditory–linguistic

TABLE 6.1. Means and Standard Deviations for Selection Variables

	Group 1		Group 2		Group 3	
Selection variables	M	SD	M	SD	M	SD
Age (months)	97.73	5.28	98.73	5.51	101.13	4.49
WISC FSIQ	94.73	5.50	97.66	5.64	98.53	6.99
WRAT						
Reading (centile)	6.86	3.46	7.53	3.26	79.33	9.68
Spelling (centile)	7.40	2.39	7.86	2.80	67.40	12.29
Arithmetic (centile)	9.00	3.61	25.33	5.16	25.66	6.93

Note. Sex ratios (boys : girls) in the groups were 11 : 4 for Group 1, 13 : 2 for Group 2, and 7 : 8 for Group 3.

variables. Statistically significant differences were found in 9 of the 10 variables, and the performance of Group 3 consistently exceeded that of Groups 1 and 2.

It was hypothesized that similar results would obtain when the younger children were compared on the same variables: it was expected that Group 3 children would perform in a superior manner to Group 1 and Group 2 children on auditory–linguistic variables.

MEASURES

The auditory–linguistic measures consisted of the following:

1. WISC VIQ, a composite score indicative of overall "verbal" functioning.
2. WISC Information subtest, which assesses a child's ability to retrieve verbal information.
3. WISC Similarities subtest, a measure of verbal associations.
4. WISC Vocabulary subtest, which requires the child to define words.
5. WISC Digit Span subtest, which was designed to assess short-term auditory memory for digits.
6. PPVT IQ (Dunn, 1965), an estimate of verbal intelligence based on a measure of recognition vocabulary.
7. Number of errors on the linguistic items of the Halstead–Wepman Aphasia Screening Test—Younger Children's Version (Reitan, 1984), a screening test for aphasia.
8. The first 30 items of the Speech-Sounds Perception Test—Children's Version (Reitan & Davison, 1974), a measure of the ability to recognize the printed versions of spoken stimulus sounds.

9. Auditory Closure Test (Kass, 1964), a measure of the ability to blend into words progressively longer chains of sound elements presented on a tape recording.
10. Sentence Memory Test (Benton, 1965), a measure of verbatim auditory memory for words in a meaningful context.

There were a small number of children with missing data on some of the variables: six had not received the Speech-Sounds Perception Test, and one had not received the Auditory Closure Test and the Sentence Memory Test. ANOVAs for unbalanced data were computed for these tests.

RESULTS AND DISCUSSION

Means and standard deviations for the performance of the three groups on auditory–linguistic variables are displayed in Table 6.2. The observed direction of effect was consistent with that predicted for the 10 auditory–linguistic measures, as Group 3 consistently performed in a manner superior to Groups 1 and 2 on these tests. A one-way miltivariate analysis of variance (MANOVA) for groups across the auditory–linguistic measures yielded a significant main effect for group, $F(20,54) = 7.32$, $p <$ .001, and one-way ANOVAs yielded significant group effects on 8 of the 10 variables. Simple effects across group were tested using the Duncan Multiple-Range Test, with the criterion for statistical significance set at the .05 level. In view of the fact that specific hypotheses were entertained prior to data analyses, *"a priori"* comparisons among means (Winer, 1962) were also carried out to compare the mean scores for Groups 1 and 2 with the mean scores of Group 3. This planned comparisons technique revealed a significant group difference on the Vocabulary subtest in addition to differences on the eight variables delineated by the ANOVA results. A summary of the MANOVA, ANOVA, and the group mean comparison results for the auditory–linguistic measures is presented in Table 6.3. Although the VIQ score is highly correlated with the four WISC Verbal subtests used in this study, its inclusion in the MANOVA did not result in a singular error matrix. A MANOVA excluding VIQ was also carried out; this analysis yielded results virtually identical to those reported with VIQ included.

The MANOVAs excluded children with missing data. Therefore, in order to maximize the number of children in each group, separate ANOVAs were computed for each variable. These analyses yielded somewhat higher F values (with p values all less than .01). However, the only change in significance value from those reported for the MANOVA results was that the VIQ for Group 3 was significantly superior to that for Group 2.

TABLE 6.2. Means and Standard Deviations for Dependent Variables

	Group 1		Group 2		Group 3	
	M	SD	M	SD	M	SD
Auditory–linguistic variables						
WISC VIQ	90.86	7.07	94.60	8.34	101.00	8.01
WISC Information (scaled score)	6.73	1.66	7.06	1.70	9.86	3.15
WISC Similarities (scaled score)	10.86	2.61	11.33	2.74	12.26	2.40
WISC Vocabulary (scaled score)	10.20	1.61	10.40	2.19	11.66	2.22
WISC Digit Span (scaled score)	6.60	1.91	7.73	1.66	8.66	2.02
PPVT IQ	93.86	11.33	95.26	10.97	106.80	12.91
Aphasia Screening Test (errors)	3.86	1.40	3.46	1.72	1.60	1.63
Speech-Sounds Perception Test (number correct)	10.28	4.02	13.16	2.12	21.53	2.47
Auditory Closure Test (number correct)	6.00	2.77	6.93	2.05	13.14	3.23
Sentence Memory Test (number correct)	9.46	2.87	8.60	3.26	11.57	2.24
Visual–spatial–organizational variables						
WISC PIQ	99.80	7.83	101.66	7.22	96.13	10.50
WISC Picture Completion (scaled score)	10.40	3.54	11.20	2.78	10.20	2.51
WISC Picture Arrangement (scaled score)	9.40	2.94	10.53	2.29	9.60	2.13
WISC Block Design (scaled score)	10.60	2.02	10.06	1.43	9.86	2.77
WISC Object Assembly (scaled score)	10.93	1.83	10.60	1.24	8.73	2.52
Target Test (number correct)	9.93	3.33	11.20	3.56	12.76	2.95
Motor, psychomotor, and tactile–perceptual variables						
Tapping, right hand (number of taps)	28.20	6.07	30.12	3.50	29.64	2.62
Tapping, left hand (number of taps)	26.52	4.68	27.64	4.41	26.73	2.70
Grip, right hand (kg)	11.04	2.49	11.33	3.72	10.53	1.82
Grip, left hand (kg)	10.31	1.94	10.82	2.88	9.55	2.17
Mazes, right hand (seconds)	5.05	3.49	6.93	5.54	4.00	2.29
Mazes, left hand (seconds)	12.99	7.29	14.15	7.73	8.84	5.56
Pegs, right hand (seconds)	36.20	7.52	36.93	6.62	37.40	8.20
Pegs, left hand (seconds)	40.66	10.08	41.40	12.25	44.26	8.23
TPT, right hand (minutes)	6.54	3.10	6.02	2.62	7.19	3.67
TPT, left hand (minutes)	5.50	4.14	4.23	1.87	4.86	3.43
TPT, both hands (minutes)	2.58	1.36	2.11	1.07	3.39	3.81
Tactile, right hand (number of errors)	7.60	5.60	4.13	2.92	5.86	3.66
Tactile, left hand (number of errors)	7.06	3.95	5.13	3.29	6.13	4.62
Concept-formation variables						
Category subtest 1 (number of errors)	0.20	0.56	0.20	0.41	0.33	0.48
Category subtest 2 (number of errors)	5.40	4.23	5.73	2.31	4.46	2.87
Category subtest 3 (number of errors)	5.93	2.60	5.20	3.54	4.46	2.09
Category subtest 4 (number of errors)	12.00	5.25	8.60	6.40	4.20	4.61
Category subtest 5 (number of errors)	1.93	1.03	1.93	1.33	1.60	0.98
Category total (number of errors)	25.46	9.59	21.66	10.95	15.06	4.93

(*continued*)

TABLE 6.2. (Continued)

	Group 1		Group 2		Group 3	
	M	SD	M	SD	M	SD
Behavioral variables						
BPC Conduct Problem subscale (centile scores)	33.13	26.85	44.13	27.20	54.76	32.69
BPC Personality Problem subscale (centile scores)	48.64	19.04	46.86	27.86	50.76	22.89
BPC Inadequacy–Immaturity subscale (centile scores)	39.00	17.77	42.20	25.18	41.92	20.24
BPC total score (centile scores)	39.80	15.37	44.66	24.01	50.76	21.97

The hypothesis that Groups 1 and 2 would perform in a manner inferior to Group 3 on tests of auditory–perceptual and linguistic functioning was strongly supported. The groups of young children in this study performed on these variables in a manner highly similar to that exhibited by older children classified in the same manner (Rourke & Finlayson, 1978). The results support the notion that children with reading and spelling problems, regardless of their level of mechanical arithmetic, also tend to have significant auditory–perceptual and linguistic-processing deficiencies.

The WISC Similarities subtest was the only measure in this category on which significant group differences were not found. It is common to find performance on the Similarities subtest "spared" in children with psycholinguistically based learning disabilities (Rourke, 1981). Children in all groups performed within the average to above-average range on this measure, suggesting that complex linguistic skills may not be a prerequisite for successful performance on this task. Rather, it appears that young children can perform adequately on this task by making simple associations and stating verbal analogies.

Study 2: Visual–Spatial–Organizational Variables

Groups of 9- to 14-year-old children were also compared on their performance on six visual–spatial–organizational measures in the Rourke and Finlayson (1978) investigation. In this study, statistically significant differences were found on five of these six measures: Group 3 children performed in a consistently inferior manner to Group 1 and Group 2 children. Therefore, it was hypothesized that the 7- and 8-year-old Group 3 children would also perform in an inferior manner to young Group 1 and Group 2 children on these measures.

TABLE 6.3. Summary of MANOVA, ANOVA, and Simple Effects Results for Dependent Variables

	ANOVA	Duncan Multiple-Range Test		
		1 versus 2	1 versus 3	2 versus 3
Auditory–linguistic variables				
WISC VIQ	**	ns	*	ns
WISC Information	**	ns	*	*
WISC Similarities	ns			
WISC Vocabulary	ns			
WISC Digit Span	*	ns	*	ns
PPVT IQ	*	ns	*	*
Aphasia Screening Test	**	ns	*	*
Speech-Sounds Perception Test	***	*	*	*
Auditory Closure Test	***	ns	*	*
Sentence Memory Test	*	ns	ns	*
MANOVA	***			
Visual–spatial–organizational variables				
WISC PIQ	ns			
WISC Picture Completion	ns			
WISC Picture Arrangement	ns			
WISC Block Design	ns			
WISC Object Assembly	**	ns	*	*
Target Test	ns	ns	*	ns
MANOVA	*			
Motor, psychomotor, and tactile–perceptual variables				
Tapping, right hand	ns			
Tapping, left hand	ns			
Grip, right hand	ns			
Grip, left hand	ns			
Mazes, right hand	ns			
Mazes, left hand	ns			
Pegs, right hand	ns			
Pegs, left hand	ns			
TPT, right hand	ns			
TPT, left hand	ns			
TPT, both hands	ns			
Tactile, right hand	ns			
Tactile, left hand	ns			
MANOVA	ns			

(continued)

TABLE 6.3. (Continued)

	ANOVA	Duncan Multiple-Range Test		
		1 versus 2	1 versus 3	2 versus 3
Concept-formation variables				
Category subtest 1	ns			
Category subtest 2	ns			
Category subtest 3	ns			
Category subtest 4	***	ns	*	*
Category subtest 5	ns			
Category total	**	ns	*	ns
MANOVA	ns			
Behavioral variables				
BPC Conduct Problem subscale	ns	ns	*	ns
BPC Conduct Problem subscale (males)	**	ns	*	*
BPC Personality Problem subscale	ns			
BPC Inadequacy–Immaturity subscale	ns			
BPC total score	ns			
BPC total score (males)	*	ns	*	ns
MANOVA	ns			

Note. *p < .05, **p < .01, ***p < .001.

MEASURES

The measures consisted of the following:

1. WISC PIQ, a composite score indicative of overall "nonverbal" functioning.
2. WISC Picture Completion subtest, a measure of visual discrimination and visual memory.
3. WISC Picture Arrangement subtest, a measure of visual sequencing.
4. WISC Block Design subtest, a measure of visual–spatial–constructional skills.
5. WISC Object Assembly subtest, a measure of visual–spatial functioning.
6. Target Test (Reitan & Davison, 1974), a measure of (immediate) visual memory involving the capacity to reproduce patterns of dots in a specified sequence after a brief delay period.

RESULTS AND DISCUSSION

Means and standard deviations for the performance of the three groups on visual–spatial–organizational variables are displayed in Table 6.2.

The observed direction of effect was consistent with that predicted on four of the six visual–perceptual measures, with Group 3 performing in an inferior manner to Groups 1 and 2. A one-way MANOVA for group yielded a significant main effect across the six dependent variables in this category, $F(12,72) = 1.99$, $p < .03$. A one-way ANOVA revealed a significant effect for group on the WISC Object Assembly subtest, $F(2,42) = 5.62$, $p < .006$. Comparisons between means with the Duncan Multiple-Range Test indicated that Group 3 performed in a manner significantly inferior to Groups 1 and 2 on this variable. A summary of the MANOVA, ANOVA, and group mean comparison results is presented in Table 6.3. Although the PIQ score is highly correlated with the four WISC Performance subtests used in this study, its inclusion in the MANOVA did not result in a singular error matrix. A MANOVA excluding PIQ was also carried out; this analysis yielded results virtually identical to those reported with PIQ included.

Thus, the results of this study provide some support for the hypothesis that Group 3 children perform in a manner inferior to the other learning-disabled children on visual–spatial–organizational measures. Several previous studies have also reported that children with "specific" arithmetic disabilities exhibit inferior scores on the Object Assembly subtest (Badian, 1983; Rourke & Finlayson, 1978). That this relationship exists even at the relatively tender ages of children in the present study suggests that certain levels of visual–perceptual and visual–spatial skills may be essential for the mastery of very basic arithmetic concepts for this subtype of learning-disabled children but not for their performance in word recognition and spelling.

The expected pattern of group differences was not found on the Target Test; in fact, Group 3 children performed in a manner superior to Group 1 children on this measure. However, in comparison to the normal population, all three groups performed in a significantly inferior manner on the Target Test. It is possible that the three groups did poorly on this test for completely different reasons: Although the verbal requirements involved in understanding the task and in guiding behavior may account for the low performance of Groups 1 and 2, Group 3 may have had difficulty on this test because of its visual–spatial requirements. Moreover, it is possible that the attentional requirements on this task were a major factor limiting the performance of all three groups of learning-disabled children.

Additional information regarding group performance on both auditory–linguistic and visual–perceptual variables has been presented recently (Ozols & Rourke, 1988).

Study 3: Motor, Psychomotor, and Tactile–Perceptual Variables

Differences among the three subtypes of 9- to 14-year-old children on motor, psychomotor, and tactile–perceptual abilities were investigated by Rourke and Strang (1978). Group differences were not found on measures of simple motor skill (such as finger tapping and grip strength), and there were no significant group × hand interaction effects in evidence. However, Group 1 and Group 2 children performed in a superior manner to Group 3 children on two measures of psychomotor coordination (the Maze Test and the Grooved Pegboard Test) as well as on a composite measure of tactile–perceptual skills. These differences were found for both the right-hand and left-hand performances of the children. On a complex measure requiring problem-solving skills as well as psychomotor coordination (the Tactual Performance Test), Group 3 children performed in an inferior manner, relative to Group 1 and Group 2 children, on the trial in which they were required to utilize both hands simultaneously when solving the task.

In the current investigation with 7- and 8-year-old children, it was hypothesized that Group 3 children would perform in an inferior manner, relative to Group 1 and Group 2 children, on the psychomotor and tactile–perceptual variables.

MEASURES

The six motor, psychomotor, and tactile–perceptual measures used in this study were the same as or very similar to (i.e., younger children's versions) those employed in the Rourke and Strang (1978) investigation. These were as follows:

1. Finger-Tapping Test (Reitan & Davison, 1974), a simple motor task that requires the child to depress a lever with his/her index finger as many times as possible within a 10-second time period. The average number of taps in the best three of four trials was used as the dependent measure.
2. Strength of Grip Test (Reitan & Davison, 1974), a simple motor task that requires the child to squeeze the Smedley Hand Dyna-

mometer three times with each hand. The average pressure (measured in kilograms) that the child exerts was used as the dependent measure.

3. Maze Test (Kløve, 1963; Knights & Moule, 1968), in which the child is asked to move a stylus through a maze without touching the sides of the maze. The total amount of time during which the stylus contacts the side of the maze was recorded (in seconds) and used as the dependent measure.
4. Grooved Pegboard Test (Kløve, 1963; Knights & Moule, 1968), in which the child is asked to place keyhole-shaped pegs into similarly shaped holes as rapidly as possible. The dependent measure was the length of time (in seconds) required to complete the task.
5. Tactual Performance Test (TPT; Reitan & Davison, 1974), in which the child is blindfolded and then is asked to place blocks in their proper spaces on a formboard. The dependent measure was the length of time (in minutes) required to complete the task.
6. The total number of errors obtained on four tests for sensory-perceptual disturbances: Tactile Perception, Finger Agnosia, Fingertip Number-Writing Recognition, and Tactile Forms Recognition (Reitan & Davison, 1974).

Performances with the right hand and with the left hand were recorded separately for each of these measures. In addition, children's performances using both hands simultaneously were recorded on the TPT. Thus, a total of 13 scores were recorded for this set of variables.

RESULTS AND DISCUSSION

Means and standard deviations obtained by the three groups on the motor, psychomotor, and tactile–perceptual variables can be found in Table 6.2.

Two-factor analyses of variance with repeated measures on the second factor (i.e., right- and left-hand performance on all measures; right-, left-, and both-hand performance on the TPT) were conducted in order to analyze differences among and within groups. The patterns of group performance varied considerably across the six tests and the 13 test scores. However, on 11 of these 13 measures, the performance of Group 3 children was inferior to that of Group 2 children.

A one-way MANOVA for group across the six dependent variables was not statistically significant, $F(12,72) = 1.28$, $p < .25$. The ANOVA results for group effect on each of the measures also did not yield statistically significant results.

There was no significant overall group $\times$ hand interaction effect revealed with the MANOVA, $F(12,72) = 0.66$, $p < .77$, and the separate ANOVAs investigating this effect were also nonsignificant. However, the expected effect for hand was in evidence, $F(6,37) = 15.25$, $p < .0001$, indicating that children in each group performed better with their right hand than with their left hand. The only ANOVA that did not reveal a highly significant effect for hand was on the composite tactile–perceptual measure, where the subjects made as many errors with the right hand as with the left hand.

Previous studies examining subtype differences on these variables with older learning-disabled children have also reported that significant group differences were not found on measures of simple motor skills, such as finger tapping and grip strength (Rourke & Strang, 1978; Rourke & Telegdy, 1971). Furthermore, the studies with older children have not revealed statistically significant group $\times$ hand interaction effects, and the results of a recent factor-analytic study suggest that dominant/nondominant sensorimotor measures lack discriminant validity for the learning-disabled population (Francis, Fletcher, & Rourke, 1988).

The performance of younger learning-disabled children on both simple and complex motor measures had been investigated in an earlier study that involved three groups of learning-disabled children selected on the basis of WISC VIQ–PIQ discrepancies (Rourke et al., 1973). Although clear differences on complex motor measures had been found using this method of classification with older learning-disabled children (Rourke & Telegdy, 1971), the results for the younger children did not bear any resemblance to the distinct patterns found with groups of older learning-disabled children.

Results of the present study also did not reveal statistically significant group differences. The large degree of subject variability within each task, as indicated by the standard deviations for each group, served to reduce the differentiation between groups on the motor and psychomotor variables. However, the finding that Group 3 children performed in an inferior manner to Group 2 children on 11 of the 13 motor, psychomotor, and tactile–perceptual measures certainly suggests that further analysis of this trend is warranted.

Study 4: Concept-Formation Variables

Differences in concept formation between 9- to 14-year-old Group 2 and Group 3 children have been examined using the older children's version of the Halstead Category Test (Strang & Rourke, 1983). This test involves nonverbal abstract reasoning, hypothesis testing, and the ability to benefit from positive and negative informational feedback. Although no significant group differences were found on the first three subtests of this task, Group 2 children were found to perform in a superior manner to Group 3 children on the final three subtests; Group 2 also exhibited significantly fewer errors overall on this test.

It is important to recognize that the younger children's version of the Halstead Category Test is quite different from the form of the test employed with older children. Successful performance on the older children's version requires a systematic problem-solving approach and is considered to be a rather difficult and complex task. In contrast, the concepts involved in the younger children's version are concrete rather than abstract, and children can likely perform this task successfully by using matching skills or simple associations. It was expected that Group 3 children would experience difficulty, relative to Group 1 and Group 2 children, on this test.

MEASURES

The younger children's version of the Category Test consists of five subtests comprising 80 items. Test items are presented individually on a small screen, below which lies an answer panel consisting of red, blue, yellow, and green lights. The child is instructed to try to find the principle or idea that is presented in each subtest and that can be deduced from the information on the screen. A pleasant bell sounds after each correct response, and a harsh buzzer sounds after each incorrect response. The principles operating in the first four subtests are color, quantity, oddity, and color prominence, while the final subtest contains items already seen in earlier subtests. The scores for the test include the number of errors on each of the five subtests as well as a total error score.

RESULTS AND DISCUSSION

The means and standard deviations for the subtypes on these variables are presented in Table 6.2.

A one-way MANOVA for group across the five subtests and total error score of the Category Test did not yield a significant main effect for group, $F(10,74) = 1.65$, $p < .10$. However, one-way ANOVAs indicated significant group effects on subtest 4, $F(2,42) = 7.66$, $p < .001$, and on the total error score, $F(2,42) = 5.13$, $p < .01$.

Testing for simple effects with the Duncan Multiple-Range Test indicated that Group 3 performed in a significantly superior fashion to Groups 1 and 2 on subtest 4 and that the Group 3 performance was significantly superior to the performance of Group 1 children on the total error score. A summary of the MANOVA, ANOVA, and group mean comparison results is presented in Table 6.3.

Thus, the hypothesis that 7- and 8-year-old Group 3 children would experience relative difficulty on the Category Test was not supported, and the pattern of group performance was the opposite of that predicted. It is possible that the younger children's version of the Category Test taps quite different abilities than those assessed in the older children's version of this test. Whereas abstraction and reasoning skills may be necessary for successful performance on the older children's version, more basic matching skills may be the prerequisite for successful performance at young ages. In this connection it is important to note that all three groups of young learning-disabled children performed within age-appropriate limits on this test.

Study 5: Behavioral Variables

It has been hypothesized that the pattern of neuropsychological deficits seen in Group 3 children is likely to put them at risk for the development of socioemotional problems (Strang & Rourke, 1985; Rourke, 1988, 1989). A number of studies have already demonstrated that Group 3 children experience difficulties in the social realm. It has been found that children with nonverbal learning disabilities obtain significantly lower ratings on measures of peer popularity and social behavior than do children with verbal learning disabilities (Badian & Ghublikian, 1983; Wiener, 1980). We have also found group differences in a study comparing a language disorder group to a spatial disorder group on four exploratory measures of social sensitivity (Ozols & Rourke, 1985). A group of children with visual–spatial–organizational deficits was also found to obtain significantly elevated scores on the Psychopathology–Internalization factor of the Personality Inventory for Children (Strang, 1981). Finally, Stewart (1986) has reported that, in comparison to children with the Group 1 pattern, children with the Group 3 pattern of academic achievement exhibit significant elevations on the Maladaptive Behavior Scale of the Vineland Adaptive Behavior Scales (Sparrow, Balla, & Cicchetti, 1984).

The fifth study in this series was designed to investigate whether differences would be evident in the social behavior of young Group 1, Group 2, and Group 3 children. The Behavior Problem Checklist (BPC; Quay & Peterson, 1979) was used to address this question. The basic validity of this scale has been demonstrated (Lahey & Piacentini, 1985). It was hypothesized that Group 3 children would exhibit elevated scores on the BPC, indicating a larger number of problems.

MEASURES

Items of the BPC have been classified into three subscales: the Conduct Problem subscale, consisting of 17 items, the Personality Problem subscale, consisting of 14 items, and the Inadequacy–Immaturity subscale, consisting of eight items. A large number of parents had failed to respond to all items on the checklist. Therefore, each child's subscale score was converted to a centile score based on the number of items endorsed divided by the number of items answered. A subject's subscale or factor score was excluded from the group analyses if more than half of the items in the subscale were not answered.

RESULTS AND DISCUSSION

Means and standard deviations obtained by the three groups on these variables are contained in Table 6.2. The standard deviations evident for each group on the three factor scales of the BPC indicate a large degree of variability within each group.

A one-way MANOVA for group effect on the three factor scales did not yield significant group differences, $F(6,72) = 1.06$, $p < .39$. One-way ANOVAs computed on the Personality Problem factor, the Inadequacy–Immaturity factor, and the BPC total score also did not reach commonly accepted levels of statistical significance. Although the ANOVA for group effect on the Conduct Problem factor did not reach the .05 level of statistical significance, $F(2,39) = 2.64$, $p < .08$, testing for simple effects revealed that Group 3 differed significantly from Group 1 on this variable, with Group 3 children obtaining higher scores (reflecting more behavioral problems) on this factor.

Separate ANOVAs for males and females were conducted. In the all-male analyses, Group 3 children were found to have significantly higher scores on the BPC Conduct Problem subscale than did either the Group 1 or the Group 2 children. In addition, the BPC total score was significantly higher for Group 3 male children than for Group 1 male children. There were no significant group differences found in the all-female analyses. A summary of the MANOVA, ANOVA, and group mean comparison results is presented in Table 6.3.

These results provide some support for the hypothesis that Group 3 children will be described as having more social and behavior problems than their learning-disabled peers in Groups 1 and 2. Although a study involving older children with visual–spatial–organizational deficits found that their social behavior consisted primarily of withdrawal and depression (Strang, 1981), results from the present study suggest that younger children with the Group 3 pattern may be more likely to "act out" rather than withdraw. Items endorsed on the Conduct Problem factor scale indicate that these children exhibit attention-seeking, disruptive, restless, and noncompliant types of behavior. Insofar as Group 3 reflects a group of children with nonverbal learning disabilities (NLD), these different results are consistent with the NLD model proposed by Rourke (1989) as these apply to the hyperactivity/conduct-disorder dimension. In this model, it is proposed that the young NLD child is likely to be characterized as exhibiting some form of externalized psychopathology (e.g., hyperactivity, conduct disorder, acting out), whereas the developmental course for such youngsters is expected to involve a gradual lessening of hyperactivity and other forms of externalized psychopathology. In late childhood and early adolescence, such children typically exhibit internalized forms of psychopathology (characterized by excessive intrapsychic conflict, anxiety, social withdrawal and isolation, and depression). (See Casey & Rourke, Chapter 13, this volume, for additional data relating to this issue.)

A Note on Sex Differences

The sex of the children was not evenly distributed across the groups: the boy:girl ratio within Group 3 was approximately equal (7:8), whereas within Groups 1 and 2 the boy:girl ratio was significantly larger (11:4 and 13:2, respectively), as is typically the case for samples of learning-disabled children. An unequal sex distribution was also reported in the earlier studies with older children (Group 1, 13:2; Group 2, 15:0; Group 3, 11:4). However, the differences in ratios were of a lesser magnitude, and additional analyses did not reveal any sex differences among the groups of older learning-disabled children.

In the present study, t-test analyses for the complete sample revealed significant sex differences on two of the selection variables and on nine of the dependent variables. Separate t-tests and ANOVAs by group indicated that most of the overall differences could be attributed to the sex differences within Group 3. Sex differences on selection variables were found on the WISC FSIQ and the WRAT Reading subtest. Girls tended to perform more poorly than boys on WISC FSIQ, $t(13,30) = 3.14$, $p < .01$, although scores obtained by girls were superior to those obtained by boys on the WRAT Reading subtest, $t(13,30) = -2.21$, $p < .05$.

The performance of boys was superior to that of girls on six of the nine dependent variables on which sex differences were found: WISC VIQ, $t(13,30) = 2.05$, $p < .05$; WISC Picture Completion subtest, $t(13,30) = 2.08$, $p < .05$; WISC Picture Arrangement subtest, $t(13,30) = 2.29$, $p < .05$; Grip Strength, right hand, $t(13,30) = 3.49$, $p < .01$; Grip

Strength, left hand, $t(13,30) = 5.38$, $p < .01$; and Tactual Performance Test, both hands, $t(13,30) = -2.09$, $p < .05$. On only one of these variables (WISC VIQ) was a significant group effect found: Group 3 children were found to perform in a superior manner to Group 1 children. However, this significant Group effect was not the result of sex differences, as the girls, in general, performed more poorly than the boys on WISC VIQ, and Group 3 contained a larger number of girls.

The performance of girls was superior (i.e., fewer errors and fewer problems) to that of boys on three dependent variables: Category Test subtest 2, $t(13,30) = 2.77$, $p < .01$; BPC—Conduct Problem subscale, $t(12,29) = 2.57$, $p < .01$; and BPC—total score, $t(12,29) = 2.55$, $p < .01$. Although group differences were not found on subtest 2 of the Category Test, significant differences between groups were reported for the Conduct Problem subscale and the total score of the BPC. Thus, the difficulties reported for Group 3 children on the BPC may be more reflective of the functioning of the boys within that group.

Summary of Findings

The results of the five studies reported here constitute an attempt to extend the validity of one method of classification of learning-disabled children. This method, which groups children according to patterns of academic achievement, has been successful in demonstrating differences between groups of 9- to 14-year-old learning-disabled children. We were interested in seeing whether young (7- and 8-year-old) learning-disabled children would perform in a similar manner to the older children on the same or similar variables.

The following are the principal findings that emerge from this exercise:

1. Group 1 and Group 2 children consistently performed in an inferior manner to Group 3 children on auditory–linguistic variables.
2. Group 3 children performed in an inferior manner to Groups 1 and 2 on some of the visual–spatial–organizational variables.
3. Statistically significant group differences were not found on motor, psychomotor, and tactile–perceptual abilities, although Group 3 children performed in an inferior manner to Group 2 children on 11 of the 13 measures.
4. On the test of elementary concept formation, Group 3 children performed in a significantly superior manner to the other groups.

5. On the BPC, Group 3 children exhibited elevated scores (indicative of more problems) on the Conduct Problem subscale.

On auditory–linguistic and visual–perceptual measures, the younger groups of children performed in a manner that was highly similar to that exhibited by the older children studied by Rourke and Finlayson (1978). In order to illustrate these comparisons, the group means on the dependent variables employed in Studies 1 and 2 were converted to T-scores based on the sample data. The T-scores were adjusted so that good performance is represented in one direction (above 50) and poor performance is represented in the opposite direction (below 50). The mean group T-scores obtained on selected auditory–linguistic and visual–perceptual measures are presented in Figure 6.1 and are compared to the T-scores obtained on the same measures in the Rourke and Finlayson (1978) study. This visual comparison highlights the clear parallels in the patterns of performance exhibited by the two age groups on these measures.

Graphs constructed in an analogous manner for Study 3 (Figure 6.2) reveal that there were fewer similarities between the younger and older groups on the motor, psychomotor, and tactile–perceptual measures. In Figure 6.2, the mean group T-scores obtained on these measures in the present study are contrasted with those obtained in the Rourke and Strang (1978) study. Although few parallels can be drawn between the age groups, it is still clear that Group 2 performance in Study 3 is superior to the Group 3 performance on most of these measures, as was the case in Rourke and Strang (1978).

On the test of concept formation the younger learning-disabled children performed in a manner quite different from the older learning-disabled children. While Group 3 children were found to have difficulty (relative to Group 1 and Group 2 children) on the older children's version of this test (Strang & Rourke, 1983), younger Group 3 children performed in a superior manner to Group 1 and Group 2 children on several subtests of the younger children's version of this test. One interpretation of this finding is that the younger children's version of the Category Test is, in the main, a measure of linguistic rather than higher-order concept-formation skills. Further studies will be needed in order to test this hypothesis.

Finally, the finding that young Group 3 children obtained elevated scores on the BPC is consistent with the reports that Group 3 children have psychosocial difficulties (Rourke, 1988, 1989). Results of the current study suggest that young Group 3 children are more likely to exhibit "externalized" types of personality disorders. A sex difference was found on the Conduct Problem subscale, indicating that Group 3 boys tend to be seen as behavior problems more than Group 3 girls.

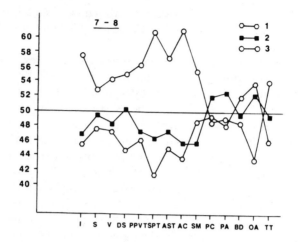

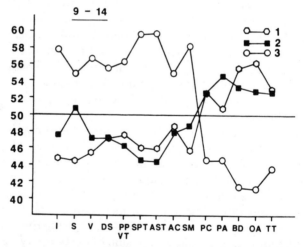

FIGURE 6.1. Mean *T*-scores obtained on selected auditory–linguistic and visual-perceptual measures for Groups 1, 2, and 3. Top = 7- to 8-year-olds; bottom = 9- to 14-year-olds. Abbreviations: I, Information; S, Similarities; V, Vocabulary; DS, Digit Span; PPVT, Peabody Picture Vocabulary Test; SPT, Speech-Sounds Perception Test; AST, Aphasia Screening Test; AC, Auditory Closure Test; SM, Sentence Memory Test; PC, Picture Completion; PA, Picture Arrangement; BD, Block Design; OA, Object Assembly; TT, Target Test.

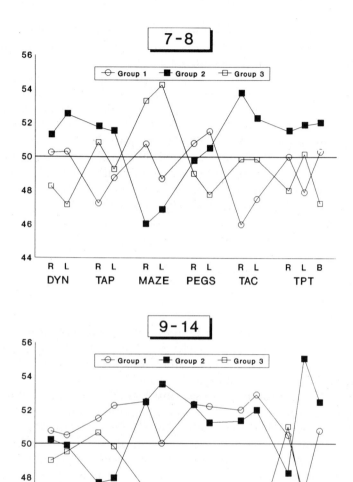

FIGURE 6.2. Mean *T*-scores for each age group on selected motor, psychomotor, and tactile–perceptual measures. Abbreviations: R, right hand; L, left hand; B, both hands; DYN, Strength of Grip Test; TAP, Finger-Tapping Test; MAZE, Maze Test; PEGS, Grooved Pegboard Test; TAC, tactile–perceptual composite measure; TPT, Tactual Performance Test.

The principal merits of this work relate to the developmental dimension that it suggests in the typology under consideration. It seems that classifying learning-disabled children according to their patterns of academic achievement will lead to somewhat different conclusions, depending on the age (developmental stage) of the child. For example, while young Group 3 children exhibit difficulties with visual–spatial and visual–perceptual skills, they do not perform poorly on tests of psychomotor development at these young ages, whereas older Group 3 children show deficits in visual–spatial–organizational skills and psychomotor skills. In contrast, Group 2 children seem to exhibit similar neuropsychological profiles at young ages (7 to 8 years) as they do at older ages (9 to 14 years). It is abundantly clear that most children with reading and spelling problems (Groups 1 and 2) also tend to have significant auditory–perceptual and linguistic processing deficiencies.

Future Directions

It will be important to cross-validate these results in other settings and with larger groups of children. Longitudinal studies designed to follow children with these patterns of academic achievement over time would be of considerable interest. Also, sex differences will need to be taken into consideration in future studies with Group 3 children.

The representativeness of these three specific subtypes to the learning-disabled population as a whole is an important issue. Several investigators have stressed the relevance of a large-scale epidemiological study of the learning-disabled population. The goal of such a study would be to present descriptive data regarding the prevalence of learning-disabled children that meet criteria for inclusion in various classifications. In addition to questions of incidence, both within the learning-disabled population and within the general population, we need to examine the neuropsychological profile of each subtype in relation to normative data. Similarities need to be studied and elucidated as carefully as we have studied the differences between these subtypes.

Finally, the important questions of the incidence and type of socioemotional problems in the learning-disabled population need to be studied in a systematic manner. The definition most commonly used to define a child as learning-disabled excludes those children with emotional disturbance. Thus, it has been difficult to obtain a comprehensive understanding of emotional problems seen in learning-disabled children. Future studies could be designed to focus on the larger group of children with "learning problems" and attempt to find measures and methods that can differentiate the "emotional problem" subgroup from the "learning disability" subgroup.

References

Badian, N. A. (1983). Dyscalculia and nonverbal disorders of learning. In H. R. Myklebust (Ed.), *Progress in learning disabilities* (Vol.. 5, pp. 235-264). New York: Grune & Stratton.

Badian, N., & Ghublikian, M. (1983). The personal-social characteristics of children with poor mathematical computation skills. *Journal of Learning Disabilities, 16*, 154-157.

Benton, A. L. (1965). *Sentence Memory Test.* Iowa City, IA: Author.

Dunn, L. M. (1965). *Expanded manual for the Peabody Picture Vocabulary Test.* Minneapolis: American Guidance Service.

Fletcher, J. M. (1983, April). *Verbal and spatial selective reminding in learning disability subtypes.* Paper presented at the meeting of the Society for Research in Child Development, Detroit, MI.

Fletcher, J. M. (1985). External validation of learning disability typologies. In B. P. Rourke (Ed.), *Neuropsychology of learning disabilities: Essentials of subtype analysis* (pp. 187-211). New York: Guilford Press.

Francis, D. J., Fletcher, J. M., & Rourke, B. P. (1988). Discriminant validity of lateral sensorimotor tests in children. *Journal of Clinical and Experimental Neuropsychology, 10*, 779-799.

Goodstein, H., & Kahn, H. (1974). Patterns of achievement among children with learning difficulties. *Exceptional Children, 41*, 47-49.

Jastak, J. F., & Jastak, S. R. (1965). *The Wide Range Achievement Test.* Wilmington, DE: Guidance Associates.

Kass, C. E. (1964). Auditory Closure Test. In J. J. Olson & J. L. Olson (Eds.), *Validity studies on the Illinois Test of Psycholinguistic Abilities.* Madison, WI: Photo Press.

Kløve, H. (1963). Clinical neuropsychology. In F. M. Forster (Ed.), *The medical clinics of North America* (pp. 1647-1658). New York: Saunders.

Knights, R. M., & Moule, A. D. (1968). Normative data on the Motor Steadiness Battery for Children. *Perceptual and Motor Skills, 26*, 643-650.

Knights, R. M., & Norwood, J. A. (1980). *Revised smoothed normative data on the neuropsychological test battery for children.* Unpublished manuscript, Carleton University, Ottawa, Ontario.

Lahey, B. B., & Piacentini, J. C. (1985). An evaluation of the Quay-Peterson Revised Behavior Problem Checklist. *Journal of School Psychology, 23*, 285-289.

Nolan, D. R., Hammeke, T. A., & Barkley, R. A. (1983). A comparison of the patterns of the neuropsychological performance in two groups of learning disabled children. *Journal of Clinical Child Psychology, 12*, 22-27.

Ozols, E. J., & Rourke, B. P. (1985). Dimensions of social sensitivity in two types of learning disabled children. In B. P. Rourke (Ed.), *Neuropsychology of learning disabilities: Essentials of subtype analysis* (pp. 281-301). New York: Guilford Press.

Ozols, E. J., & Rourke, B. P. (1988). Characteristics of young learning disabled children classified according to patterns of academic achievement: Auditory-perceptual and visual-perceptual abilities. *Journal of Clinical Child Psychology, 17*, 44-52.

Quay, H. D., & Peterson, D. R. (1979). *Manual for the behavior problem checklist.* Available from author.

Reed, J. C. (1967). Reading achievement as related to differences between WISC Verbal and Performance IQs. *Child Development, 38,* 835–840.

Reitan, R. M. (1984). *Aphasia and sensory-perceptual deficits in children.* Tucson, AZ: Neuropsychology Press.

Reitan, R. M., & Davison, L. A. (Eds.). (1974). *Clinical neuropsychology: Current status and applications.* New York: John Wiley & Sons.

Rourke, B. P. (1981). Neuropsychological assessment of children with learning disabilities. In S. B. Filskov & T. J. Boll (Eds.), *Handbook of clinical neuropsychology* (pp. 453–478). New York: Wiley-Interscience.

Rourke, B. P. (1983). Reading and spelling disabilities: A developmental neuropsychological perspective. In U. Kirk (Ed.), *Neuropsychology of language, reading and spelling* (pp. 209–234). New York: Academic Press.

Rourke, B. P. (1988). Socioemotional disturbances of learning disabled children. *Journal of Consulting and Clinical Psychology, 56,* 801–810.

Rourke, B. P. (1989). *Nonverbal learning disabilities: The syndrome and the model.* New York: Guilford Press.

Rourke, B. P., Dietrich, D. M., & Young, G. C. (1973). Significance of WISC Verbal-Performance discrepancies for younger children with learning disabilities. *Perceptual and Motor Skills, 36,* 275–282.

Rourke, B. P., & Finlayson, M. A. J. (1978). Neuropsychological significance of variations in patterns of academic performance: Verbal and visual–spatial abilities. *Journal of Abnormal Child Psychology, 6,* 121–133.

Rourke, B. P., Fisk, J. L., & Strang, J. D. (1986). *Neuropsychological assessment of children: A treatment-oriented approach.* New York: Guilford Press.

Rourke, B. P., & Strang, J. D. (1978). Neuropsychological significance of variations in patterns of academic performance: Motor, psychomotor, and tactile–perceptual abilities. *Journal of Pediatric Psychology, 3,* 62–66.

Rourke, B. P., & Telegdy, G. A. (1971). Lateralizing significance of WISC Verbal-Performance discrepancies for older children with learning disabilities. *Perceptual and Motor Skills, 33,* 875–883.

Rourke, B. P., Young, G. C., & Flewelling, R. W. (1971). The relationships between WISC Verbal-Performance discrepancies and selected verbal, auditory–perceptual, visual–perceptual, and problem-solving abilities in children with learning disabilities. *Journal of Clinical Psychology, 27,* 475–479.

Satz, P., & Morris, R. (1981). Learning disability subtypes: A review. In F. J. Pirozzolo & M. C. Wittrock (Eds.), *Neuropsychological and cognitive processes in reading* (pp. 109–141). New York: Academic Press.

Siegel, L. S., & Linder, A. (1984). Short-term memory processes in children with reading and arithmetic disabilities. *Developmental Psychology, 20,* 200–207.

Sparrow, S. S., Balla, D. A., & Cicchetti, D. B. (1984). *The Vineland Adaptive Behavior Scales: A revision of the Vineland Social Maturity Scale by Edgar A. Doll.* Circle Pines, MN: American Guidance Services.

Stewart, M. L. (1986). *The adaptive behavior characteristics of learning disabled children classified by patterns of academic achievement.* Unpublished master's thesis, University of Windsor.

Strang, J. D. (1981). *Personality dimensions of learning disabled children: Age and subtype differences.* Unpublished doctoral dissertation, University of Windsor.

Strang, J. D., & Rourke, B. P. (1983). Concept-formation/non-verbal reasoning abilities of children who exhibit specific academic problems with arithmetic. *Journal of Clinical Child Psychology, 12,* 33–39.

Strang, J. D., & Rourke, B. P. (1985). Adaptive behavior of children who exhibit specific arithmetic disabilities and associated neuropsychological abilities and deficits. In B. P. Rourke (Ed.), *Neuropsychology of learning disabilities: Essentials of subtype analysis* (pp. 302–328). New York: Guilford Press.

Wechsler, D. (1949). *Manual for the Wechsler Intelligence Scale for Children*. New York: Psychological Corporation.

Wiener, J. R. (1980). A theoretical model of the acquisition of peer relationships of learning disabled children. *Journal of Learning Disabilities, 13*, 506–511.

Winer, B. J. (1962). *Statistical principles in experimental design*. New York: McGraw-Hill.

CHAPTER 7

Biopsychological Validation of L- and P-Type Dyslexia

Dirk J. Bakker, Robert Licht, and Jan van Strien

Evidence is accumulating that dyslexia encompasses a heterogeneous group of reading problems that are differentially tied with the brain and that require different therapeutic interventions (Hooper & Willis, 1989; Bakker & van der Vlugt, 1989). The heterogeneity of factors related to dyslexia is documented by the outcomes of taxonomic research (Rourke, 1985). That the cerebral correlates of dyslexia may vary is suggested by the neuroanatomic findings of Rosen, Sherman, and Galaburda (1986) and is discussed by both Kinsbourne (1989) and Morris (1989).

We have developed a neuropsychological model that accounts for two types of dyslexia, an L and P type (Bakker, 1990). Before discussing the validity of this classification, it is necessary to touch on the etiology of L and P dyslexia.

Etiology of L- and P-Type Dyslexia

Reading concerns the left and right cerebral hemispheres in a balanced fashion. Whether the balance dips more to the left or to the right depends on the phase of the learning-to-read process. Neuropsychological and electrophysiological evidence is available to show that initial and advanced reading are predominantly mediated by the right and left hemisphere, respectively (Fletcher & Satz, 1980; Silverberg, Gordon, Pollack, & Bentin, 1980; Licht, Bakker, Kok, & Bouma, 1988).

The predominance of right hemispheric participation in initial reading has been argued to result from the requirements of perceptual feature analysis (Bakker, 1979). The novice reader is faced with new shapes (letters and clusters of letters) that have no correlates in daily life in that these letter shapes fail to show shape constancy. Constancy refers to the property of objects and shapes in keeping their meaning irrespective of their position in space. Thus, a chair is called a chair, and it does not matter whether the chair is shown in an upright or upside-down position. But, turning around and/or mirroring the letter "b" makes it a "d," "p," or "q." On the other hand, "b," "B," and "*B*" do have the same meaning, although they are different in shape. Whether one gets "amen," "name," "mean," or "mane" is dependent on the left–right arrangement of the constituent letters. But "amen" is the same as "AMEN," is the same as "Amen," and is even the same as "aMEN." The same principles hold for sentences: depending on the spatial arrangement of "home," "at," "he," and "is," one reads "he is at home," "is he at home," "at home he is." Thus, the novice reader is faced with quite a number of visuospatial demands; this is thought to induce predominantly right hemispheric involvement in early reading.

Visuoperceptual analyses become automatisms and sink below the level of consciousness during advanced stages of the learning-to-read process (Fries, 1963). Advanced readers, in order to be able to read fluently, use semantic and syntactic strategies, predominantly generated by the left hemisphere. Thus, the balance of hemispheric participation in reading swings to the left during advanced reading, after having dipped to the right during initial reading.

Some children, for whatever reason, may not be able to make this shift. They continue to rely primarily on right hemispheric reading strategies; this induces an oversensitivity to the perceptual features of text. These P-type dyslexics read relatively slowly, in a fragmented fashion, albeit rather accurately. Some other children may begin the learning-to-read process wrongly, that is, by premature reliance on the left hemisphere, as reflected in efforts to generate semantic and syntactic strategies. These L-type dyslexics read in a hurried fashion and produce many substantive errors.

The classifications of L- and P-type dyslexia are based on the distinction of fast/inaccurate reading (L types) versus slow/fragmented reading (P types). A number of studies on the validity of the L/P classification have been conducted in an effort to show that L and P dyslexics differ with regard to (1) electrophysiological parameters, (2) cognitive performance, (3) cognitive performance of their biological parents, and (4) responses to the same treatment. Some of these studies have yielded clues regarding the mechanisms that underlie the L and P strategies of reading.

Electrophysiological Parameters

Early Studies

L and P dyslexia presumably correlate with the predominant generation of left and right hemispheric reading strategies, respectively. As a consequence, L and P dyslexics should show differential hemispheric activity during reading. Figure 7.1 shows word-elicited potentials at left (T3) and right (T4) temporal locations by L and P types of dyslexia (the words to read were flashed in the central visual field). Analyses of variance revealed L dyslexics to show larger N1 (N1b) amplitudes in the left than in the right temporal area, and P dyslexics to show the reverse pattern ($p < .01$; Bakker & Licht, 1986).

Frequency analyses revealed the N2 latencies to be relatively larger on the right than on the left parietal side in 77% of the P dyslexics and in 37% of the L dyslexics ($p < .005$; Bakker, 1986). Figure 7.1 indicates that the N1 complex shows two peaks rather than one. More L dyslexics showed single rather than double parietal N1 peaks, whereas more P dyslexics showed double rather than single parietal N1 peaks ($p < .05$, two-tailed; Linstra, 1983).

In conclusion, the results indicate that L and P dyslexics differ with regard to the lateral distribution of certain brain responses to flashed words.

A New Study

Stimulation of the right hemisphere in L dyslexics through the flashing of words in the left visual field has been shown to result in slower and more accurate reading (Bakker, Moerland, & Goekoop-Hoefkens, 1981; Bakker & Vinke, 1985). A concomitant change in hemispheric asymmetry of a positive event-related potential (ERP) component around 240 msec (P240) was also found. These results may indicate that the treatment caused better right hemispheric processing of words in L-type dyslexics. Such an effect may either be the result of increased efficiency in information processing of word features or of changes in the lateral distribution of attentional mechanisms. Kinsbourne (1975) has argued that the presentation of stimuli in a visual field activates the contralateral hemisphere, resulting in enhanced processing capacity of that hemisphere and an attentional bias to stimuli presented in that field.

In the current study, we sought to find out whether the treatment effects that had been found previously are associated with differences between L- and P-type children in attending to spatial locations and in

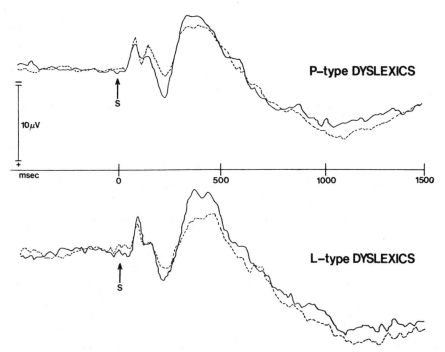

FIGURE 7.1. Visual evoked responses elicited by words presented in the central visual field of P- and L-type dyslexics. ———— T3; ------- T4. From Bakker and Licht (1986). Copyright 1986 by John Wiley & Sons, Ltd. Reprinted by permission.

selective processing of target stimuli presented at these locations. To investigate these attentional processes, a selective attention task was presented to P- and L-type dyslexics and normal control children while electrophysiological responses (ERPs) were recorded simultaneously over the left and right hemispheres. Attending to a particular spatial location has been associated with increased amplitudes of early negative peaks in the ERP waveform (100–150 msec) over the contralateral hemisphere, whereas the processing of targets that are embedded in series of background stimuli is characterized by a large positive wave over parietal areas (P3, P300, or P3b). For backgrounds, this positive wave generally is absent or small.

It was predicted that if dyslexic children have problems in attending to spatial locations and in selecting targets, this would be reflected in reduced amplitude effects for early negative and late positive ERP components, respectively.

A group of 16 L-type and 20 P-type children (selected on the basis of reading errors and lagging 1.5 years or more on reading achievement) and 20 normal readers, all children aged 9 to 12 years, participated in the experiment. A selective attention task was administered that required the children to respond (push-button) only to target letter stimuli presented at a relevant location that had to be attended and to neglect all other stimuli. The locations to be attended were the left and right visual fields (blockwise). Target stimuli were presented on 33% of the trials and were, as the backgrounds, evenly distributed over the fields. Stimulus duration was 100 msec, and the visual angle was 4.5°. Eye fixation was controlled by recording horizontal and vertical EOG. Children were instructed to fixate on a central cross, and stimuli were only presented if the eyes were within an area less than 1° from the fixation point.

ERPs were recorded from the left and right frontal (F3, F4), central (C3, C4), temporal (T3, T4), parietal (P3, P4), posterior temporal (T5, T6), and occipital (O1, O2) locations during 1,500 msec starting 250 msec prior to stimulus presentation and were referenced against linked earlobes.

The reaction times to attended targets were found to be slower (around 100 msec) in L and P dyslexics than in normal readers (Table 7.1). No differences between the left and right visual fields were found, neither in dyslexic nor in normal readers. L-type children tended to make more omission errors than did P-type and control children.

The ERP waveform, averaged across groups, was characterized by a large positive wave that was maximal over parietooccipital areas and that peaked around 500 msec (P500). Comparable late positive waves in children have also been reported by Courchesne (1983) and by Friedman, Sutton, Putnam, Brown, and Erlenmeyer-Kimling (1988). Analyses of attend–unattend difference amplitudes revealed an increase in early negativity (10–200 msec) at parietal locations contralateral to the attended field. Although no group differences were found in hemispheric distribution of this negativity, an interesting finding was that L-type children showed larger negativity over frontal sites and that P-types showed more

TABLE 7.1. Mean Response Times for Targets and Percentage of Omissions and False Positives in the Left and Right Visual Fields as a Function of Group

	P type			L type			Normal		
	RT	OM	FP	RT	OM	FP	RT	OM	FP
Left	689	3.0	0.6	693	4.7	1.0	595	0.7	0.7
Right	681	2.0	0.7	679	4.3	1.0	585	1.8	0.5

Note. RT, response time (msec); OM, omissions (%); FP, false positives (%).

positivity at occipital locations (Figure 7.2). Tentatively, these findings may indicate that P-type children have more posterior (visuoperceptual) control of orienting to spatial cues than do L-type children.

For both L-type and P-type children as well as for normal readers increased P500 positivity was found for attended targets, suggesting that the dyslexic children are capable of selecting and processing of target stimuli. Interestingly, the hemispheric involvement in this stage of processing seems to be different for the L- and P-type children compared with the normal readers. Normal children showed more attention-related positivity over the left hemisphere, whereas L-type children tended to show similar effects over the right hemisphere. P-type children showed more positivity over the hemisphere contralateral to the field of presentation (Figure 7.2). Future analyses have to reveal the functional significance of these group-specific hemispheric asymmetry patterns.

Cognitive Performance

Study 1

It has been argued that words can be read along an indirect or a direct route (Barron, 1986; Reitsma, 1983). The indirect or phonological route provides for the identification of words through the stepwise translation of graphemes into phonemes. This word-reading strategy is expected to be found in the majority of beginning readers. Through the direct or lexical route, words can be identified directly on the basis of word-specific features that are stored in word memory (lexicon). This route is expected to be used by fluent readers when reading familiar words.

As has already been described, L- and P-type dyslexic children are classified on the basis of reading speed and type of errors made. P-type dyslexics are slow readers who make relatively many fragmentation errors, whereas L-type dyslexics read hastily and inaccurately. Similar types of reading disability have also been proposed by Van der Leij (1983), who labeled them "spellers" and "guessers," respectively. Van der Leij assumes that "guessers" prefer a direct word-recognition strategy but that they have to guess at word meaning because of insufficient processing of the visuoperceptual features of words. In contrast, "spellers" keep relying on the slower, stepwise (grapheme-to-phoneme) translation strategy in reading. In view of their hurried and inaccurate style of reading, it is likely that L-type dyslexics may be considered "guessers" and P-type dyslexics "spellers." If this assumption is valid, one might expect L- and P-type children to differ on tasks measuring strategies of word recognition. To investigate this prediction, different reading and reading-related

130 / *Content Areas*

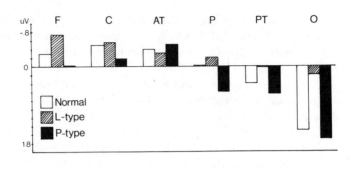

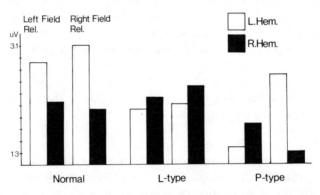

FIGURE 7.2. Attend–unattend difference amplitudes in the 110–200 msec period as a function of group and electrode location (upper panel) and in the 400–600 msec period (P500) as a function of group, field, and hemisphere (lower panel). F, frontal; C, central; AT, anterior–temporal; P, parietal; PT, posterior–temporal; O, occipital.

tasks were administered to a group of 29 P-type and 28 L-type dyslexic children who were 8.5 to 12 years old. The results of four tasks are discussed.

The first task was the Revised Underlining Test (UNDERL), which taps accuracy in that targets have to be picked out from a series of background letters or shapes (Rourke & Petrauskas, 1977). The second task (JOUK) was composed of three simple texts that had to be read under different conditions: a standard condition (STAND), an auditory-noise condition (AUD), and a visual-noise condition (VIS). The auditory noise was meant to interfere with a phonological reading strategy, and the visual noise was designed to disrupt direct visual recognition strategies. The third task (WDT) required the child to read regular (REG), irregular (IRREG), and pseudowords (PSEUD) (van Aarle & Volleberg, 1986). It is assumed that irregular words are identified better with a lexical strategy and pseudowords better if a phonological route is used. The fourth task was the Stroop interference task (STROOP). This task requires the child to read color names (A), to name colors (B), and to name the color in which color names are printed (C). It is expected that children with fast, direct word recognition strategies will experience the most interference in the last condition.

It was found (Figure 7.3) that (1) L-type dyslexics were better than P-type dyslexics in underlining normal and nonsense words; (2) L-type dyslexics were faster than P-type dyslexics in reading on the JOUK tasks. When auditory noise was presented, only P-types slowed down (11%), whereas in the visual-noise condition both P- and L-type dyslexics decreased in reading speed (26% and 24%, respectively); (3) L dyslexics made the most errors in reading pseudowords, whereas P dyslexics had most difficulty reading irregular words; and (4) L-type dyslexics were slower than P-type dyslexics in naming the color of printed words in the STROOP interference condition. However, they were faster than P types in reading color names (see also Licht, 1989, and Licht & van der Meer, 1989).

The present results suggest several differences between P- and L-type dyslexic children regarding the way in which they recognize words. L types seem to have fewer reading problems than P types: on almost all reading tasks, L types are faster readers than P types. This finding suggests that the two reading disability subtypes differ quantitatively rather than qualitatively in reading performance. However, there are several findings in support of the inference that L dyslexics rely on a direct word recognition strategy and that P dyslexics, in contrast, prefer an indirect word recognition strategy. L-type dyslexics showed strong interference in the STROOP task in that word meaning, while generated almost automatically, interferes with the learning of the color of print. L-type children also made fewer errors reading irregular words than in reading pseudowords, which require an indirect approach. In addition, these children slowed down reading in the perceptual-load (VIS) condition of the JOUK task. In contrast, P-type children had less interference in the STROOP task, had more difficulty with irregular than with pseudowords, and showed a decrease in reading speed in the auditory-noise (AUD) condition of the JOUK task.

If our interpretation of the differences between L- and P-type dyslexic children in terms of word recognition strategies is valid, then the results may indeed indicate (1) that L-type dyslexics show inadequate perceptual processing of words, leading to the guessing of word meaning, and (2) that P-type dyslexics show difficulty in storing and retrieving word-specific knowledge required to speed up reading. P dyslexics, as a consequence, have to rely on a stepwise reading strategy (Reitsma, 1983).

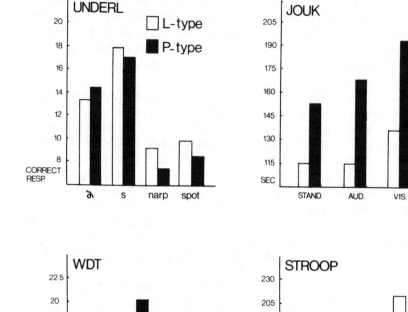

FIGURE 7.3. The average number of correct responses on the four subtests of the Underlining Test, the mean reading times in the JOUK and STROOP conditions, and the average number of errors for regular and irregular and pseudowords in the WDT for P- and L-type dyslexic children.

Study 2

A second study that was conducted concerning cognitive performance further validates the L and P typology (van Strien, Bakker, Bouma, & Koops, 1988). L-dyslexic, P-dyslexic, and normal-reading boys were tested in two sessions. In the first session, each subject completed a series of cognitive tasks. In the second session, each subject received a verbal dichotic listening task, a tachistoscopic bilateral word-reading task, and a lexical-decision task. All subjects were right-handed and had normal IQ scores (>90). Dyslexics had reading scores at least 1.5 years below their age-expectancy level. Control subjects were matched for age (mean age of entire sample, 10 years; range, 8–13 years).

A multivariate analysis of variance on the scores of the *cognitive tasks* revealed that both L and P dyslexics performed more poorly than did normal readers on verbal tasks such as Verbal Fluency, Digit Span, and Verbal Learning. With regard to nonverbal tasks, it was found that (1) dyslexics and normal readers performed equally well on Incomplete Pictures, (2) both L and P dyslexics performed worse than normal readers on Block Design and Corsi Block Tapping, and (3) L dyslexics displayed a poorer performance than both P dyslexics and normal readers on Figure Rotation. In sum, both L and P dyslexics gave evidence of a cognitive impairment on a range of tasks. Interestingly, P dyslexics and L dyslexics performed differently on the figure-rotation task, with L dyslexics showing substantial impairment. This task, in which the subject has to decide whether rotated figures are identical to a given target figure or whether they are a mirror image of it, closely resembles the problem a novice reader is faced with—the discrimination between letter shapes (e.g., "d" and "b"). The figure-rotation results thus support the hypothesis that L dyslexics have specific difficulties with the processing of visuospatial text features.

The results on the *verbal dichotic listening task* (four digit pairs per trial; free recall) revealed (1) the dyslexics to show poorer overall performance than the normal readers and (2) a significant right-ear advantage for all subjects. The lower overall performance of both L and P dyslexics on this task may indicate that these subjects have limited memory capacity. The right-ear advantage in P dyslexics suggests that the inferred overinvolvement of their right hemisphere in the process of learning to read is not reflected in auditory asymmetry.

The *bilateral word-reading task* required the subject to read familiar three-letter or four-letter words that were flashed bilaterally for 160 msec. Across visual fields, L dyslexics (mean correct = 41%) and P dyslexics (31%) recognized significantly fewer words correctly than did normal readers (64%). This result indicates that dyslexics, the slow-reading P dyslexics in particular, had great difficulty recognizing the briefly exposed words. In none of the groups was a visual field preference observed.

The *lexical decision task* required the subject to decide whether a word was a real word or a pseudoword. The length of these words varied: half of the presentations concerned three-letter words and half four-letter words. A significant main effect was found for group, and significant interactions were found for group by word length and for group by type of word (normal/pseudo). Normal readers displayed much faster RTs ($M = 1,090$ msec) than did L dyslexics ($M = 1,877$ msec) and P dyslexics ($M = 2,257$ msec). The effect of word length was largest for the group of P dyslexics, with the four-letter words resulting in a 215-msec-longer mean RT than for 3-letter words. For L dyslexics, this difference was 135 msec, and for normal readers it was 30 msec. The fact that P dyslexics displayed the largest effect of word length can be explained by their slow, "spelling" way of reading. The effect of type of word was also largest in the group of P dyslexics. It took them 660 msec longer to give the right response in the case of a pseudoword than in the case of a correct word. For L dyslexics, the difference between pseudo- and correct words was 455 msec, and for normal readers it was 154 msec. This result indicates a linguistic deficit in dyslexics, which is most pronounced in P dyslexics. It may be that P dyslexics (and to a lesser extent L dyslexics) have diminished/decreased access to their lexicon. A common-sense explanation could be that (P) dyslexics are afraid of misreading the word and, in the case of a pseudoword, perform addtional checks before giving the response.

Cognitive Performance of Biological Parents

Evidence for familial components in the etiology of dyslexia has been obtained from both genetic and familial studies (Childs & Finucci, 1983). As the influence of familial antecedents on reading disabilities has been demonstrated, the question arises whether L- and P-type dyslexias show differential familial antecedents. To examine this problem, the biological parents of L and P dyslexic and normal-reading boys were invited to participate in a study concerning cognitive performance. All boys and their parents received a number of tests that were supposed to assess primarily either left or right hemispheric functions. Principal component analyses, for boys and parents separately, indicated that Verbal Fluency, Digit Span, Verbal Learning, and Corsi Block Tapping loaded highly on a Verbal Memory factor and that Incomplete Pictures and Block Design loaded highly on a Visuospatial factor. Figure Rotation, which loaded highly on the Visuospatial factor in boys, yielded a distinct third factor only for the parents. Because of this inconsistent PCA result, Figure Rotation was excluded from the analyses of parent–child resemblances. For all subjects, two composite measures were calculated: (1) a composite measure for the Verbal/Memory factor (by averaging the z-transformed test scores of Verbal Fluency, Digit Span, Verbal Learning, and Corsi Block Tapping) and (2) a composite measure for the Visuospatial factor (by averaging the z-transformed test scores of Incomplete Pictures and Block Design).

Parent-child resemblance for cognitive performances can be expressed as the regression of the child score on midparental value (Plomin, DeFries, & McClearn, 1980). The midparental value is the average of the scores of both parents on a particular test. It should be stressed that this index is a measure of familiality rather than a measure of heritability, since genetic influences and influences of the family environment cannot be dissected (this index is called *the upper limit* of heritability). In addition to the regressions of child on midparent, direct father-son and mother-son effects were determined by means of path analysis (see van Strien, Bakker, Bouma, & Koops, in press, for details). The direct father-son and mother-son effects are estimates of the upper limit of *half* of the heritability. The regressions of child on midparent and the direct single-parent-child effects for each group and composite measures are displayed in Table 7.2.

From Table 7.2 it can be seen that, for both composite measures, the regressions of child on midparent were rather low in families of normal-reading boys and rather high in families of L dyslexics. In families of P dyslexics, a low regression for the Verbal/Memory factor and a high regression for the Visuospatial factor was found. The direct single-parent-child effects indicate that, in families of L dyslexics, the familial resemblance for the Verbal/Memory factor, as well as for the Visuospatial factor, is attributable to both a father-son and a mother-son effect. In families of P dyslexics, the familial resemblance for the Visuospatial factor is mainly attributable to the father-son effect.

In conclusion, we found evidence for differential familial resemblances among families of the three types of children, with a high father-son effect for visuospatial abilities (in the absence of a mother-son effect)

TABLE 7.2. Regressions of Child on Midparent and Single-Parent-Child Estimates

	L families	P families	C families
Verbal/Memory			
Midparent-child	.61	.18	.22
Father-son	.37	.07	.04
Mother-son	.27	.13	.16
Visuospatial			
Midparent-child	.66	.69	.24
Father-son	.28	.56	.21
Mother-son	.26	.04	.05

Note. L, L dyslexics; P, P dyslexics; C, normal readers.

in families of P dyslexics and with moderate single-parent–child effects for both the Verbal/Memory factor and the Visuospatial factor in families of L dyslexics.

Dyslexia Type × Treatment Interaction

A different response of L and P dyslexics to the same treatment would validate the L/P classification. In one of our studies (Bakker & Vinke, 1985), L and P dyslexics received different experimental treatments, but one of the control treatments was the same for both groups in that the children of these groups stayed in their (special) classroom at the time when the other children were receiving experimental treatment. Prior to and following a treatment period of 8 months (one session/week), visual evoked responses (VER) to centrally flashed words were recorded at left and right hemispheric locations, and between-hemispheric VER differences (BHD) were established. During the 8-month period, the P250 component of these BHDs appeared to have changed differently in the L and P dyslexics who had received the same control treatment. Parietal electrophysiological activity had "leftened" (i.e., had increased at left hemispheric relative to right hemispheric locations) in L dyslexics and had "rightened" in P dyslexics. Thus, the lateral distribution of physiological responses to flashed words showed an opposite development in L and P dyslexics who had received the same (control) treatment.

In another study (Bakker, van Leeuwen, & Spyer, 1987), an L- and a P-type dyslexic child received the same drug (piracetam) treatment. In accordance with the predictions, this treatment was found to affect the reading performance of the P dyslexic but not the reading performance of the L dyslexic. Performance on a maze-learning control task was not affected in either the L or the P dyslexic. This dyslexia type × treatment interaction is presently being investigated in a group experiment.

Summary and Conclusions

The L/P typology of dyslexia is based in an etiological model of learning to read. The external validity of the L/P classification has been investigated with both physiological and psychological variables. The lateral distribution of brain responses evoked by words to be read was found to be different in L and P dyslexics in that either the morphology, amplitudes, or latencies of the negative VER components showed dissimilar right–left differences in these groups. The lateral distribution of another VER component (P250) appeared to develop differently in L and P

dyslexics. To date, little evidence is available that these electrophysiological differences between dyslexia types are related to hemisphere-specific
attentional processing. However, the research in this domain has only
recently begun, so that the prediction that attentional mechanisms are
associated with the L/P classification awaits verification or falsification.
A number of cognitive and neuropsychological variables appeared to
discriminate between L- and P-type dyslexic children, whereas significant
associations were found between P-type boys' and P-type fathers' visuospatial performance as well as between L-type boys' and L-type fathers'
verbal-memory performance. The various findings regarding the type-
differentiating cognitive tasks may indicate that L-type dyslexics predominantly use direct, lexical routes when they read and that P-type
dyslexics use predominantly indirect, phonological routes. The use of a
direct or indirect route would be compatible with the fast/inaccurate
reading style of L dyslexics and with the slow/accurate reading style of P
dyslexics.

Acknowledgment

The authors would like to thank Ginny Spyer, M.A., for reviewing and processing the manuscript.

References

Bakker, D. J. (1979). Hemispheric differences and reading strategies: Two dyslexias?
    Bulletin of the Orton Society, 29, 84–100.
Bakker, D. J. (1986). Electrophysiological validation of L- and P-type dyslexia. *Journal of
    Clinical and Experimental Neuropsychology, 8,* 133.
Bakker, D. J. (1990). *Neuropsychological treatment of dyslexia.* New York: Oxford Univer-
    sity Press.
Bakker, D. J., & Licht, R. (1986). Learning to read: Changing horses in mid-stream. In G. T.
    Pavlidis & D. F. Fisher (Eds.), *Dyslexia: Neuropsychology and treatment* (pp. 87–95).
    London: John Wiley & Sons.
Bakker, D. J., Moerland, R., & Goekoop-Hoefkens, M. (1981). Effects of hemisphere-specific
    stimulation on the reading performance of dyslexic boys: A pilot study. *Journal of
    Clinical Neuropsychology, 3,* 155–159.
Bakker, D. J., & van der Vlugt, H. (Eds.). (1989). *Learning disabilities, Vol. 1: Neuropsycho-
    logical correlates and treatment.* Lisse, Netherlands: Swets and Zeitlinger.
Bakker, D. J., van Leeuwen, H. M. P., & Spyer, G. (1987). Neuropsychological aspects of
    dyslexia. In D. J. Bakker, C. Wilsher, H. Debruyne, & N. Bertin (Eds.), *Developmental
    dyslexia and learning disorders* (pp. 30–39). Basel: S. Karger.
Bakker, D. J., & Vinke, J. (1985). Effects of hemisphere-specific stimulation on brain activity
    and reading in dyslexics. *Journal of Clinical and Experimental Neuropsychology, 7,*
    505–525.

Barron, R. W. (1986). Word recognition in early reading: A review of the direct and indirect access hypotheses. *Cognition, 24,* 93–119.

Childs, B., & Finucci, J. M. (1983). Genetics, epidemiology, and specific reading disability. In M. Rutter (Ed.), *Developmental neuropsychiatry* (pp. 507–519). New York: Guilford Press.

Courchesne, E. (1983). Cognitive components of the ERP: Changes associated with development. In A. W. K. Gaillard & W. Ritter (Eds.), *Tutorials in ERP research: Endogenous components* (pp. 329–344). Amsterdam: North-Holland Publishing Company.

Fletcher, J. M., & Satz, P. (1980). Developmental changes in the neuropsychological correlates of reading achievement: A six year longitudinal follow up. *Journal of Clinical Neuropsychology, 2,* 23–37.

Friedman, D., Sutton, S., Putman, L., Brown, C., & Erlenmeyer-Kimling, L. (1988). ERP components in picture matching in children and adults. *Psychophysiology, 25,* 570–590.

Fries, C. C. (1963). *Linguistics and reading.* New York: Holt, Rinehart and Winston.

Hooper, S. R., & Willis, W. G. (1989). *Learning disability subtyping.* New York: Springer.

Kinsbourne, M. (1975). The mechanism of hemispheric cotnrol of the lateral gradient of attention. In P. M. A. Rabbitt & S. Dornic (Eds.), *Attention and performance V* (pp. 81–97). New York: Academic Press.

Kinsbourne, M. (1989). Neuroanatomy of dyslexia. In D. J. Bakker & H. van der Vlugt (Eds.), *Learning disabilities, Vol. 1: Neuropsychological correlates and treatment* (pp. 105–122). Lisse, Netherlands: Swets and Zeitlinger.

Licht, R. (1989). Reading disability subtypes: Cognitive and electrophysiological differences. In D. J. Bakker & H. van der Vlugt (Eds.), *Learning disabilities, Vol 1: Neuropsychological correlates and treatment* (pp. 81–103). Lisse, Netherlands: Swets and Zeitlinger.

Licht, R., Bakker, D. J., Kok, A., & Bouma, A. (1988). The development of lateral event-related potentials (ERPs) related to word naming: A four year longitudinal study. *Neuropsychologia, 26,* 327–340.

Licht, R., & van der Meer, D. J. (1989). Differences in word recognition between P- and L-type reading disability. *Journal of Clinical and Experimental Neuropsychology, 11,* 359.

Linstra, A. (1983). *Event-related potentials and the assessment of brain function.* Master's thesis, Free University, Amsterdam.

Morris, R. (1989). Remediation and treatment of learning disabilities from a neuropsychological framework. In D. J. Bakker & H. van der Vlugt (Eds.), *Learning disabilities, Vol. 1: Neuropsychological correlates and treatment* (pp. 183–190). Lisse, Netherlands: Swets and Zeitlinger.

Plomin, R., DeFries, J. C., & McClearn, G. E. (1980). *Behavioral genetics: A primer.* San Francisco: W. H. Freeman.

Reitsma, P. (1983). *Phonemic and graphemic codes in learning to read.* Doctoral dissertation, Free University, Amsterdam.

Rosen, G. D., Sherman, G. F., & Galaburda, A. M. (1986). Biological interactions in dyslexia. In J. E. Obrzut & G. W. Hynd (Eds.), *Child neuropsychology, Vol. 1: Theory and research* (pp. 155–173). New York: Academic Press.

Rourke, B. P. (Ed.). (1985). *Neuropsychology of learning disabilities: Essentials of subtype analysis.* New York: Guilford Press.

Rourke, B. P., & Petrauskas, R. J. (1977). *Underlining Test (Revised).* Windsor, Ontario: Authors.

Silverberg, R., Gordon, H. W., Pollack, S., & Bentin, S. (1980). Shift in visual field preference for Hebrew words in native speakers learning to read. *Brain and Language, 1,* 99–105.

van Aarle, E. J. M., & Volleberg, M. J. (1986). Raders en spellers: Wat is de betekenis van dit onderscheid in de groep zwakke lezers? *Pedagogische Studiën, 4,* 339–346.

Van der Leij, D. A. V. (1983). *Ernstige leesproblemen.* Doctoral dissertation, Free University, Amsterdam.

van Strien, J. W., Bakker, D. J., Bouma, A., & Koops, W. (1988). Familial antecedents of P- and L-type dyslexia. *Journal of Clinical and Experimental Neuropsychology, 10,* 323.

van Strien, J. W., Bakker, D. J., Bouma, A. & Koops, W. (in press). Familial resemblance for cognitive abilities in families with P-type or L-type dyslexic boys and families with normal reading boys. *Journal of Clinical and Experimental Neuropsychology.*

CHAPTER 8

Neuropsychological Validation Studies of Learning Disability Subtypes: Verbal, Visual-Spatial, and Psychomotor Abilities

Harry van der Vlugt

In the past it has been demonstrated that groups of learning-disabled learners and controls differ from each other on a wide variety of neuropsychological, cognitive, mnestic, and social measures (Benton, 1975; Fletcher, 1981; Rourke, 1978; Vellutino, 1978). This contrasting-groups paradigm is still very popular. Frequently, groups of learning-disabled children and controls are compared on a measure of some psychological construct, and, if the groups differ, it is often concluded that this specific construct has some explanatory value with regard to the learning disability. This resulted in a large number of variables appearing to differentiate between learning-disabled children and controls and resulted in considerable controversy concerning the underlying cause(s) of learning disabilities.

However, controversy is an inevitable consequence of applying a research strategy based on a univariate contrasting-groups paradigm when the experimental group is not homogeneous and the basis for the disability is multivariate in nature. The multiple sources of variability inherent in learning disability studies stem from at least two sources (Fletcher & Satz, 1984). The first source concerns the construct validity of the dependent variables, which rarely represent pure measures of the underlying construct (Doehring, 1978; Satz & Fletcher, 1980). The second source of variability relates to the heterogeneity of disabled learners, who can vary according to academic problems, cognitive problems, and a variety of other attributes (intelligence, socioeconomic status, etc.). In order to deal with this intrasubject variability, researchers (e.g., Boder, 1973; Doehring & Hoshko, 1977; Fisk & Rourke, 1979; Lyon, 1982; Mattis,

French, & Rapin, 1975; Petrauskas & Rourke, 1979; Rourke, 1985, 1989; Satz & Morris, 1981) developed typologies by grouping together disabled learners who share common attributes.

Specific Developmental Dyslexia

The definition of "specific developmental dyslexia" developed by the World Federation of Neurology is as follows:

> A disorder manifested by difficulty in learning to read despite conventional instruction, adequate intelligence, and sociocultural opportunity. It is dependent upon fundamental cognitive disabilities which are frequently of constitutional origin. (Critchley, 1970, p. 11)

By accepting this definition, one also adopts a theory of how learning-disabled children should be classified. A number of studies have shown, however, that children with the defining attributes cannot be differentiated from other disabled learners with poor intelligence, cultural deprivation, and other problems (Satz & Fletcher, 1980; Taylor & Fletcher, 1983).

The abovementioned problem was tested by Taylor, Satz, and Friel (1979). For this study, the World Federation of Neurology definition of dyslexia was used to select a group of "dyslexic" disabled learners ($n = 40$) meeting the exclusionary criteria. These white male children were compared with a group of same-age "nondyslexic" disabled learners ($n = 40$) who failed to meet one or more of these criteria (e.g., low IQ, low socioeconomic status). Two groups of nondisabled learners were also included in this study. These four groups were compared along seven dimensions on which patterns specific to the "dyslexic" group could potentially emerge: (1) neuropsychological tests, (2) other academic tests, (3) severity of reading problems, (4) reversal and letter confusions, (5) parental reading proficiency, (6) neurological examinations, and (7) personality questionnaires. The results of the study revealed that while both the "dyslexic" and "nondyslexic" groups differed from controls along each of these seven dimensions, there were no differences between "dyslexic" and "nondyslexic" disabled learners. Consequently, this study challenged traditional exclusionary definitions of learning disabilities. This is one of the major reasons why classification research is necessary.

Apparently, the concept of "dyslexia," as it was formulated by the World Federation of Neurology, is not a unique and specific entity. This encouraged us to develop another approach to the problem of so-called "learning-disabled" children.

Statistical versus Clinical Approaches

In the past, learning disability taxonomies have been developed through clinical inspection of psychometric protocols (Boder, 1973; Mattis et al., 1975). We did not favor the clinical methods for our studies because of the difficulty of establishing the reliability and validity of the emergent typologies. Hence, statistical methods were chosen so that systematic studies of the reliability and validity of the typology could be conducted.

Cluster Analysis versus *Q*-Type Factor Analysis

When researchers choose among statistical methods, a variety of techniques are available. Two general classes or methods involve either *Q*-type factor analysis or cluster analysis, both of which present problems. The problems with *Q*-type factor analysis have been amply summarized by Fleiss and Zubin (1969). On the other hand, clustering methods are complex, and many decisions must be made when these techniques are employed (Bashfield, 1980; Morris, Blashfield, & Satz, 1981). For a more extensive discussion of these problems see Fletcher and Satz (1985).

Applying Cluster Analysis to the Dutch Data

Background

Because our study was meant to serve as a replication and a cross-cultural validation of the initial Florida study by Satz and Morris (1981), cluster-analytic techniques were employed. Furthermore, the nature of the data and our approach to classification research were more suited to cluster analysis. Validity studies were planned prior to the initiation of this series of studies. In this connection it should be noted that a good typology must exhibit both internal and external validity (Skinner, 1981). "Internal validity" concerns the reliability of the typology. In order to demonstrate that a typology is not method- or sample-dependent, additional internal validity studies should explore the adequacy of the clustering solution. The many methods available for cluster analysis provide an opportunity to replicate results across techniques. Monte Carlo studies have also been conducted to address the reliability of the clustering solutions (Morris et al., 1981). "External validity" concerns the issue of whether the subtypes are truly distinct through systematic comparisons of subgroups on variables not used to develop the typology. We had available a variety of variables that could be employed to evaluate external validity, including the Dichotic Listening Test (van der Vlugt, 1979) and the Underlining Test (Rourke & Petrauskas, 1977).

In both of the studies reported here, all children were quite homogeneous in terms of age, sex, and race. It was decided to include normal as well as disabled learners in order to allow the use of statistical procedures to identify the learning-disabled group. This way of separating disabled and nondisabled learners dictated the need to use similarity coefficients that incorporated elevation information. Furthermore, we wished to restrict the number of variables in an effort to reduce test redundancy and increase subtype interpretability.

Two sets of variables were employed in these studies. The first set represented the Reading, Spelling, and Arithmetic subtests from the Wide Range Achievement Test (WRAT; Jastak, & Jastak, 1978); these were cluster-analyzed to determine whether academic achievement subgroups could be defined in both overall samples. The second set of variables was employed with the subgroups of disabled learners that emerged from the achievement classification. The results of factor-analytic studies of the Florida investigation indicated that measures of visual–spatial and verbal skills were of particular importance (Fletcher & Satz, 1980). The visual–spatial measures included the Developmental Test of Visual–Motor Integration (Beery & Buktenica, 1967), a perceptual–motor copying test, and Recognition–Discrimination Test (Fletcher & Satz, 1984), a geometric-figure-matching task. Verbal measures included the Verbal Fluency Test (Spreen & Benton, 1969), which requires children to give words beginning with different letters of the alphabet under timed conditions, and the Wechsler Intelligence Scale for Children—Revised (WISC-R) Similarities subtest, a measure of verbal reasoning. These tests were chosen because they were the best measures of these skills in the Florida battery and because they exhibit high levels of reliability (Fletcher & Satz, 1984). In the next section, a series of cluster-analytic studies parallelling the Florida study and based on the two Dutch projects are summarized.

The Initial Study

Very often subtyping research attempts to classify children according to achievement dimensions (e.g., Boder, 1973; Doehring & Hoshko, 1977; Rourke & Finlayson, 1978; Rourke & Strang, 1978) or processing deficiencies based on a battery of cognitive–neuropsychological tests (e.g., Fisk & Rourke, 1979; Lyon, 1982; Mattis et al., 1975; Petrauskas & Rourke, 1979). As was done in the initial Florida studies (Satz & Morris, 1981), we chose to attempt both types of classification by clustering first on achievement variables and then on processing-deficiency variables. All analyses were completed using CLUSTAN (Wishart, 1975), a general-purpose softward package for cluster analysis.

Classification on Achievement Variables

As in our previous study (van der Vlugt, Satz, & Morris, 1983), we again identified a group of learning-disabled children by testing two large samples of an older and a younger age group with the WRAT (van der Vlugt & Satz, 1985). Both groups consisted of 250 boys. The younger group was aged 7 years, 6 months (SD = 4 months), and the older group was aged 11 years, 6 months (SD = 5 months). For both groups, the WRAT Reading, Spelling, and Arithmetic subtest scores were first converted into discrepancy scores by comparing a child's grade level with the grade-equivalent score obtained on each subtest. For both groups, the scores were then subjected to cluster analysis in order to group individuals most similar to each other on these discrepancy scores.

The WRAT data were subjected to an average-linkage, hierarchical agglomerative clustering method, utilizing a squared euclidean distance measure of similarity. The average-linkage method combined with the euclidean distance measure was used because of the high correlation among the WRAT subtests and because of its sensitivity to elevation in a data set. This method was thought likely to eventuate in clusters that differed in their levels of achievement. After we calculated the clusters for both age groups, we subjected them to a k-means iterative partitioning method of clustering. This additional method was used in view of the fact that an individual, once placed in a given cluster by a hierarchical agglomerative method, cannot be reassigned to a later-forming cluster, even if his similarity to the members of the later-forming cluster would be greater. (During each iterative partitioning phase, each individual is statistically removed from his parent cluster, and his similarity to members of all other clusters is computed. If the individual's similarity to members of another cluster is greater, he is placed in that cluster.) This method, which attempts to reduce within-cluster variance while increasing between-cluster variance, has been recommended by Morris et al. (1981) as an important prevalidation check on the cluster solution.

For the younger boys, the five-cluster solution, which included 242 subjects, revealed the following patterns and levels of performance. (Note that the coverage was extremely high, 97%, with only eight subjects resisting incorporation into the primary clusters. Following the recommendation of Everitt, 1980, these "outliers" were dropped from further analyses.) The results for each of the five subgroups are presented in Figure 8.1, where the discrepancy scores on each WRAT subtest are

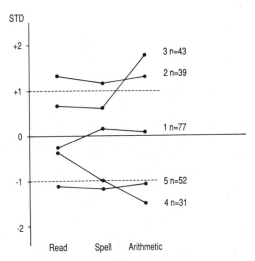

FIGURE 8.1. WRAT discrepancy scores for achievement subgroups; mean based on younger Dutch schoolboys (age: 7 years, 6 months).

expressed on a scale with a population mean of 0 and a *SD* of 1. This method permits visualization of the subgroups in terms of both pattern and elevation.

Several patterns of reading, spelling, and arithmetic skills can be seen in Figure 8.1 Subgroups 2 ($n = 39$) and 3 ($n = 43$) both obtained superior scores in arithmetic, reading, and spelling. Subgroup 1 ($n = 77$) exhibited average performance in reading, spelling, and arithmetic. Subgroup 4 ($n = 31$) emerged as a group with average reading and severely depressed spelling and arithmetic. Subgroup 5 ($n = 52$) contained a large number of children severely dificient on all three WRAT subtests.

A tentative comparison can be made between these results and those of Bakker's P and L subtypology (Bakker, 1990). According to Bakker's "balance model," the P-type dyslexic is characterized by an analytic-perceptual, spelling, reading style, making relatively many time-consuming errors. The L-type dyslexic, however, is characterized by fast reading and the production of many substantive errors. Specifically, children in subgroup 4 read more words correctly on the reading subtest than did subgroup 5. However, a close examination of the data indicates that the subjects in subgroup 4 also read more words erroneously than did subgroup 5 subjects. This suggests that subgroup 4 (L-type dyslexia) reads faster and more inaccurately than subgroup 5 and that subgroup 5 (P-type dyslexia) reads more slowly but more accurately than subgroup 4.

For the older boys eight clusters (subgroups) emerged. As for the younger age group, k-means iterative partitioning method of clustering was used. The eight subgroups included 244 of the 250 subjects. Six "outliers" were dropped from the analysis. The data were transformed in the same manner as was done for the younger age group. The patterns of the reading, spelling, and arithmetic performance for each subgroup are presented in Figure 8.2.

Subgroup 1 ($n = 16$) obtained superior scores in reading, spelling, and arithmetic. Subgroup 2 ($n = 21$) exhibited superior scores in reading but only slightly above-average scores for spelling and arithmetic. Subgroup 3 ($n = 41$) achieved high scores for reading and arithmetic and slightly above-average scores in spelling. Subgroup 4 ($n = 32$) obtained average scores for all three variables. Subgroup 5 ($n = 47$) exhibited average scores for reading and spelling and an above-average score for arithmetic. Subgroup 6 ($n = 22$) exhibited the same pattern for spelling and reading as subgroup 5 but was below average for arithmetic. Subgroups 7 ($n = 27$) and 8 ($n = 33$) each contained a large number of children who exhibited a severe deficiency on all three subtests of the WRAT. Subgroup 7 performed slightly better in arithmetic than did subgroup 8. These findings for subgroups 6, 7, and 8 are particularly interesting, since similar subgroups have been investigated or have emerged in other studies (Fletcher & Satz, 1985; Rourke, 1982; van der Vlugt & Satz, 1985). For example, Rourke and Finlayson's (1978) Group 1

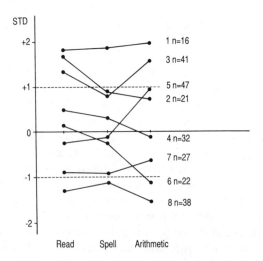

FIGURE 8.2. WRAT discrepancy scores for achievement subgroups; mean based on older Dutch schoolboys (age: 11 years, 6 months).

was uniformly deficient on all three subtests of the WRAT, similar to our subgroups 7 and 8; Group 2 was very poor in reading and spelling but significantly better (although still impaired relative to age norms) in arithmetic, a pattern at least comparable with our subgroup 5; Group 3 was composed of children who were at least average in reading and spelling but poor in arithmetic, similar to subgroup 6. A comparison of these results with those of Fletcher and Satz (1985) and van der Vlugt and Satz (1985) indicates that our current subgroup 1 (with superior scores in reading, spelling, and arithmetic skills) is highly comparable to subgroup 1 of the Fletcher and Satz study and subgroup 2 of the van der Vlugt and Satz study. Subgroup 2 (with superior scores in reading and average scores in spelling and arithmetic skills) is almost identical to subgroup 2 and subgroup 4, respectively of these studies. Again, subgroup 3 is represented in all three studies about equally. With respect to the learning disability subgroups, we see that subgroup 6 (with average scores in reading and spelling and poor scores in arithmetic skills) is comparable to subgroup 5 of the Fletcher and Satz study and subgroup 7 of the van der Vlugt and Satz study. All three studies also identify two subgroups with very inferior performance on all three WRAT subtests.

Validation: Type of School

For the younger age group, three of the five subgroups were characterized by average to superior achievement (subgroups 1, 2, and 3), and two subgroups were characterized by specific and/or general delays in achievement (subgroups 4 and 5). If one compares these subgroup classifications (predictions) with the actual school settings in which the children resided (external criteria), one could determine the accuracy or validity of the clustering solution.

Inspection of Table 8.1 reveals that, of 159 younger children classified in subgroups 1, 2, and 3, 13 were misclassified as mildly learning disabled; this represents a valid negative rate of 92% (146/159) and a false positive rate of 8% (13/159). Conversely, of the 83 younger children who were classified as belonging to subgroups 4 and 5, 16 were misclassified as average students; these outcomes represent a valid positive rate of 81% (67/83) and a false negative rate of 19% (16/83). For the older age groups, the outcomes were as follows. In the average to superior subgroups (subgroups 1, 2, 3, 4, and 5) there was a valid negative rate of 94% (148/157) and a false positive rate of 6% (9/157). In the below-average subgroups (subgroups 6, 7, 8, and 9), there was a valid negative rate of 91% (79/87) and a false positive rate of 9% (8/87). In terms of overall classification accuracy, the clustering solution for the younger age group, based on

TABLE 8.1. Validation of Classification Method Using WRAT
Subtests, by Type of School

Cluster	n	Type of school		
		Regular	Mild LD	Severe LD
Younger children[a]				
1	77	64	13	0
2	39	39	0	0
3	43	43	0	0
4	31	9	19	3
5	52	7	9	36
Older children[b]				
1	16	16	0	0
2	21	21	0	0
3	41	41	0	0
4	32	29	3	0
5	47	41	6	0
6	22	8	12	2
7	27	0	18	9
8	38	0	2	36

Note. LD, learning disabilities.
[a]Five-cluster solution.
[b]Eight-cluster solution.

the three WRAT subtests, correctly classified 88% of the total sample (213/
242). For the older age group, the correct classification rate was 93% for
the total sample (227/244).

Subtype Classification

In a previous study (van der Vlugt & Satz, 1985) and in the one reported
above, we used the same neuropsychological measures as clustering variables in the investigation of the younger (subgroups 4 and 5) and the
older (subgroups 6, 7, and 8) learning disability subgroups. All of these
subgroups were severely impaired on at least one of WRAT subtests.
    Data for the subjects in the two subgroups of younger children (n =
83) and the three subgroups of older children (n = 87) were then subjected
to cluster-analytic techniques based on their performance on the four
neuropsychological tests mentioned before. A discussion of the tests and

the factor analysis can be found in Fletcher and Satz (1980). The rationale for this procedure was to restrict the number of tests to a few highly independent factors in an effort to reduce test redundancy and random error variance and, thereby, the increase subtype interpretability. Reliable variables were, therefore, expected to yield a reliable classification. The variables also provided the opportunity to employ a number of clustering techniques to insure that the subtypes were replicable across different clustering methods. Replication at this level was felt to be mandatory in view of the controversy surrounding the potential uses and misuses of cluster analysis (Everitt, 1980).

The four-cluster solution for the younger age group (see Figure 8.3) and the four-cluster solution for the older age group (see Figure 8.4) appeared to be highly replicable. The subtypes are based on performances on the four neuropsychological tests, which have been converted to standard scores with a population mean of 0 and a *SD* of 1 for the control groups (*n* = 50 for both age groups).

Comparing the four-cluster solution for the younger children with that of a more or less identical study (Morris, Blashfield, & Satz, 1986), it is obvious that subtype 1 (*n* = 17) represents a group of learning-disabled children that is well known to neuopsychologists and educators. They have relatively poor verbal and visual–perceptual–motor skills and are highly comparable with subtype C of the Morris et al. (1986) study. For subtype 2 (*n* = 24), visual–perceptual–motor abilities are clearly

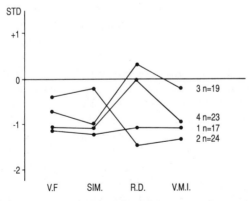

FIGURE 8.3. Neuropsychological test discrepancy scores for learning disability subtypes; mean based on young Dutch schoolboys (age: 7 years, 6 months). V.F., Verbal Fluency Test; SIM., WISC Similarities subtest; R.D., Recognition–Discrimination Test; V.M.I., Developmental Test of Visual–Motor Integration.

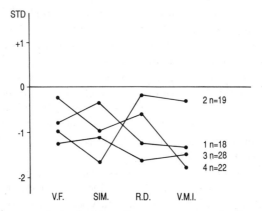

FIGURE 8.4. Neuropsychological test discrepancy scores for learning disability subtypes; mean based on older Dutch schoolboys (age: 11 years, 6 months). For key to abbreviations, see Figure 8.3.

deficient, while verbal abilities are about average. This subtype is comparable with subtype B of the Morris et al. (1986) study. Subtype 3 (n = 19) demonstrates a clear verbal deficiency where visual–perceptual–motor abilities are average or above average. This subtype 3 is comparable with the Morris et al. (1986) subtype A, demonstrating the same pattern. Apart from the three previous subtypes, we identified subtype 4 (n = 23), which was deficient in all domains except for an average score on the Recognition Discrimination Test. This subtype did not emerge in the Morris et al. (1986) study. However, this is a well-recognized clinical group of learning-disabled children who have problems in the organization of their expressive skills (perhaps caused by a maturational lag).

Comparing the four-cluster solution of the older children with that of the previous Dutch study (van der Vlugt & Satz, 1985) and with the Florida study (Satz & Morris, 1983), it is obvious that the visual–spatial–motor subtype (subtype 1, n = 18) is highly similar to subtype 7 of the Dutch study and the visual–perceptual–motor subtype of the Florida study. Also, the general verbal deficiency subtype (subtype 2, n = 19) shows a strong resemblance to subtypes 1 and 3 of the Dutch study and the general deficiency subtype of the Florida study. Subtype 3 (n = 28) of this study is highly similar to subtypes 4 and 5 of the Dutch study and to the general deficiency subtype of the Florida study. Subtype 4 (n = 22) exhibits deficiencies on Similarities and Visual–Motor Integration and is comparable with subtype 2 of the Dutch study.

Comments

The results reported above are quite similar to findings reported in other studies. The results regarding the younger age group closely approximate the findings by Morris et al. (1986). The results of the older age group demonstrate a striking resemblance with previous studies by Satz and Morris (1983) and van der Vlugt and Satz (1985).

In the younger as well as in the older age group, the subtypes are comparable to those established in other studies, which have reported a relatively poor verbal and/or poor visual–perceptual–motor subtype of learning-disabled children (Doehring & Hoshko, 1977; Mattis, 1978; Mattis et al. 1975; Petrauskas & Rourke, 1979). In the present study, 71% (59/83) of the younger age group and 80% (69/87) of the older age group evidenced some type of language difficulty on the neuropsychological tests. However, 29% of the younger age group and 20% of the older age group demonstrated some kind of learning disability without any impairment of language skills. The identification of this subtype of learning-disabled children who continue to show selective cognitive deficiencies in processing visual information should give pause to those who postulate a unitary language deficit in learning-disabled children (Vellutino, 1978). Although this subtype is more prominent at a younger age, to ignore the pattern of abilities and deficits exhibited by them might lead to the adoption of and subject them to inappropriate methods of remediation (Strang & Rourke, 1985).

External Validation Based on
Other Neuropsychological Variables

In addition to the tests mentioned earlier in the chapter, the children in both age groups were administered the Dichotic Listening Test (assessing lateralization, auditory information processing, and auditory verbal memory), the Underlining Test (attention to and discrimination of verbal and nonverbal stimuli), the Peabody Picture Vocabulary Test (PPVT: matching verbal information to pictorial patterns, and a verbal IQ estimate), and a reading test in which the types of reading errors were analyzed. The outcomes of this part of the study are summarized in Table 8.2. Since three patterns for the younger and older age groups were essentially the same (only the proportions of the different subtypes differed; that is, a higher percentage of the younger age group showed visual–spatial deficiencies), we summarize the outcomes in Table 8.2 only for the three different subtypes that both age groups have in common: a general deficiency subtype (GD) (subtype 1 younger and subtype 3 older

TABLE 8.2. Validation of Classification of Three Learning Disability Subtypes Using the Dichotic Listening Test, the Underlining Test, the PPVT, and a Reading Test

	GD	VD	SD
Dichotic listening, right ear	−	−	+
Dichotic listening, left ear	−	Average	−
Dichotic listening, total	− −	−	Average
Dichotic listening, right–left	−	No difference or left-ear advantage	Strong right-ear advantage
Underlining	− −		
PPVT	−		+/−
Reading errors			
Time-consuming	Variable	− −	
Substantive	Variable		− −

Note. GD, general deficiency; VD, verbal deficiency; SD, visual–spatial deficiency; −, between 1 and 2 standard deviations below average; +, between 1 and 2 standard deviations above average.

boys), a verbal deficiency subtype (VD) (subtype 3 younger and subtype 2 older boys), and a visual–spatial deficiency subtype (SD) (subtype 2 younger and subtype 1 older boys).

In the table, there are data that can be seen as relating to the work of Fletcher, Satz, Morris, Rouke, and Bakker. For example, in the GD subtype, we see a lowered level of performance without any specific kind of pattern of language disturbance. In this sense, the pattern is quite unstable. The characteristics of the GD subtype seem to be a lower score on the PPVT (which fits well with the type of school they are attending) but also problems with the recall of verbal information (low score on the Dichotic Listening Test R + L) and a limited attention span (low score on the Underlining Test). The VD subtype is more explicit and shows some relationship with other subtypes mentioned in the literature. The significantly lower score for the right-ear dichotic listening, the lower total score (R + L) on that same test, and the lower score on the Underlining Test might suggest some kind of general deficiency in which left hemisphere functions in particular tend to be lowered, suggesting a specific left hemisphere dysfunction. The SD subtype exhibits a higher score for the right ear and a lower score for the left ear on the Dichotic Listening Test, resulting in a strong right-ear advantage. Visual attention span is limited, and these children's reading strategy is characterized by substantive errors.

Although one could propose speculations regarding how much these profiles resemble other profiles, we prefer to stick to a comparison with the studies by Bakker who used more or less the same variables. (Bakker, 1986, 1990; Bakker, Licht, Kok, & Bouma, 1980; Bakker & Vinke, 1985). Bakker's L and P subtypes of dyslexia were first identified from ear asymmetry data of children on dichotic listening tasks. A child who consistently showed a large left-ear advantage (P type) for verbal materials was considered to exhibit a less effective left hemisphere. On the other hand, a child who consistently showed a large right-ear advantage (L type) might be considered to have a less effective right hemisphere. Bakker suggests that reading is primarily mediated by the right hemisphere early in the learning-to-read process and by the left hemisphere during advanced reading development. He considers the need for early right hemisphere involvement to result from the visual–spatial nature of beginning script analysis.

Problems may arise during the early or later phases in the learning-to-read process. Some children may generate predominantly left hemispheric reading strategies right from the beginning of the learning-to-read process (L type), whereas others may fail to shift to left hemispheric strategies and stick to the visual–perceptual approach (P type). According to Bakker's "balance model," L-type dyslexics can also be differentiated from P-type dyslexics on the basis of speed and accuracy of reading. L-type children are characterized by fast reading and the production of many substantive errors, whereas P-type dyslexics read slowly and make relatively many time-consuming errors.

If we compare Bakker's "balance model" with our validation study variables in Table 8.2, we see that the VD subtype is almost identical with Bakker's P type of dyslexics. Both subtypes have no ear advantage or a left-ear advantage on the Dichotic Listening Test, and both show time-consuming errors during a reading task. The only difference is the cause of the lateralization outcome on the Dichotic Listening Test. Bakker's outcome results from a higher left-ear score because of overactivation of the right hemisphere, whereas in our study, the outcome results from a lowered right-ear score, suggesting a possible left hemisphere dysfunction. The SD subtype is very similar to Bakker's L type of dyslexics. Both types exhibit a strong right-ear advantage on the Dichotic Listening Test, and both make substantive errors during a reading task.

Validation by Means of Eye Movement Registration

In order to test the abovementioned similarities with the Bakker subtypes, we recorded the eye movements of younger and older good and poor readers. When we examine the eye movements of a good young reader (see Figure 8.5) we see the spelling-reading strategy. One can clearly see the

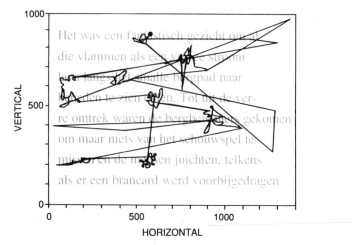

FIGURE 8.5. Full eye movement recordings during reading in a younger good reader.

many fixations, the short jumps between fixations, the numerous back-and-forth alternations over the separate letters of a word. This is exactly what Bakker predicted in the "balance model." The eye movements of an older good reader also fit Bakker's model (see Figure 8.6). One can clearly see that the advanced reader jumps through the text with much larger lapses and fewer fixations. When we examine the eye movements of an

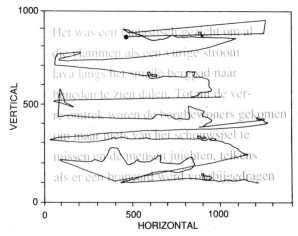

FIGURE 8.6. Full eye movement recordings during reading in an older good reader.

older poor reader from our VD subtype (see Figure 8.7), we can see that he appears to be reading in a fashion identical to that seen in a young good reader (see Figure 8.5); that is, he exhibits many fixations at the grapheme and phoneme level. Hence, our VD subtype appears to match Bakker's P type of dyslexia. Finally, if we look at the eye movements of the young poor reader, the L type of dyslexic of Bakker and the VD subtype in our study, we are unable to confirm predictions based on Bakker's model (see Figure 8.8). All we can see from our eye movement recordings are more or less random eye movements. The young child is looking everywhere except at the text. Basically, one can say that the child does not use any strategy at all. It seems that the child is unable to pay adequate attention to the text he is supposed to read.

Conclusion

By means of eye movement recordings, several predictions derived from Bakker's "balance model" could be confirmed. It could be that he is partially correct. Perhaps another interpretation of his outcomes is needed, as Morris (1989) has recently suggested. It may be the case that his model should be explained in terms of the relationship between right hemisphere and novelty (Goldberg & Costa, 1981) and the shift from right

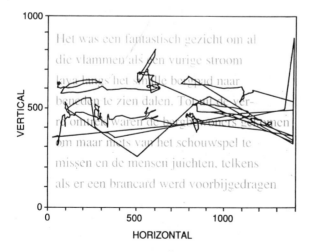

FIGURE 8.7. Full eye movement recordings during reading in an older poor reader.

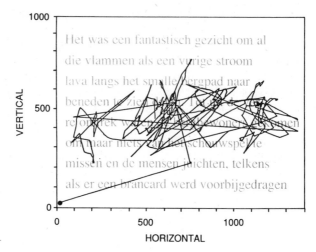

FIGURE 8.8. Full eye movement recordings during reading in a younger poor reader.

to left as a shift in hemispheric attentional mechanisms (Kinsbourne, 1975) when novelty wears off during the learning-to-read process.

Based on his theory, Bakker developed a hemisphere-specific stimulation treatment. By stimulating the "deficient" hemisphere, Bakker produced improved reading across both L and P types, but the results were much clearer for L types. Future subtype research combing the notion of novelty, attentional mechanisms, Bakker's developmental model, lateralized deficiencies, and eye-view monitoring, psychophysiological, and treatment validation outcomes might prove to be a fruitful way to approach the problems in dyslexia research.

References

Bakker, D. J. (1986). Electrophysiological validation of L- and P-type dyslexia. *Journal of Clinical and Experimental Neuropsychology, 8,* 133.

Bakker, D. J. (1990). *Neuropsychological treatment of dyslexia.* New York: Oxford University Press.

Bakker, D. J., Licht, R., Kok, A., & Bouma, A. (1980). Cortical responses to word reading in right- and left-eared normal and reading-disturbed children. *Journal of Clinical Neuropsychology, 6,* 1–18.

Bakker, D. J., & Vinke, J. (1985). Effects of hemisphere-specific stimulation on brain activity and reading in dyslexics. *Journal of Clinical and Experimental Neuropsychology, 7,* 505–525.

Beery, K., & Buktenica, N. A. (1967). *Developmental Test of Visual-Motor Integration.* Chicago: Follet Education Company.

Benton, A. L. (1975). Developmental dyslexia: Neurological aspects. In W. J. Friedlander (Ed.), *Advances in neurology* (Vol. 7, pp. 1–47). New York: Raven Press.

Blashfield, R. K. (1980). Propositions regarding the use of cluster analysis in clinical research. *Journal of Consulting and Clincial Psychology, 3.* 456–459.

Boder, E. (1973). Developmental dyslexia: A diagnostic approach based upon three atypical reading-spelling patterns. *Developmental Medicine and Child Neurology, 15,* 663–687.

Critchley, M. (1970). *The dyslexic child.* Springfield, IL: Charles C. Thomas.

Doehring, D. G. (1978). The tangled web of behavioral research on developmental dyslexia. In A. L. Benton & D. Pearl (Eds.), *Dyslexia: An appraisal of current knowledge* (pp. 123–135). New York: Oxford University Press.

Doehring, D. G., & Hoshko, I. M. (1977). Classification of reading problems by the *Q*-technique of factor analysis. *Cortex, 13.* 281–294.

Everitt, B. (1980). *Cluster analysis.* London: Heinemann Educational Books.

Fisk, J. L., & Rourke, B. P., (1979). Identification of subtypes of learning disabilities at three age levels: A Neuropsychological, multivariate approach. *Journal of Clinical Neuropsychology, 1.* 289–310.

Fleiss, J. L., & Zubin, J. (1969). On the methods and theory of clustering. *Multivariate Behavioral Research, 4.* 235–250.

Fletcher, J. M. (1981). Linguistic factors in reading acquisition: Evidence for developmental changes. In F. J. Pirozzolo & M. C. Wittrock (Eds.), *Neuropsychological and cognitive processes in reading* (pp. 261–294). New York: Academic Press.

Fletcher, J. M., & Satz, P. (1980). Developmental changes in the neuropsychological correlates of reading achievement: A six-year longitudinal follow-up. *Journal of Clinical Neuropsychology, 2.* 23–37.

Fletcher, J. M., & Satz, P. (1984). Preschool prediction of reading failure. In M. Levin & P. Sata (Eds.), *Middle childhood: Development and dysfunction* (pp. 153–182). Baltimore: University Park Press.

Fletcher, J. M., & Satz, P. (1985). Cluster analysis and the search for learning disability subtypes. In B. P. Rourke (Ed.), *Neuropsychology of learning disabilities: Essentials of subtype analysis* (pp. 40–64). New York: Guilford Press.

Goldberg, E., & Costa, L. (1981). Hemispheric differences in the acquisition and use of descriptive systems. *Brain and Language, 14.* 144–173.

Jastak, J., & Jastak, S. (1978). *The Wide Range Achievement Test,* Wilmington, DE: Guidance Associates.

Kinsbourne, M. (1975). The mechanisms of hemispheric control of the lateral gradient of attention. In P. M. A. Rabbitt & S. Dornic (Eds.), *Attention and performance* (pp. 81–97). London: Academic Press.

Lyon, R. (1982). Subgroups of LD readers: Clincial and empirical identification. In H. R. Myklebust (Ed), *Progress in learning disabilities* (Vol. 5, pp. 103–133). New York: Grune & Stratton.

Mattis, S. (1978). Dyslexia syndromes: A working hypothesis that works. In A. L. Benton & D. Pearl (Eds.), *Dyslexia: An appraisal of current knowledge* (pp. 45–58). New York: Oxford University Press.

Mattis, S., French, J. H., & Rapin, I. (1975). Dyslexia in children and adults: Three independent Neuropsychological syndromes. *Developmental Medicine and Child Neurology, 119.* 121–127.

Morris, R. (1989). Treatment of learning disabilities from a neuropsychological framework. In D. J. Bakker & H. Van der Vlugt (Eds.), *Learning disabilities, Vol. 1: Neuropsychological correlates and treatment* (pp. 183–189). Lisse: Swets and Zeitlinger.

Morris, R., Blashfield, R. K., & Satz, P. (1981). Neuropsychology and cluster analysis: Problems and pitfalls. *Journal of Clinical Neuropsychology, 3.* 79-99.

Morris, R., Blashfield, R., & Satz, P. (1986). Developmental classification of reading-disabled children. *Journal of Clinical and Experimental Neuropsychology, 8.* 371-392.

Petrauskas, R., & Rourke, B. P. (1979). Identification of subgroups of retarded readers: A neuropsychological, multivariate approach. *Journal of Clinical Neuropsychology, 1.* 17-37.

Rourke, B. P. (1978). Neuropsychological research in reading retardation. In A. L. Benton & D. Pearl (Eds.), *Dyslexia: An appraisal of current knowledge* (pp. 139-171). New York: Oxford University Press.

Rourke, B. P. (1982). Central processing deficiences in children: Toward a developmental neuropsychological model. *Journal of Clinical Neuropsychology, 4.* 1-18.

Rourke, B. P. (Ed.). (1985). *Neuropsychology of learning disabilities: Essentials of subtype analysis.* New York: Guilford Press.

Rourke, B. P. (1989). *Nonverbal learning disabilities: The syndrome and the model.* New York: Guilford Press.

Rourke, B. P., & Finlayson, M. A. J. (1978). Neuropsychological significance of variations in patterns of academic performance: Verbal and visual-spatial abilities. *Journal of Abnormal Child Psychology, 6.* 121-133.

Rourke, B. P., & Petrauskas, R. J. (1977). *Underlining Test (Revised).* Windsor, Ontario, Canada: Author, Department of Psychology, University of Windsor.

Rourke, B. P., & Strang, J. D. (1978). Neuropsychological significance of variations in patterns of academic performance: Motor, Psychomotor, and tactile-perceptual abilities. *Journal of Pediatric Psychology, 3.* 62-66.

Satz, P., & Fletcher, J. M. (1980). Minimal brain dysfunctions: An appraisal of research concepts and methods. In H. Rie & E. Rie (Eds.). *Handbook of minimal brain dysfunctions* (pp. 669-714). New York: Wiley-Interscience.

Satz, P., & Morris, R. (1981). Learning disability subtypes: A review. In F. J. Pirozzolo & M. C. Wittrock (Eds.) *Neuropsychological and cognitive processes in reading* (pp. 109-141). New York: Academic Press.

Satz, P., & Morris, R. (1983). The search for subtype classification in learning-disabled children. In R. Tarter (Ed.), *The child at risk* (pp. 128-150). New York: Oxford University Press.

Skinner, H. A. (1981). Toward the integration of classification theory and methods. *Journal of Abnormal Psychology, 90.* 68-87.

Spreen, O., & Benton, A. L. (1969). *Spreen-Benton Language Examination Profile.* Iowa City: University of Iowa.

Strang, J. D., & Rourke, B. P. (1985). Adaptive behavior of children who exhibit specific arithmetic disabilities and associated neuropsychological abilities and deficits. In B. P. Rourke (Ed.), *Neuropsychology of learning disabilities: Essentials of subtype analysis* (pp. 302-331). New York: Guilford Press.

Taylor, H. G., & Fletcher, J. M. (1983). Biological foundations of "specific developmental disorders": Methods, findings, and future directions. *Journal of Clinical Child Psychology, 12.* 46-65.

Taylor, H. G., Satz. P., & Friel, J. (1979). Developmental dyslexia in relation to other childhood reading disorders: Significance and clinical utility. *Reading Research Quarterly, 15.* 84-101.

van der Vlugt, H. (1979). *Lateralisatie van Hersenfunkties* [Lateralization of brain function]. Lisse: Swets and Zeitlinger.

van der Vlugt, H., & Satz, P. (1985). Subgroups and subtypes of learning-disabled and normal children: A cross-cultural replication. In B. P. Rourke (Ed.), *Neuropsychology of learning disabilities: Essentials of subtype analysis* (pp. 212–227). New York: Guilford Press.

van der Vlugt, H., Satz, P., & Morris, R. (1983). Supgroepen en subtypen leergestoorde kinderen [Subgroups and subtypes of learning-disabled children]. In R. Godijns & F. Loncke (Eds.), *Leerproces en taalverwerving bij kinderen, Vol. 2: Neuropsychologische benadering van het leren* (pp. 11–50). Leuven: Acco.

Vellutin. F. R. (1978). Toward an understanding of dyslexia: Psychological factors in specific reading disability. In A. L. Benton & D. Pearl (Eds.), *Dyslexia: An appraisal of current knowledge* (pp. 61–111). New York: Oxford University Press.

Wishart, D. (1975). *CLUSTAN user manual* (3rd ed.). London: University of London.

CHAPTER 9

Validation of Psychosocial Subtypes of Children with Learning Disabilities

Darren R. Fuerst and Byron P. Rourke

For some time it has been widely held that learning difficulties and pathological socioemotional functioning are intimately related. Although the relationships between learning disabilities (LD) and psychosocial functioning have been extensively investigated, a coherent and meaningful pattern of psychosocial characteristics of children with LD has not emerged from the literature (Rourke, 1988a). We suspect that this is, in large part, the result of the use of variants of the simple contrasting-groups design, in which an undifferentiated group of LD children is compared to an equally undifferentiated group of normal-achieving children. The assumption underlying such an approach is that children with LD may be prone to developing a particular pattern of psychosocial dysfunction and that within-group differences are of little concern. This method can only be justified if the assumption that children with LD comprise a homogeneous group with respect to psychosocial functioning is valid.

In our laboratory we have undertaken a research program with the immediate aim of more precisely describing the psychosocial functioning of children with LD. This chapter provides an overview of a series of four studies in which we have explored patterns of personality and psychosocial functioning in such children. In these studies, we have applied multivariate statistical subtyping methods, Q-factor analysis, and/or some of the many variants of cluster analysis to selected scales of the Personality Inventory for Children (PIC; Wirt, Lachar, Klinedinst, & Seat, 1977) in an attempt to derive both reliable and valid psychosocial subtypes of children with LD. Questions that we have tried to address in these studies include the following: (1) Are children with LD homogeneous or heterogeneous in terms of psychosocial functioning? (2) If heterogeneity exists, are there psychosocial subtypes that can be reliably identified? (3) What are the characteristics of these subtypes? (4) Do these subtypes differ in a predictable manner on other measures of interest to neuropsychologists?

For the most part, our research program has followed the sequence of these four central questions. However, in the two most recent studies, issues related both to reliability and to validity were considered in a concurrent manner. Indeed, because reliability (internal validity) is a necessary precondition for external validity, the two are difficult to separate. However, in the interests of clear exposition, we deal with them sequentially in this chapter. First, we outline the typology that has emerged as our research has progressed and describe the characteristics of the subtypes we have found. Following this, we discuss the results of our first efforts to establish the external validity of this typology.

Reliability (Internal Validity)

Study 1

In the first study of this series, Porter and Rourke (1985) applied Q-factor analysis to the PIC scores of 100 children with LD. The children ranged in age from 6.5 to 15.3 years. On the basis of the resulting factor pattern, children were assigned to one of four subtypes. These subtypes were then examined in terms of the mean PIC profiles exhibited by the subjects within them.

The first and largest subtype showed no elevations on PIC scales reflecting psychosocial disturbance and had an essentially normal, well-adjusted profile (Figure 9.1). The parents of these children were most concerned with the cognitive development and academic functioning of their children. The second subtype (Figure 9.2) had a mean PIC profile that was strongly suggestive of seriously disturbed socioemotional functioning of an "internalized" type (e.g., symptoms suggestive of significant depression, withdrawal, and anxiety). The third subtype had a mean PIC profile that was suggestive of "externalized," "hyperkinetic" behavioral disturbance (Figure 9.3), with maximal elevations on the Delinquency, Hyperactivity, and Social Skills scales. The fourth, and smallest, group derived showed relatively normal psychosocial adjustment overall but evidenced a variety of somatic complaints (Figure 9.4).

Ideally, subtyping methods of any type should produce reliable, homogeneous groups that can be replicated across different samples and classification techniques (Everitt, 1980). This issue is of particular concern when multivariate subtyping techniques are applied in an explora-

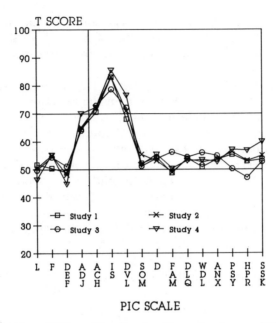

FIGURE 9.1. Mean PIC profiles for the Normal subtype. Abbreviations for Figures 9.1–9.7: L, Lie; DEF, Defensiveness; ADJ, Adjustment; ACH, Achievement; IS, Intellectual Screening; DVL, Development; SOM, Somatic Concern; D, Depression; FAM, Family Relations; DLQ, Delinquency; WDL, Withdrawal; ANX, Anxiety; PSY, Psychosis; HPR, Hyperactivity; SSK, Social Skills. Study 1 refers to Porter and Rourke (1985); Study 2 refers to Fuerst, Fisk, and Rourke (1989); Study 3 refers to Fuerst, Fisk, and Rourke (1990); and Study 4 refers to Fuerst and Rourke (in preparation).

tory fashion to data with relatively unknown statistical properties. Multivariate subtyping techniques, such as cluster analysis and Q-factor analysis, will always produce some grouping of cases, even if purely random data are used in the procedures. Furthermore, different statistical subtyping techniques can and often do produce disparate solutions when applied to the same data. Replicability of solutions across different samples from the same population and across different subtyping techniques is a crucial step in determining the validity of the subtypes so derived (Fletcher, 1985).

Study 2

Thus, in the next study (Fuerst, Fisk, & Rourke, 1989), we concentrated on establishing the reliability of the Porter and Rourke (1985) subtypes,

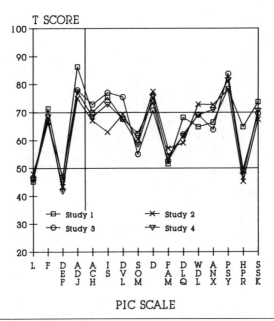

FIGURE 9.2. Mean PIC profiles for the Internalized Psychopathology subtype.

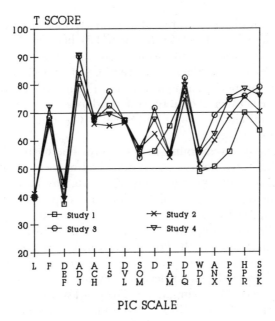

FIGURE 9.3. Mean PIC profiles for the Externalized Psychopathology subtype.

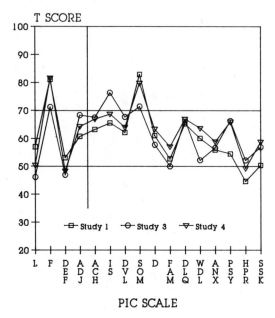

PIC SCALE

FIGURE 9.4. Mean PIC profiles for the Somatic Concern subtype.

using a new sample of children and a variety of statistical subtyping techniques. The scores of 132 children with LD, between the ages of 6 and 12 years, on nine selected PIC scales were investigated using Q-factor analysis, four hierarchical–agglomerative clustering techniques, and one iterative partitioning clustering technique. The results revealed excellent correspondence between the subtypes derived by all grouping methods in terms of both misclassifications and mean PIC profile similarity of the subtypes across techniques.

Three subtypes were found in the study. The mean PIC profile of one subtype indicated normal psychosocial adjustment. This group was almost identical to the Normal subtype reported by Porter and Rourke (1985) in terms of both general PIC profile shape and elevation and relative size (Figure 9.1). The second subtype exhibited evidence of significant internalized psychopathology and was very similar to the corresponding children found in the Porter and Rourke (1985) study, with only minor discrepancies in mean profiles that were overshadowed by overall similarity of shape and general elevation (Figure 9.2). The relative sizes of the two groups were also comparable. The third subtype had a mean PIC profile suggestive of externalized, "hyperkinetic" psychopathology and was very similar to the corresponding Porter and Rourke (1985) subtype

(Figure 9.3). The profile of this group also bore a striking resemblance to one reported by Breen and Barkley (1983) in a study of 26 children diagnosed as hyperactive or as having attention deficit disorder with hyperactivity. Indeed, the two profiles were found to correlate .89, confirming substantial similarity of profile shape. The fourth, "Somatic Concern" subtype of Porter and Rourke (1985) was not found in this study.

The results of the Porter and Rourke (1985) and Fuerst et al. (1989) studies led to three important conclusions. First, children with LD are heterogeneous in terms of psychosocial functioning; that is, there is no unique LD personality type. Second, statistical subtyping techniques can produce reliable and interpretable subgroups of children that are replicable across samples. Third, LD children seem to fall into three broad psychosocial subtypes, namely, Normal, Internalized Psychopathology, and Externalized Psychopathology. About half of the children we studied demonstrated the first pattern of psychosocial functioning, with the remainder being divided between the latter two patterns.

Study 3

Although these three general patterns of psychosocial functioning are consistent with patterns of PIC profiles seen in clinical practice, experience suggests that a greater diversity of psychosocial functioning is, in fact, presented by children with LD. In the next study in this series (Fuerst, Fisk, & Rourke, 1990), we attempted to develop a more "fine-grained" typology of psychosocial functioning through the application of more sophisticated clustering techniques. We also used a slightly wider range of PIC scales in the cluster analysis to ensure that subtypes were formed on the basis of relatively complete, comprehensive PIC profiles. In this study we used the same 132 children that took part in the Fuerst et al. (1989) investigation.

In the Fuerst et al. (1990) study we found six, rather than three, subtypes within the sample that could be readily replicated using a variety of clustering methods. One subtype exhibited a mean PIC profile that suggested normal psychosocial functioning, with elevations only on scales related to academic and intellectual functioning, and was very strongly related to the Fuerst et al. (1989) Normal group (Figure 9.1). A second subtype was also relatively normal, with some indications of mild hyperactive or acting-out forms of behavior (Figure 9.5). A third subtype was characterized chiefly by elevation of the Somatic Concern scale (Figure 9.4). This subtype was not related to any of the three found in the Fuerst et al. (1989) study but was very similar to the Somatic Concern group found by Porter and Rourke (1985). Two of the subtypes were

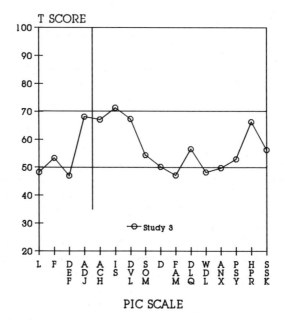

FIGURE 9.5. Mean PIC profile for the Mild Hyperactivity subtype.

related to the internalized psychopathology group found by Fuerst et al. (1989): one subtype showed evidence of mild anxiety and depression (Figure 9.6), whereas the other showed evidence of severe internalized psychopathology (Figure 9.2). Finally, an Externalized Psychopathology or hyperactive subtype, very similar to the one found in the Fuerst et al. (1989) study (Figure 9.3), was in evidence.

Study 4

The last set of data to be reviewed here are actually the preliminary results of a more comprehensive investigation still in progress (Fuerst & Rourke, in preparation). One purpose of this study was to replicate the subtypes found by Fuerst et al. (1990) in a large and diverse sample of children. In this study, we selected 500 children between the ages of 6 and 12 years with normal psychometric intelligence and, to ensure an adequate sample of psychopathology, at least one PIC clinical scale score greater than 70 *T*. The subjects were clustered by the *k*-means method using the same PIC scales that were employed by Fuerst et al. (1990). Six subtypes emerged in this investigation, five of which were extremely similar to the subtypes found in the Fuerst et al. (1990) study (Normal, Somatic Concern, Mild Anxiety, Internalized Psychopathology, and Externalized Psychopathology or Hyperactive). In the Fuerst and Rourke (in preparation) study, a Mild Hyperactive group was not found; however, a sixth subtype did have a mean PIC profile suggestive of conduct disorder (Figure 9.7).

Summary of Studies 1 through 4

The results of the four studies reviewed above are summarized schematically in Figure 9.8. Each box on the chart represents a subtype derived from the study noted in the leftmost column of the figure. Within each box is a descriptive label that characterizes the mean PIC profile of the subtype, a single digit that refers to the subtype number in that particular study (for use when referring to the original paper), and, in the lower right corner, the relative size of the subtype expressed as a percentage of the subjects classified within the study. Correlations between corresponding subtypes across studies appear on the connecting lines. Note that although some of the subtypes are arranged hierarchically, this order is based on the temporal course or our research and is not meant to imply

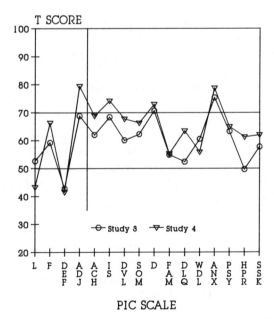

FIGURE 9.6. Mean PIC profiles for the Mild Anxiety subtype.

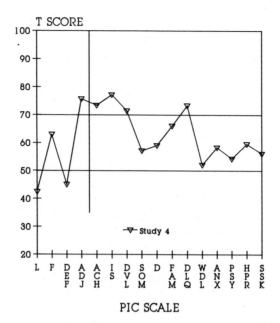

PIC SCALE

FIGURE 9.7. Mean PIC profile for the Conduct Disorder subtype.

that such a hierarchical division does, in fact, exist. Whether certain broad categories of psychosocial functioning can be usefully and accurately divided into subcategories, as implied by the figure, can only be determined by further research.

When the results of the four studies are considered, it is apparent that three, or perhaps four, of the subtypes are readily replicable using different samples, statistical techniques, and selection of PIC scales. Perhaps the most reliable subtype we have found is the Externalized Psychopathology or hyperactive group. This subtype has been found in all four studies, and, in all four studies, the subtype has been quite consistent in terms of both profile shape and relative size. The second most consistent subtype has been the Internalized Psychopathology group. Although this group has been quite consistent in terms of relative size across studies, there have been some very minor variations in mean PIC profile shape.

The third most consistent subtype has been the Normal group. Although the PIC profile shape of this group has been very consistent across studies, the relative size of the group decreases markedly when (1) more PIC scales are used to form subtypes and, as a result, (2) a greater number of subtypes are formed. (It is also clear that adding the requirement of at least one PIC scale elevation above 70 *T*, as we did in the Fuerst

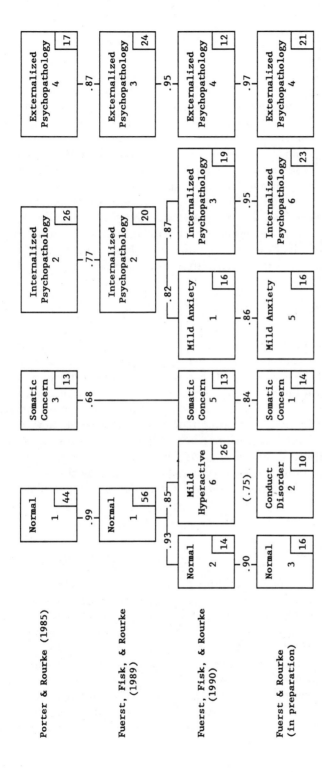

FIGURE 9.8. Summary of the psychosocial typologies developed in the Porter and Rourke (1985), Fuerst, Fisk, and Rourke (1989), Fuerst, Fisk, and Rourke (1990), and Fuerst and Rourke (in preparation) studies.

and Rourke [in preparation] study, has the effect of reducing the relative size of the Normal group.) This suggests that as finer discriminations are made between patterns of psychosocial functioning, subjects who might be classified as Normal in relatively coarse typologies do show some differences, perhaps contributing (to an as yet unknown extent) to Mild Hyperactive, Conduct Disorder, or Mild Anxiety groups. Finally, although a Somatic Concern subtype was not found in the Fuerst et al. (1989) study, this group has been found in three separate samples of children and may be reliable. However, in a previous study (Rourke, Pohlman, Fuerst, Porter, & Fisk, 1985), we found that the Normal and Somatic Concern subtypes of Porter and Rourke (1985) could not be differentiated on the basis of PIC factor scales. Greater confidence in the reliability of this subtype will depend on replication in yet another sample of children.

External Validity

Although demonstrating the reliability of a typology is a crucial step in subtyping research, reliability *per se* provides little information on which to evaluate a typology. It is possible to develop statistical typologies that are extremely reliable yet provide no useful information about the phenomena under investigation. A useful typology must provide a framework within which existing hypotheses can be tested, new relationships discerned, and conclusions reached that have at least some degree of clinical significance (Fletcher, 1985). Quite simply, a useful typology is one that is meaningful. The following are a series of observations that would lead us to the conclusion that the typologies that we have developed are valid.

Clinical Interpretability

One relatively simple manner in which external validity can be assessed is determining whether subtypes are interpretable and consonant with patterns of behavior observed in clinical settings (Del Dotto & Rourke, 1985). In this respect, the groups derived in the studies reviewed above appear to be valid. The mean PIC profiles of all groups are readily interpretable within the guidelines set forth in the PIC manual (Wirt et al., 1977). In addition, these profiles are consistent with general patterns of PIC profiles seen in clinical practice. The similarity between the Hyperactive subtype and the Breen and Barkley (1983) PIC profiles also provides modest additional evidence for the external validity of that subtype.

Concurrent Validity

Of course, such a cursory examination of a typology provides only limited support for external validity. To establish the external validity of a typology, it is necessary to demonstrate that subtypes differ in a meaningful and predictable manner on measures outside the domain of those used to develop the typology (Fletcher, 1985). For example, if subtypes are developed from patterns of reading, spelling, and arithmetic achievement, there is little point to demonstrating that the subtypes differ on the same, or similar, measures of reading, spelling, and arithmetic performance. Instead, evidence for external validity must be obtained by demonstrating subtype differences on measures of behaviors that (1) might reasonably be assumed to be independent of those used to derive the typology and (2), for theoretical reasons, might be related.

The Strang and Rourke (1985) Study

This investigation provides an example of external validation that is both interesting and relevant to the topic of this chapter. In this study, the investigators selected children with LD so as to comprise three subtypes of a previously derived, *a priori* typology based on patterns of Wide Range Achievement Test (WRAT; Jastak & Jastak, 1965) performance. One subtype showed uniformly deficient WRAT Reading, Spelling, and Arithmetic (Group 1). A second subtype had poor Reading and Spelling scores relative to Arithmetic (Group 2). The third subtype demonstrated deficient Arithmetic scores relative to their Reading and Spelling performance (Group 3). Based on their clinical experience and previous studies (see Rourke, 1989, and Strang & Rourke, 1985, for details), the investigators predicted that the Group 3 children would show greater evidence of psychopathology than would either Group 1 or Group 2 children.

Mean PIC profiles for the three groups were then calculated and compared. The mean PIC profiles of Group 1 and Group 2 subjects were typical of the majority of children with LD and suggested normal psychosocial adjustment and functioning. The mean PIC profile of Group 3, however, showed a significant elevation on the Adjustment and Psychosis scales and lesser but noteworthy elevations on those scales comprising the Psychopathology–Internalization factor identified by Wirt et al. (1977). It should be noted that the PIC profile of Group 3 was quite similar to the PIC profiles of the Internalized Psychopathology subtype identified in the studies reviewed above, whereas the profiles of Group 1 and Group 2 were very similar to the Normal subtype derived in those studies.

Clearly, a child's performance on WRAT Reading, Spelling, and Arithmetic bears no direct relationship to the caretaker's responses on the PIC: The domains measured are quite different. However, "different," in this instance, does not mean entirely independent. Strang and Rourke (1985) demonstrated the external validity of the WRAT-derived subtypes by showing that the subtypes differed on measures of psychosocial functioning and, as a consequence, demonstrated that psychosocial functioning and performance on academic, and perhaps cognitive, measures might be related in some manner.

Studies 3 and 4

This issue was a central concern in both the Fuerst et al. (1990) and Fuerst and Rourke (in preparation) investigations. However, in these studies we took the opposite approach to that employed in the Strang and Rourke (1985) investigation in that we first attempted to develop a psychosocial typology (using the PIC and statistical methods) and then examined the manner in which these subtypes differed on cognitive and academic measures. In Fuerst et al. (1990), the subjects were selected so as to comprise three (equal-sized) groups with distinctly different patterns of Wechsler Intelligence Scale for Children (WISC; Wechsler, 1949), Verbal IQ (VIQ), and Performance IQ (PIQ) scores. One group had VIQ greater than PIQ by at least 10 points (VIQ > PIQ), a second had VIQ less than PIQ by at least 10 points (VIQ < PIQ), and a third had VIQ–PIQ scores within 9 points of each other. The frequencies of these three groups within each psychosocial subtype were calculated and compared (see Figure 9.9).

We found that within the Normal subtype, children with VIQ > PIQ were found at a much lower frequency (roughly 6% of the subtype) than either children with the opposite pattern of VIQ–PIQ discrepancy or those with no significant difference between VIQ and PIQ. This was also the case in the Mild Anxiety subtype. In this subtype, subjects with VIQ > PIQ were found at a rate significantly below expectation (about 5% of the subtype). In the Mild Hyperactivity subtype, the frequencies of subjects from the three VIQ–PIQ groups were approximately equal. These results indicated that, overall, within normal and mildly disturbed subtypes of children with LD, there was a tendency for VIQ > PIQ children to occur at lower frequencies than do VIQ = PIQ or VIQ < PIQ children. There were only about half as many VIQ > PIQ children in these three groups as there were VIQ = PIQ or VIQ < PIQ children.

In the Internalized Psychopathology subtype, subjects with VIQ = PIQ were found at significantly lower than expected frequencies (about

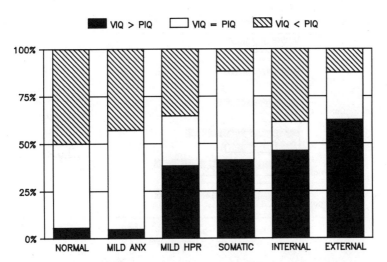

FIGURE 9.9. Proportions of subjects with VIQ > PIQ, VIQ = PIQ, and VIQ <
PIQ in the subtypes developed in the Fuerst, Fisk, and Rourke (1990) study.

15% of the subtype). On the other hand, subjects with VIQ > PIQ were
found at a higher frequency than would be expected (roughly 46% of the
subtype) and at a higher frequency than VIQ < PIQ subjects (39%).
Within the Externalized Psychopathology subtype, subjects with VIQ >
PIQ were found at a much higher frequency (about 63%) than were children with either VIQ = PIQ or VIQ < PIQ. Thus, unlike the normal and
mildly disturbed groups, within subtypes showing severe psychosocial
disturbance, there was a tendency for VIQ > PIQ subjects to be found at
higher frequencies than either the VIQ = PIQ or VIQ < PIQ subjects. In
total there were about twice as many VIQ > PIQ children in these two
groups as there were VIQ = PIQ or VIQ < PIQ children.

In the Fuerst and Rourke (in preparation) investigation, we examined the differences between subtypes on WRAT Reading, Spelling, and
Arithmetic standard scores (Figure 9.10). Overall, the six subtypes were
indiscriminable on WRAT Arithmetic. However, there were significant
differences between some of the groups on WRAT Reading and Spelling.
The Externalized Psychopathology and Internalized Psychopathology
groups had mean WRAT Reading scores that were significantly higher
than the scores of the Somatization and Normal groups. Similarly, the
Externalized and Internalized Psychopathology subtypes scored higher
on WRAT Spelling than did the Conduct Disorder and Normal groups,
and the Internalized Psychopathology group also scored higher than did
the Somatization group.

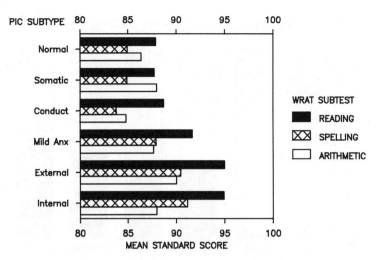

FIGURE 9.10. Mean WRAT Reading, Spelling, and Arithmetic scores for the subtypes found in Fuerst and Rourke (in preparation).

These findings were echoed when WRAT Reading, Spelling, and Arithmetic were simultaneously considered in a canonical discriminant analysis. The first canonical function was significant, providing better than chance discrimination between the groups. When the standardized scoring coefficients for this function were considered, it was apparent that scores on this variable were virtually simple sums of WRAT Reading and Spelling scores (i.e., approximately equal weights), with Arithmetic playing a trivial role. Examination of group means on the canonical variables (Figure 9.11) indicated that the Normal, Somatization, and Conduct Disorder groups were indistinguishable on this variable. These three groups were, however, clearly separated from the higher-scoring Externalized and Internalized Psychopathology groups, which appeared to form a second "clump" on their own. The Mild Anxiety group fell about midway between these two sets of groups.

These results suggest that clinic-referred, primarily LD children with relatively well-developed reading and spelling skills are more likely to appear in PIC subtypes with profiles suggestive of severe psychopathology, be it of the internalizing or externalizing type. On the other hand, children with relatively mild somatization or conduct disorder problems are indistinguishable from normal children on the basis of academic skills. Children with symptoms of mild anxiety and depression appear to fall between these two extremes and cannot be clearly distinguished from either of these two sets of groups using these academic measures.

We also compared the groups on differences between WRAT Reading (R) and Spelling (S) versus Arithmetic (A) scores (R — A and S — A). Overall, the Internalized Psychopathology group showed not only the largest absolute difference on each measure but also deficient Arithmetic relative to both Reading and Spelling. Specifically, on the R — A measure, the Internalized Psychopathology group was significantly different from the Somatization group; on the S — A measure they were significantly different from the Normal group. None of the other subtypes could be differentiated on either R — A or S — A.

The implications of the results of the Fuerst et al. (1990) and Fuerst and Rourke (in preparation) studies appear to be fairly straightforward. First, as patterns of WRAT scores are also known to be associated with patterns of WISC VIQ–PIQ discrepancies in children with LD (Rourke, Dietrich, & Young, 1973; Rourke & Finlayson, 1978; Rourke, Young, & Flewelling, 1971), it is not surprising that the results of the Fuerst and Rourke (in preparation) study are consistent with the findings of the Fuerst et al. (1990) study. Considering the results of the two studies, it appears that psychosocial functioning of children with LD is indeed related to cognitive functioning and that children with relatively well-developed psycholinguistic skills may be at greater risk for serious socio-

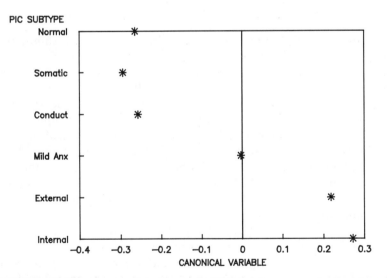

FIGURE 9.11. Mean scores of the Fuerst and Rourke (in preparation) subtypes on a canonical discriminant function derived from WRAT Reading, Spelling, and Arithmetic standard scores.

emotional problems than are children who are relatively less adept in linguistic skills. Contrary to a commonly held notion, relatively deficient linguistic skills do not appear to be related to seriously disordered psychosocial functioning in children with LD. However, the certainty with which this assertion can be made is dependent on the degree to which psycholinguistic abilities are associated with WISC Verbal IQ and with WRAT Reading and Spelling scores. Although from previous research we know that WRAT Reading and Spelling measures are associated with verbal and auditory–perceptual skills of children with LD (Rourke et al., 1971, 1973; Rourke & Finlayson, 1978), further investigation using more direct and detailed measures of auditory–perceptual and linguistic functioning is required in order to have greater confidence in this conclusion.

Second, our finding that the Internalized Psychopathology subtype showed the largest R − A and S − A values, with Arithmetic always being the lower score, suggests that *patterns* of cognitive strengths and deficits may be associated with type of pathology in addition to level of pathology as discussed above. This particular result is in accord with previous findings (Strang & Rourke, 1985) and lends some support to clinically and theoretically based arguments that nonverbal learning disabilities may eventuate in pathological psychosocial functioning of that type (Rourke, 1982, 1987, 1988a, 1988b, 1989).

Conclusions and Future Directions

The results of the four studies reviewed in this chapter can be summarized in the following eight points:

1. Children with LD are heterogeneous in terms of psychosocial functioning. There is no unique LD personality type.

2. Statistical subtyping techniques can produce reliable and interpretable subgroups of children that are replicable across samples.

3. LD children seem to fall into three broad psychosocial subtypes, namely, Normal, Internalized Psychopathology, and Externalized Psychopathology. However, within this broad framework more subtle distinctions can be made. Additional subtypes characterized as Somatic Concern, Mild Anxiety, Mild Hyperactivity, and Conduct Disorder have been found in our samples.

4. Children with VIQ > PIQ by at least 10 points are (1) less likely to be found in normal or mildly disturbed psychosocial subtypes than are children with VIQ < PIQ or no substantial difference in IQ scores and (2) much more likely to be found in significantly disturbed psychosocial subtypes as compared to children with VIQ < PIQ or children showing no substantial difference in IQ scores.

5. Children with LD in significantly disturbed psychosocial subtypes tend to have higher WRAT Reading and Spelling standard scores than do children in relatively normal psychosocial subtypes. Children in the Mild Anxiety subtype tend to have WRAT Reading and Spelling scores about midway between these two sets of subtypes.

6. Considering points 4 and 5, children with LD having relatively well-developed linguistic skills seem to be at greater risk for the development of significant psychopathology than are children with less well-developed linguistic skills.

7. Children showing significant internalized psychopathology tend to have a larger discrepancy between WRAT Reading and Spelling versus Arithmetic, with the latter measure being lower relative to the other two, than do children in other subtypes.

8. Considering points 4 and 7, patterns of cognitive strengths and deficits appear to be related to *type* of psychopathology as well as to level of pathology. A pattern of good language skills (WRAT Reading and Spelling) but relatively poor arithmetic skills (WRAT Arithmetic) is associated with internalized psychopathology. This is consistent with expectations based on the Rourke (1989) nonverbal learning disabilities model.

Clearly, these four studies are only the initial steps on the road toward a full understanding of the psychosocial functioning of children with LD. There are many issues and avenues of investigation that have not yet been explored in our research. Some of these include the following:

1. Replication of the typology within a more diverse socioeconomic and cultural milieu is required. The children used in our studies have been relatively homogeneous in these respects.

2. There should be replication and validation using psychosocial measures other than the PIC. Although the PIC is an excellent clinical and investigative tool, other measures (such as behavior checklists, structured interviews, teacher reports, direct observation), perhaps used in conjunction with the PIC, might produce a typology that is more comprehensive and ecologically valid.

3. External validation using more precise measures of cognitive and neuropsychological functioning should be examined. The WISC and WRAT scales are complex multidetermined measures. The use of other, more specific neuropsychological instruments might allow for a more precise delineation of the relationships between cognitive and psychosocial functioning.

4. Development and validation of a psychosocial typology that includes the developmental dimension is required. To date, our studies have used subjects covering a relatively large age range; however, it is

clear that psychosocial functioning and manifestation of pathology can change with age (see Rourke, 1989, for detailed examples within the context of nonverbal learning disabilities). This might be addressed either with cross-sectional studies (i.e., the development of typologies at different age levels, as we are currently attempting to do) or, preferably, with longitudinal studies studying change in psychosocial status over time.

References

Breen, M. J., & Barkley, R. A. (1983). The Personality Inventory for Children (PIC): Its clinical utility with hyperactive children. *Journal of Pediatric Psychology, 8*, 359–366.
Del Dotto, J. E., & Rourke, B. P. (1985). Subtypes of left-handed learning-disabled children. In B. P. Rourke (Ed.), *Neuropsychology of learning disabilities: Essentials of subtype analysis* (pp. 89–130). New York: Guilford Press.
Everitt, B. (1980). *Cluster analysis.* New York: Halsted.
Fletcher, J. M. (1985). External validation of learning disabilities typologies. In B. P. Rourke (Ed.), *Neuropsychology of learning disabilities: Essentials of subtype analysis* (pp. 187–211). New York: Guilford Press.
Fuerst, D. R., Fisk, J. L., & Rourke, B. P. (1989). Psychosocial functioning of learning-disabled children: Replicability of statistically derived subtypes. *Journal of Consulting and Clinical Psychology, 57*, 275–280.
Fuerst, D. R., Fisk, J. L., & Rourke, B. P. (1990). Psychosocial functioning of learning-disabled children: Relationships between WISC Verbal IQ–Performance IQ discrepancies and personality subtypes. *Journal of Consulting and Clinical Psychology, 58*.
Fuerst, D. R., & Rourke, B. P. (in preparation). *Psychosocial functioning of learning-disabled children: Relationships between personality subtypes and achievement test scores.*
Jastak, J. F., & Jastak, S. R. (1965). *The Wide Range Achievement Test.* Wilmington, DE: Guidance Associates.
Porter, J. E., & Rourke, B. P. (1985). Socioemotional functioning of learning-disabled children: A subtypal analysis of personality patterns. In B. P. Rourke (Ed.), *Neuropsychology of learning disabilities: Essentials of subtype analysis* (pp. 257–279). New York: Guilford Press.
Rourke, B. P. (1982). Central processing deficiencies in children: Toward a developmental neuropsychological model. *Journal of Clinical Neuropsychology, 4*, 1–18.
Rourke, B. P. (1987). Syndrome of nonverbal learning disabilities: The final common pathway of white-matter disease/dysfunction?. *The Clinical Neuropsychologist, 1*, 209–234.
Rourke, B. P. (1988a). Socio-emotional disturbances of learning-disabled children. *Journal of Consulting and Clinical Psychology, 56*, 801–810.
Rourke, B. P. (1988b). The syndrome of nonverbal learning disabilities: Developmental manifestations in neurological disease, disorder, and dysfunction. *The Clinical Neuropsychologist, 2*, 293–330.
Rourke, B. P. (1989). *Nonverbal learning disabilities: The syndrome and the model.* New York: Guilford Press.
Rourke, B. P., Dietrich, D. M., & Young, G. C. (1973). Significance of WISC Verbal-

Performance discrepancies for younger children with learning disabilities. *Perceptual and Motor Skills, 36,* 275–282.

Rourke, B. P., & Finlayson, M. A. J. (1978). Neuropsychological significance of variations in patterns of academic performance: Verbal and visual-spatial abilities. *Journal of Abnormal Child Psychology, 6,* 121–133.

Rourke, B. P., Pohlman, C. L., Fuerst, D. R., Porter, J. E., & Fisk, J. L. (1985). Personality subtypes of learning-disabled children: Two validation studies. *Journal of Clinical and Experimental Neuropsychology, 7,* 157.

Rourke, B. P., Young, G. C., & Flewelling, R. W. (1971). The relationships between WISC Verbal–Performance discrepancies and selected verbal, auditory, perceptual, and problem-solving abilities in children with learning disabilities. *Journal of Clinical Psychology, 27,* 475–479.

Strang, J. D., & Rourke, B. P. (1985). Adaptive behavior of children with specific arithmetic disabilities and associated neuropsychological abilities and deficits. In B. P. Rourke (Ed.), *Neuropsychology of learning disabilities: Essentials of subtype analysis* (pp. 302–328). New York: Guilford Press.

Wechsler, D. (1949). *Wechsler Intelligence Scale for Children. Manual.* New York: Psychological Corporation.

Wirt, R. D., Lachar, D., Klinedinst, J. K., & Seat, P. D. (1977). *Multidimensional description of child personality: A manual for the Personality Inventory for Children.* Los Angeles: Western Psychological Services.

CHAPTER 10

Subtypes of Arithmetic-Disabled Children: Cognitive and Personality Dimensions

John W. DeLuca, Byron P. Rourke, and Jerel E. Del Dotto

As do disorders of reading and spelling, arithmetic disabilities pose significant barriers to the continued development of academic abilities in children. In many cases, investigators have chosen to focus on and enumerate isolated deficits associated with poor arithmetic performance (Badian, 1983; Badian & Ghublikian, 1983; McLeod & Crump, 1978; Siegel & Linder, 1984; Webster, 1979, 1980). In contrast, other investigators have described more global syndromes that include poor arithmetic skills as one symptom in the context of other strengths and weaknesses. For example, both the nonverbal learning disability (NLD; Rourke, 1987, 1988, 1989) and the developmental output failure (DOF; Levine, Oberklaid, & Meltzer, 1981) syndromes are associated with a poor capacity for mechanical arithmetic and intact reading (word recognition) skills.

Over the course of several years, Rourke and his associates (Rourke, 1982, 1987, 1988, 1989; Rourke & Finlayson, 1978; Rourke & Strang, 1978; Rourke, Young, & Leenaars, 1989; Rourke, Young, Strang, & Russell, 1986; Strang & Rourke, 1983, 1985a, 1985b) have written extensively on the nature of the NLD child. Academically, these children are defined by impoverished arithmetic abilities in the context of well-developed word recognition and written spelling skills. They exhibit a constellation of neuropsychological deficits involving the following: poorer Performance IQ relative to Verbal IQ on the Wechsler Intelligence Scale for Children (WISC) or the Wechsler Intelligence Scale for Children—Revised (WISC-R); bilateral tactile–perceptual deficits and psychomotor coordination difficulties, both of which are often more marked on the left side of the body; outstanding deficiencies on tasks involving visual–spatial organization and synthesis; clear deficits in nonverbal concept formation, hypothesis testing, ability to benefit from immediate feedback, and problem solving; and very well-developed rote verbal capacities and rote verbal memory skills.

The appreciation of cause–effect relationships, humor, and the ability to adapt to novel or otherwise abstract or complex situations are also problematic for the NLD child (Rourke, 1982, 1987, 1988, 1989). For example, Ozols and Rourke (1985) reported that children classified in a manner that reflected some significant dimensions of the NLD syndrome had difficulties in interpreting visual–perceptual input relevant to social perception, comprehension, and interaction (e.g., nonverbal cues such as facial expressions, hand movements, body postures, and other physical gestures). Although the verbal skills of NLD children are relatively well developed, their verbal expressions tend to be of a repetitive, straightforward, and rote nature. Their language is characterized by poor psycholinguistic content, pragmatics, and speech prosody. These children often overrely on language as their principal means for social relating, information gathering, and relief from anxiety. Social isolation and poor self-concept are common. NLD children are often considered to be at risk for emotional disturbances and "internalized" forms of psychopathology (e.g., depression, withdrawal, isolation, and anxiety; Rourke, 1989; Rourke et al., 1989; Strang & Rourke, 1985a, 1985b).

Other investigators have offered somewhat different descriptions of arithmetic-disabled children with intact reading skills. For example, Levine et al. (1981) identified a type of learning disability referred to as developmental output failure. Twenty-six children (10 to 14 years of age) were selected on the basis of the following criteria: (1) complaints of low productivity in school by parents and teachers; (2) average to above-average level of intellectual functioning; and, (3) reading skills at or near grade level. The mean age of the children was 12 years, 10 months; there were 23 males and 3 females in the group. Very few of the children experienced difficulty in the mechanics of reading, such as decoding, word analysis, sight vocabulary, or speed of reading. Delays of less than 12 months in reading were evidenced by slightly more than one-half of the group. However, problems in mechanical arithmetic, spelling, and reading comprehension were often more pronounced. All children exhibited difficulties in writing and/or written expression (Levine et al., 1981).

The following deficiencies (and percentages of children exhibiting them) were found to characterize DOF children (Levine et al., 1981): poor fine-motor and pencil control skills (72%); finger agnosia (50%); poor visual retrieval skills (80%); difficulties in sequential memory (36%); deficiencies in expressive language (36%); and poor selective attention and concentration skills (60%).

Problems in visual retrieval were considered to be associated with deficiencies in the following areas: visual recall, the revisualization of patterns and shapes, and the accurate and automatic retrieval of letter and/or word configurations. Levine et al. (1981) consider the latter skills to be essential for fast and effective spelling and writing. Difficulties in sequential memory included problems in storing and retrieving sequences of information, in arranging letters in the appropriate order, in carrying out series of processes in arithmetic calculation, and/or in remembering and following multiple-step instructions.

Levine et al. (1981) contend that DOF is not meant to describe a new syndome but is a framework for delineating a heterogeneous group of unproductive middle-school children. According to Levine et al. (1981), a transition occurs at about the fourth grade level (at approximately 9 years of age). Prior to this age, learning is fairly passive and relies heavily on the decoding of symbols and ideas. However, as the children progress to the later grades, they encounter increased demands for output and encoding (e.g., writing tasks, oral reports, organization of projects, complex arithmetic assignments, and the integration of information from multiple sources). DOF children are often unable to respond effectively to these increased demands. Instead, they develop poor work and study habits, organizational difficulties, an inefficient use of time, a loss of interest in school, an inability or reluctance to complete homework, and lowered self-esteem and/or self-confidence (Levine et al., 1981). As a result, these children are often misdiagnosed as being lazy, poorly motivated, emotionally disturbed, or as exhibiting attitudinal problems (Levine, 1984).

Siegel and Feldman (1983) described a group of 29 children between 7 and 13 years of age whom they believe exhibit DOF. All children obtained WISC-R Full Scale IQs above 79 and Wide Range Achievement Test (WRAT) Arithmetic centile scores less than 26. These children evidenced a constellation of symptoms including the following: difficulty in completing assignments, trouble with written work, organizational problems, poor eye–hand coordination, visuomotor and graphomotor problems, and compromised short-term memory capabilities. Reading skills were age-appropriate. However, the degree to which spelling tasks consistently pose similar problems for this particular group of children is less clear. Siegel and Feldman (1983) contend that arithmetic disability is an underestimated component of DOF. More specifically, poor eye–hand coordination (especially with respect to written work) and short-term memory skills were thought to be especially implicated.

Although the DOF children described by Levine et al. (1981) share some of the elements characteristic of the NLD syndrome (e.g., poor eye–

hand coordination, organizational problems, deficient arithmetic skills, finger agnosia, and poor self-concept), they appear to be uniquely different with respect to their patterns of academic performances. That is to say, mechanical arithmetic is the sole area of deficiency for the NLD child, while written spelling performance is typically above an age-expectancy level. In contrast, DOF children are quite likely to encounter difficulties in both arithmetic and written spelling achievement. This being the case, it may be that children who are experiencing problems in arithmetic alone are quite different with respect to their neuropsychological and personality functioning from children who are encountering problems in both mechanical arithmetic and written spelling areas.

In addition to differences evident between NLD and DOF children, the DOF syndrome itself is quite heterogeneous. For example, only 36% of the DOF children evidenced deficiencies in either sequential memory or expressive language skills (Levine et al., 1981). Moreover, the description of attention and concentration symptoms provided by Levine et al. (1981) is still quite broad: It includes distractibility, impulsivity, and overactivity as well as proneness to fatigue and a lack of persistence in completing tasks. It may be that two different DOF subgroups exist. One DOF subgroup may exhibit primary deficits in memory retrieval, in revisualization, and in spelling. They may also exhibit a lack of persistence to complete tasks and proneness to fatigue. A second subgroup might be characterized by problems in sequencing, in completing multistep operations, in planning, in verbal expression, and in visuo-motor and psychomotor skills. Poor impulse-control skills may also be apparent.

We carried out a study to determine whether these alternative formulations could be validated (DeLuca, Del Dotto, & Rourke, 1987). We reasoned that if all of these formulations were true, different subtypes of children who exhibit adequate word recognition and deficient arithmetic would emerge. The purposes of the DeLuca et al. (1987) study were as follows: (1) to determine whether a sample of arithmetic-disabled children with intact reading skills is heterogeneous with respect to their patterns of academic performances on the WRAT Reading, Spelling, and Arithmetic subtests (Jastak & Jastak, 1978); (2) if this sample of children were shown to be heterogeneous, to determine if the results are replicable using additional subjects in a split-half sample comparison; and (3) to determine if these subtypes could be validated externally by comparing their patterns of neuropsychological skills, their ratings on the Personality Inventory for Children (PIC; Lachar & Gdowski, 1979; Wirt, Lachar, Klinedinst, & Seat, 1977), and their ratings on the Behavior Problem

Checklist (Quay & Peterson, 1979) and an Activity Rating Scale (Werry, 1968). More specifically, it was hypothesized that three distinct but somewhat overlapping groups of children would emerge, as follows.

Subtypes of Arithmetic-Disabled Children

Subtype A

This group of children was expected to exhibit patterns of performance similar to those characterizing NLD children as summarized by Rourke (1987, 1988, 1989). The latter includes well-developed reading and spelling skills in the context of poor mechanical arithmetic. It was thought that they would obtain the highest ratings on the PIC Psychosis and Social Skills scales.

Subtype B

This group was expected to evidence performances similar to the DOF children described by Levine et al., 1981) who experience particular difficulty in memory retrieval, in revisualization, and in spelling. It was thought that both spelling and arithmetic performances would be compromised while reading skills would be age-appropriate. On the parental ratings of the PIC, it was thought that these children would evidence elevations on the Depression, Withdrawal, and Anxiety scales. It was thought that they would evidence low scores on both the Behavior Problem Checklist and the Activity Rating Scale.

Subtype C

This group was expected to have performances similar to the DOF children described by Levine et al. (1981) who evidenced problems in sequencing, in completing multistep operations, in planning, in verbal expression, in visuomotor and psychomotor abilities, and in impulse-control skills. It was thought that they would exhibit intact reading skills, mildly deficient spelling, and poor arithmetic skills. Significant elevations on the PIC Delinquency and Hyperactivity scales, the Behavior Problem Checklist, and the Activity Rating Scale were also expected.

Finally, several hypotheses regarding appropriate remedial strategies are offered for each subtype. The latter serves only as a heuristic framework.

Method

Subjects

A group of 156 children exhibiting WRAT Arithmetic centile scores less than 27 and Reading centile scores greater than 40 were culled from a data base of over 4,800 children who had been referred to a multiservice mental health clinic because of suspected central processing deficiencies. All 156 children were between the ages of 9 and 14 years, obtained Full Scale IQs between 85 and 115 on the WISC (Wechsler, 1949), and were free of any visual or auditory acuity deficiencies and any known or suspected environmental deprivation. All children spoke English as their primary language.

All children underwent a comprehensive neuropsychological evaluation that was administered in a standardized manner by highly trained neuropsychology technicians.

Cluster Analysis

Cluster analysis, rather than clinical-inferential subtyping, was selected as the method of choice in order to preclude the acceptance of *a priori* assumptions with respect to the degree of homogeneity present in this sample. That is, it was felt that the optimal number of clusters or subtypes should be determined more by the actual structure of the data than by some preconceived notion. WRAT subtest standard scores were chosen as cluster variables following Satz and Morris's (1981) suggestion that cluster analysis be used to identify subtypes of learning-disabled children based on patterns of academic performances prior to the analysis of neuropsychological data. They indicated that attempts to identify the hidden structure of complex data sets dictate that classification techniques be applied initially in order to provide more objective criteria for identifying subtypes based on patterns of academic performance.

In addition to concerns with respect to subject and variable selection, Morris, Blashfield, and Satz (1981) outlined several decision points important to the use of cluster analysis. These include choice of similarity measure, type of cluster method, determination of the optimal number of clusters, and validation.

Of the several types of similarity measures discussed by Aldenderfer and Blashfield (1984), only two were considered here: squared euclidean distance (SED) and correlation coefficient (CC). Advantages and disadvantages are associated with each type. For example, use of the CC tends to emphasize profile shape, while it disregards elevation. On the other hand, SED tends to emphasize level of performance and ignores, to some degree, profile shape. Moreover, distance measures may tend to emphasize level of performance even when it is not relevant (Adams, 1985).

With respect to the choice of clustering method, the consensus of most researchers is that no one clustering method can be considered the "best" in all situations. Since a single set of scores analyzed by two different methods can result in entirely different solutions, Everitt (1974) suggested the use of several clustering techniques. Several clustering methods are available, and the advantages and disadvantages of each are discussed in detail elsewhere (Blashfield & Morey, 1980; Edelbrock, 1979; Edelbrock & McLaughlin, 1980; Everitt, 1974; Mezzich, 1978; Milligan, 1980; Milligan & Cooper, 1987; Morey, Blashfield, & Skinner, 1983; Morris et al., 1981).

In this instance, the WRAT data were subjected to three hierarchical clustering techniques (i.e., complete linkage, centroid, and Ward's method) using both CC and SED as similarity measures (CLUSTAN, Version 1C2; Wishart, 1978). However, only SED was utilized in conjunction with Ward's method (Wishart, 1978). Ward's method and centroid sorting techniques (using SED) were chosen primarily because of the high correlation among the WRAT subtests and the high degree of sensitivity of these combinations of methods to elevation (or levels of performance) in the data set (Satz & Morris, 1981). More specifically, since the WRAT preselection criteria imposed strict limitations on the range of possible subtest centile scores (i.e., Reading 40–99; Spelling 0–99; and Arithmetic 0–27), it was felt that cluster techniques and similarity measures that emphasized level of performance differences would be the most appropriate. Other cluster method/similarity measure combinations were included in order to determine if the cluster solutions would be replicated across several different techniques.

For each combination of cluster method and similarity measure, an iterative relocation procedure was used in order to clarify the cluster solutions (CLUSTAN, Version 1C2, procedure RELOCATE; Wishart, 1978). This procedure reexamines each cluster solution in order to determine if any subjects should be reclassified into another cluster. Statistically, this method is used to minimize within-cluster variance and to maximize between-cluster variance. To circumvent the problem of finding a "global optimum" solution, two relocation "starting positions" were employed (Wishart, 1978): a size difference classification array and a random initial configuration. The percentage of subjects reclassified for any single method is thought to provide an index of the stability of the solution (Morris et al., 1981); however, there are some problems associated with this procedure (DeLuca, Adams, & Rourke, in press; DeLuca, Adams, & Rourke, Chapter 3, this volume).

Another problem in cluster analysis involves the difficulty in deciding the correct number of clusters for a given data set. Two commonly used techniques or indicators were employed in the present study: examination of the dendogram (or mapping of the data) and plotting of the clustering coefficients (Everitt, 1974; Morris et al., 1981).

In order to answer the first experimental question, the WRAT Reading, Spelling, and Arithmetic standard scores were subjected to several hierarchical clustering techniques using CLUSTAN (Wishart, 1978).

Internal Validity (Reliability)

Several methods were suggested by Morris et al. (1981) to determine the "internal validity" (reliability) of cluster solutions. In order to address the second experimental question, two methods were chosen for use in the present study: (1) the inclusion of additional subjects (all of which meet the constraints of the original sample selection criteria) in the data set and (2) the clustering of split-half samples. A series of cluster analyses identical to those employed with the initial sample were utilized in conjunction with split-half samples obtained from the extended data set (n = 194).

External Validity

Concurrent validation of the obtained subtypes involved the use of external criterion measures (i.e., variables not used in the initial classification): 22 neuropsychological measures and selected clinical scales for the PIC.

TEST MEASURES

Table 10.1 contains a list of the measures included in the neuropsychological test battery. The battery was composed of measures thought to represent various adaptive skill areas outlined by Reitan (1974) and has been described in detail elsewhere (Reitan, 1966; Rourke, Bakker, Fisk, & Strang, 1983; Rourke, Fisk, & Strang, 1986). These include tactile–perceptual and tactile–kinesthetic abilities; visuomotor, visual–perceptual, and visual–spatial skills; sequential processing abilities; auditory–perceptual and language related abilities; simple motor and psychomotor skills; and conceptual reasoning and nonverbal problem-solving capacities.

The criteria for selecting neuropsychological test variables were identical to those outlined by Fisk and Rourke (1979). That is, (1) the

TABLE 10.1. List of Variables by Category

Auditory-verbal
*1. WISC Information Subtest (INF)
 2. WISC Comprehension Subtest
 3. WISC Similarities Subtest
*4. WISC Vocabulary Subtest (VOC)
 5. Peabody Picture Vocabulary IQ
 6. Auditory Imperception and Suppression—Right
 7. Auditory Imperception and Suppression—Left
*8. Speech-Sounds Perception Test (SSP)
 9. Auditory Closure Test
*10. Sentence Memory Test (SEN)
*11. Verbal Fluency Test (VFL)

Sequencing
*12. WISC Arithmetic Subtest (ART)
*13. WISC Digit Span Subtest (DIG)
*14. WISC Coding Subtest (COD)
 15. Seashore Rhythm Test

Visual-spatial
*16. WISC Picture Completion Subtest (PIC)
*17. WISC Picture Arrangement Subtest (PAR)
*18. WISC Block Design Subtest (BKD)
 19. WISC Object Assembly Subtest
 20. Visual Imperception and Suppression—Right
 21. Visual Imperception and Suppression—Left
*22. Target Test (TAR)
*23. Trails A (TRA)

Tactile
 24. Tactile Imperception and Suppression—Right Hand
 25. Tactile Imperception and Suppression—Left Hand
 26. Tactile Finger Recognition—Right Hand
 27. Tactile Finger Recognition—Left Hand
*28. Tactile Finger Recognition—Mean (FGA)
 29. Fingertip Number Writing—Right Hand
 30. Fingertip Number Writing—Left Hand
*31. Fingertip Number Writing—Mean (FTW)
 32. Tactile Coin Recognition—Right Hand
 33. Tactile Coin Recognition—Left Hand
 34. Tactile Coin Recognition—Mean

 35. Tactual Performance Test—Right Hand
 36. Tactual Performance Test—Left Hand
*37. Tactual Performance Test—Mean (TPM)
*38. Tactual Performance Test—Both Hands (TPB)
 39. Tactual Performance Test—Memory
 40. Tactual Performance Test—Location

 41. Finger Tapping Test—Right Hand
 42. Finger Tapping Test—Left Hand
*43. Finger Tapping Test—Mean (TAP)
 44. Foot Tapping Test—Right Foot

(continued)

TABLE 10.1. (Continued)

45. Foot Tapping Test—Left Foot
46. Dynamometer—Right Hand
47. Dynamometer—Left Hand
48. Grooved Pegboard Test—Right Hand
49. Grooved Pegboard Test—Left Hand
*50. Grooved Pegboard Test—Mean (PEG)
51. Maze Time—Right Hand
52. Maze Counter—Right Hand
53. Maze Speed—Right Hand
54. Maze Time—Left Hand
55. Maze Counter—Left Hand
56. Maze Speed—Left Hand
*57. Maze Time—Mean (MAZ)
58. Maze Counter—Mean
59. Maze Speed—Mean
60. Holes Time—Right Hand
61. Holes Counter—Right Hand
62. Holes Time—Left Hand
63. Holes Counter—Left Hand
64. Holes Time—Mean
65. Holes Counter—Mean
66. Name Writing Speed—Right Hand
67. Name Writing Speed—Left Hand

Academic
68. WRAT Reading Subtest (READSS)
69. WRAT Spelling Subtest (SPELSS)
70. WRAT Arithmetic Subtest (ARITSS)

Abstract-conceptual; other
*71. Category Test (CAT)
*72. Trails B (TRB)

Personality/behavior
*73. PIC Lie scale (LIE)
*74. PIC Frequency scale (FREQ)
*75. PIC Defensiveness scale (DEF)
*76. PIC Adjustment scale (ADJ)
*77. PIC Achievement scale (ACH)
*78. PIC Intellectual Screening scale (IS)
*79. PIC Development scale (DVL)
*80. PIC Somatic Concern scale (SOM)
*81. PIC Depression scale (DEP)
*82. PIC Family Relations scale (FAM)
*83. PIC Delinquency scale (DLQ)
*84. PIC Withdrawal scale (WDL)
*85. PIC Anxiety scale (ANX)
*86. PIC Psychosis scale (PSY)
*87. PIC Hyperactivity scale (HPR)
*88. PIC Social Skills scale (SSK)
*89. Activity Rating Scale (ARS)
*90. Behavior Problem Checklist (BPC)

Note. * indicates variables selected for analysis.

selected variables were thought to represent the lowest possible intercorrelations between test measures within an individual skill area; (2) the number of tests selected was to be approximately the same within each adaptive skill area; and (3) the selected variables were chosen to reflect a reasonably high degree of clinical explanatory potential. Prior to any statistical analysis, all raw data were converted to T-scores (with a mean equal to 50 and a standard deviation equal to 10; higher scores are representative of better performances) based on age-appropriate normative data (Knights, 1970; Knights & Moule, 1967, 1968; Knights & Norwood, 1980).

One important consideration with respect to the choice of sensorimotor variables is the problem of having measures for both the right and left sides of the body. Francis, Fletcher, and Rourke (1988) suggested combining scores from the right- and left-hand versions of the same test in order to increase test reliability and eliminate problems of test-specific relationships caused by the inclusion of doublet scores. In the present study, composite scores for sensorimotor tests were calculated by computing a mean T-score based on the right- and left-hand measures for each test.

With respect to PIC variables, only T-score data from the clinical scales were used for subsequent analyses. The validity scales were not employed because they represent primarily the test-taking attitude of the respondent and not actual behavioral ratings of the child. In the case of the Behavior Problem Checklist and the Activity Rating Scale, raw scores were utilized; no age-appropriate normative data were available for these scales.

Two methods were employed to address the third experimental question involving the concurrent validity of the resulting subtype solutions. The first was to use separate multivariate and univariate analyses (SAS, PROC GLM; SAS Institute, 1985) of the neuropsychological, personality, and behavioral rating data. The second was a visual inspection and comparison of the mean T-score profiles for the neuropsychological and personality variables.

Results

Cluster Analysis

Initial application of the cluster-analytic technique to the data set suggested the presence of several subtypes within the target sample that differed from one another in terms of their performances on academic measures. Plots of the cluster coefficients for the several cluster methods employed suggested an optimal solution of four clusters. Cluster coefficients for the various method/similarity metric combinations are presented in Table 10.2. Table 10.3 represents the WRAT standard score means and standard deviations for the various cluster solutions using squared euclidean distance. In general, these solutions appear to be quite similar and suggest a rather stable four-cluster solution.

The results of the clustering solutions using correlation as a metric of similarity are not reported for several reasons. The results (1) were not consistent across methods, (2) were inconsistent with the clustering solutions utilizing squared euclidean distance, and (3) evidenced rather large percentages of reclassified subjects following the use of iterative relocation methods. Of the several combinations of cluster methods, similarity measures, and iterative relocation procedures utilized, the random relocation of both the centroid sorting and complete linkage clustering methods (using SED as a similarity metric) provided the most stable solutions. That is, these methods evidenced the smallest percentage of relocated subjects (see Table 10.4). However, subsequent analyses utilizing Monte Carlo data sets have shown that the measure, percentage relocated, is basically meaningless (DeLuca, Adams, & Rourke, Chapter 3, this volume). Figure 10.1 represents the WRAT Reading, Spelling, and Arithmetic subtest scores for this four-group solution.

MANOVAs for the WRAT subtests indicated that all were significant: Reading, $F(3,152) = 136.33$, $p < .0001$; Spelling, $F(3,152) = 182.96$, $p < .0001$; and Arithmetic, $F(3,152) = 5.77$, $p < .0009$. In order to determine which groups were differentiated on these variables, subsequent

TABLE 10.2. Cluster Coefficients for Each Combination of Cluster Method and Similarity Measure

Number of clusters	Complete linkage/SED	Centroid sorting/SED	Ward's method/SED	Complete linkage/CC	Centroid sorting/CC
10	162.67	47.87	266.97	.972	.989
9	167.00	45.69	408.04	.964	.986
8	181.67	50.16	411.79	.942	.983
7	209.67	61.29	442.39	.925	.981
6	219.33	63.28	577.19	.894	.974
5	317.33	72.23	881.75	.878	.951
4	335.33	67.89	1242.07	.808	.911
3	502.00	83.60	1865.62	.611	.898
2	570.67	141.32	2385.41	.382	.875
1	1437.67	211.91	9548.62	−.516	.697

TABLE 10.3. WRAT Reading, Spelling, and Arithmetic Standard Score Means and Standard Deviations for Initial and Relocated Clusters

Cluster		Centroid sorting/SED			Complete linkage/SED			Ward's method/SED	
		Initial	Random	Size	Initial	Random	Size	Initial	Random
1	n	97	78	69	59	78	69	59	78
Reading	Mean	105.66	104.10	104.10	102.34	104.10	104.10	103.08	104.10
	SD	4.79	3.73	3.68	3.45	3.73	3.68	3.45	3.73
Spelling	Mean	95.69	94.46	93.80	92.76	94.46	93.80	92.29	94.46
	SD	5.31	4.11	4.91	3.91	4.11	4.91	4.40	4.11
Arithmetic	Mean	83.44	83.36	84.00	81.69	83.36	84.00	86.08	83.36
	SD	5.12	5.56	4.90	6.43	5.56	4.90	3.96	5.56
2	n	22	33	36	49	33	36	30	33
Reading	Mean	122.18	116.33	113.61	112.47	116.33	113.61	109.47	116.33
	SD	5.46	6.57	5.71	7.19	6.57	5.71	3.57	6.57
Spelling	Mean	107.68	102.70	102.08	100.94	102.70	102.08	102.07	102.70
	SD	8.01	4.61	5.68	4.78	4.61	5.68	5.03	4.61
Arithmetic	Mean	85.82	84.61	84.89	84.73	84.61	84.89	83.23	84.61
	SD	4.39	4.20	4.28	4.12	4.20	4.28	5.22	4.20

		1	8	11	11	8	11	24	8
3	n	1	8	11	11	8	11	24	8
Reading	Mean	141.00	125.88	127.18	124.18	125.88	127.18	123.13	125.88
	SD	0.00	7.57	6.10	6.97	7.57	6.10	6.15	7.57
Spelling	Mean	116.00	116.63	111.64	113.55	116.63	111.64	106.42	116.63
	SD	0.00	5.24	8.26	6.95	5.24	8.26	8.63	5.24
Arithmetic	Mean	85.00	85.75	87.36	84.36	85.75	87.36	85.33	85.75
	SD	0.00	5.39	3.47	5.22	5.39	3.47	4.25	5.39
4	n	36	37	40	37	37	40	43	37
Reading	Mean	99.22	99.56	99.45	100.95	99.56	99.45	100.67	99.56
	SD	2.03	2.77	2.27	3.89	2.77	2.27	3.70	2.77
Spelling	Mean	81.72	81.59	83.35	82.19	81.59	83.35	84.84	81.59
	SD	6.19	5.85	7.06	6.29	5.85	7.06	8.02	5.85
Arithmetic	Mean	79.67	79.86	78.05	82.03	79.86	78.05	77.00	79.86
	SD	6.66	6.23	5.75	5.97	6.23	5.75	4.94	6.23

TABLE 10.4. Percentage of Children Relocated

	Relocation method	
Cluster method	Random	Size
Complete linkage/SED	24	30
Centroid sorting/SED	19	29
Ward's method/SED	31	—
Complete linkage/CC	27	61
Centroid sorting/CC	38	74

multiple comparisons were calculated using the Tukey–Kramer modification of Tukey's "honestly significant difference" test. Of these multiple comparison procedures, the following were significant ($p < .05$): for both reading and spelling, all groups were significantly different from each other; for arithmetic, the performance of Subtype 2 was superior to that of Subtype 4, and the performance of Subtype 3 was superior to that of Subtype 4.

Internal Validity (Reliability)

Split-half samples were obtained from an extended data set ($n = 194$) and subjected to clustering procedures identical to those used in the initial analysis. Plots of cluster coefficients obtained with sample A ($n = 97$) suggested an optimal solution of four clusters. Plots of the cluster coefficients obtained with sample B ($n = 97$) indicated an optimal solution of five clusters. However, since one of the clusters included only one subject, this cluster was considered to be an outlier and was discarded. The remaining four clusters were taken as the optimal solution. Figure 10.2 represents the WRAT Reading, Spelling, and Arithmetic standard scores of the four-group solution for split samples A and B.

External Validity

Further statistical analyses conducted on the initial data set ($n = 156$) in order to ascertain the concurrent validity of the subtypal solutions indicated that the obtained subtypes did, in fact, differ on a variety of measures and attributes not included in the initial classification process (i.e., neuropsychological and personality variables). Table 10.5 represents the means and standard deviations for the four subtypes on age, WISC IQ scores, and WRAT centile scores. Subtypes 3 and 4 differed significantly in terms of age and WISC PIQ. Table 10.6 presents the means and standard deviations for the four subtypes across all 22 neuropsychological variables, and Figure 10.3 is a graphic illustration of these data. The main effect of subtype classification was significant: Wilk's criterion, multivariate $F(66,392.06) = 1.46$, $p < .0167$.

Subsequent univariate ANOVAs were computed to assess the individual significance of the dependent measures. Of the 22 measures, 6 were significant: WISC Information, $F(3,152) = 3.27$, $p < .0230$; Verbal Fluency, $F(3,152) = 2.75$, $p < .0447$; Speech-Sounds Perception Test, $F(3,152) = 2.70$, $p < .0477$; Digit Span, $F(3,152) = 2.83$, $p < .0405$; WISC Block Design, $F(3,152) = 3.63$, $p < .0294$; and Category Test (total errors), $F(3,152) = 3.08$, $p < .0294$. In addition, two other variables approached

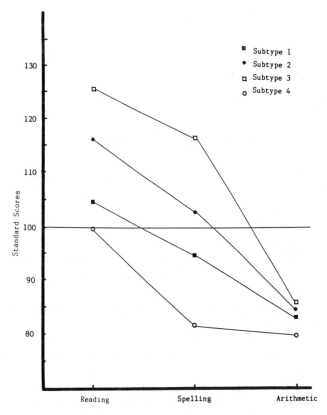

FIGURE 10.1. Plot of WRAT Reading, Spelling, and Arithmetic standard scores for the corrected cluster solution.

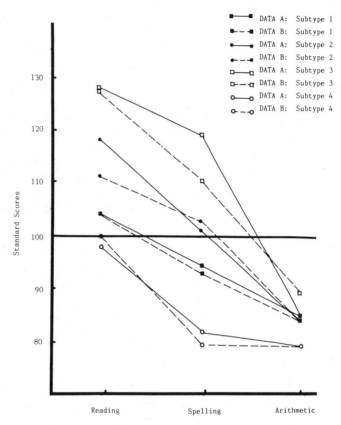

FIGURE 10.2. Plot of WRAT Reading, Spelling, and Arithmetic standard scores for the split-half cluster solutions.

significance: WISC Vocabulary, $F(3,152) = 2.18$, $p < .0933$; and Tactual Performance Test (mean of right- and left-hand trials), $F(3,152) = 2.42$, $p < .0686$. These results indicate the specific variables contributing to the overall group differences.

In order to determine which groups were differentiated in terms of these variables, subsequent multiple comparisons were calculated using the Tukey–Kramer modification of Tukey's "honestly significant difference" test. Of these multiple comparison procedures, the following were significant ($p < .05$): WISC Digit Span (Subtype 3 was superior to Subtype 1) and WISC Block Design (Subtype 4 was superior to Subtype 3). However, several other comparisons approached commonly accepted levels of statistical significance: WISC Information (Subtype 3 was superior to Subtype 4); WISC Vocabulary (Subtype 2 was superior to Subtypes 3 and 4); Verbal Fluency (Subtype 3 was superior to Subtype 1); Sentence Memory (Subtype 3 was superior to Subtype 1). Speech-Sounds Perception Test (Subtype 3 ws superior to Subtype 1); WISC Coding (Subtype 1 was superior to Subtype 3); Trail Making Test (Part A) (Subtype 3 was superior to Subtype 2). Tactual Performance Test (mean of right- and left-hand trials; Subtype 4 was superior to Subtype 2); Tactual Performance Test (both hands) (Subtype 3 was superior to Subtype 2); Tapping Test (mean of both hands; Subtype 1 was superior to Subtype 3); Grooved Pegboard Test (mean of both hands; Subtype 4 was superior to Subtype 3); and Category Test (total errors; Subtype 4 was superor to Subtype 1).

Table 10.7 presents means and standard deviations for the personality variables for each subtype. Of these 16 variables, the 12 selected variables are presented graphically for each subtype separately in Figure 10.4. The main effect of subtype classification as significant: Wilk's criterion, multivariate $F(36,175.05) = 1.70$, $p < .0130$. Thus, the significant MANOVA results for the personality variables suggest that, as for the results obtained using the set of neuropsychological variables, the four subtypes of children generated on the basis of patterns of reading, spelling, and arithmetic performances can also be differentiated on the basis of nonacademic measures.

TABLE 10.5. Raw Score Means (Standard Deviations) for Age, WISC FSIQ, VIQ, PIQ, and WRAT Reading, Spelling, and Arithmetic Centile Scores

	Cluster			
Variable	1	2	3	4
n	78	33	8	37
Age	11.53	11.49	10.70	12.25
	(1.56)	(1.55)	(0.90)	(1.60)
WISC FSIQ	98.40	100.70	98.38	101.00
	(8.17)	(6.89)	(12.01)	(7.68)
VIQ	94.72	100.85	99.38	96.05
	(8.39)	(8.46)	(9.78)	(7.54)
PIQ	102.68	100.55	97.38	106.51
	(10.57)	(10.03)	(14.78)	(10.86)
Reading (%)	60.60	84.12	94.25	48.84
	(9.33)	(8.62)	(4.13)	(7.06)
Spelling (%)	35.86	56.82	85.38	12.57
	(10.26)	(11.83)	(7.09)	(6.29)
Arithmetic (%)	14.82	16.03	18.25	10.76
	(7.44)	(6.35)	(8.15)	(7.39)

TABLE 10.6. *T*-Score Means (Standard Deviations) for Each Subtype: Neuropsychological Measures

Variable	Subtype			
	1	2	3	4
n	78	33	8	37
INF	44.53 (7.00)	47.78 (8.15)	49.16 (6.36)	43.42 (6.50)
VOC	49.15 (6.85)	52.83 (7.37)	50.42 (11.19)	49.19 (7.18)
VFL	40.11 (10.78)	45.87 (10.10)	45.92 (14.88)	40.23 (11.20)
SEN	38.56 (9.38)	42.57 (8.91)	43.64 (11.62)	40.43 (8.99)
SSP	49.02 (13.64)	54.71 (11.29)	59.36 (8.85)	52.15 (12.91)
ART	44.15 (6.95)	45.56 (7.05)	42.92 (8.25)	42.16 (7.12)
DIG	46.41 (8.63)	49.39 (8.31)	54.58 (9.25)	48.20 (8.07)
COD	50.17 (7.95)	47.68 (10.02)	44.17 (13.18)	49.28 (8.89)
PIC	51.37 (8.98)	52.02 (8.82)	53.33 (12.34)	54.50 (7.63)
PAR	50.68 (8.31)	50.61 (8.60)	48.33 (7.56)	51.17 (9.82)
BKD	51.71 (9.38)	51.21 (8.07)	47.08 (9.83)	56.40 (9.18)
TRA	45.42 (10.59)	43.85 (13.10)	50.13 (7.72)	44.49 (11.23)
TAR	42.44 (14.70)	42.93 (10.08)	39.51 (10.44)	44.93 (12.76)
FGA	33.24 (31.05)	36.29 (24.11)	33.67 (25.17)	38.50 (24.32)
FTW	38.77 (26.46)	36.71 (27.04)	47.27 (12.56)	32.36 (53.24)
TPM	46.91 (9.34)	43.70 (13.42)	49.86 (8.27)	50.01 (8.97)
TPB	40.73 (20.39)	36.60 (24.36)	49.57 (10.91)	42.21 (18.51)
TAP	51.37 (9.24)	49.06 (11.12)	45.58 (19.10)	51.10 (10.61)
PEG	45.86 (14.23)	43.99 (16.86)	37.69 (20.44)	46.48 (19.91)
MAZ	51.00 (14.97)	46.81 (23.47)	41.92 (27.22)	49.56 (21.64)
CAT	47.70 (8.23)	48.46 (8.65)	49.98 (9.47)	52.64 (7.92)
TRB	41.05 (16.15)	36.43 (21.14)	39.77 (19.78)	41.46 (12.89)

Subsequent univariate ANOVAs were calculated to assess the individual significance of the dependent measures. Of the 12 measures employed, only two were sugnificant: Psychosis, $F(3,70) = 3.36$, $p < .0234$; and Social Skills, $F(3,70) = 3.20$. $p < .0284$. In addition, one other variable approached significance: Hyperactivity, $F(3,70) = 2.21$, $p < .0951$. These results indicate the specific variables contributing to the overall group differences. Of the multiple comparison procedures, only Psychosis was significant (the elevation for Subtype 3 was higher than that of Subtype 2, $p < .05$). However, one other comparison approached significance: Somatic Concerns (Subtype 3 was higher than Subtype 2).

In addition to the above analyses, univariate ANOVAs were calculated for the PIC validity scales (i.e., Lie, Frequency, Defensiveness, and Adjustment). None of the differences for these variables was statistically significant.

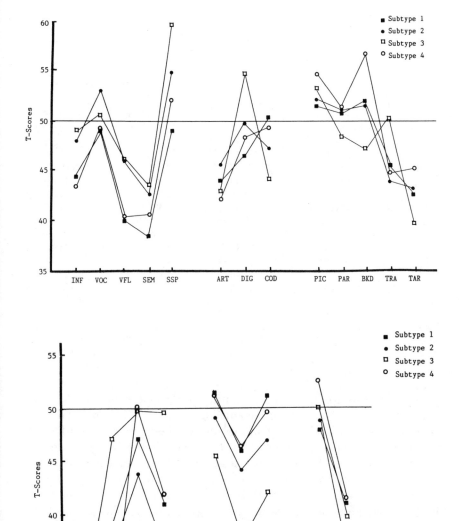

FIGURE 10.3. Plot of *T*-score means for each subtype: neuropsychological measures.

TABLE 10.7. *T*-Score Means (Standard Deviations) for Each Subtype: Personality/Behavior Measures

Variable	Subtype			
	1	2	3	4
n	42	17	3	12
LIE	41.46 (8.97)	44.06 (12.74)	49.33 (10.02)	44.50 (7.98)
FREQ	66.52 (17.34)	57.59 (12.96)	70.00 (8.89)	62.42 (19.45)
DEF	42.05 (11.50)	44.47 (9.68)	34.00 (4.36)	49.67 (12.49)
ADJ	79.71 (19.71)	75.59 (11.42)	77.67 (14.19)	79.00 (14.96)
ACH	64.19 (9.97)	59.41 (7.57)	63.33 (4.16)	68.33 (11.07)
IS	65.10 (17.00)	60.94 (13.47)	72.67 (28.57)	62.33 (21.42)
DEV	63.07 (8.57)	62.65 (10.21)	70.33 (10.26)	63.33 (4.94)
SOM	58.45 (12.44)	55.47 (10.57)	67.33 (5.13)	59.75 (9.75)
DEP	68.60 (14.88)	58.88 (11.86)	66.67 (20.40)	68.25 (13.02)
FAM	54.50 (10.95)	53.47 (8.84)	48.33 (6.11)	54.75 (10.15)
DLQ	67.79 (14.64)	65.06 (14.64)	56.33 (9.24)	62.09 (12.87)
WDL	61.50 (16.96)	53.35 (12.15)	62.67 (26.31)	59.23 (9.25)
ANX	67.43 (13.65)	58.41 (14.54)	65.33 (19.55)	62.92 (9.08)
PSY	70.02 (17.34)	56.88 (12.68)	83.00 (34.70)	65.42 (16.34)
HPR	59.45 (15.98)	61.00 (12.80)	51.33 (25.54)	48.17 (12.64)
SSK	67.86 (13.86)	56.74 (12.14)	64.00 (14.11)	62.17 (7.79)
ARS	23.00 (15.67)	22.50 (14.89)	25.60 (12.42)	16.13 (12.17)
BPC	42.45 (22.22)	36.70 (17.54)	36.20 (16.05)	32.50 (18.37)

The results for the Activity Rating Scale and Behavior Problem Checklist for each subtype are presented in Table 10.7. The main effect of subtype classification was not significant for these variables: Wilk's criterion, multivariate $F(6,240) = 1.56$, $p < .1601$. Table 10.8 presents the frequencies for the Activity Rating Scale and Behavior Problem Checklist ratings "not at all," "sometimes true," and "often true" for each subtype. Although not significant, there is a trend for Subtype 1 to have the highest frequency of ratings acknowledging problem behaviors. Subtype 3 evidenced the highest level of increased activity levels. Subtype 4 children appeared to have the lowest ratings for both activity and problem behaviors.

Discussion

The results of the cluster analysis revealed that (1) children with arithmetic difficulties and normal reading (word recognition) skills are heterogeneous with respect to their patterns of academic performance, (2) cluster analyses are replicable using a split-half method, and (3) the subtypes can be differentiated on the basis of neuropsychological and personality measures. Four subtypes were identified. The implications of these findings as they relate to classification and differential diagnosis are discussed below. However, there are some methodological considerations that should be addressed first.

Methodological Considerations

A number of methodological issues surround the use of cluster analysis, such as the selection of variables, the choice of similarity measure and clustering methods, and the determination of the optimal number of clusters. Most important, however, is the evidence supporting the validity of the derived solution. The internal validity (i.e., reliability) of the present four-cluster solution is shown not only by the similarity of results obtained across several clustering methods and relocation analyses (see Table 10.3) but also by the results of the split-half clustering solutions.

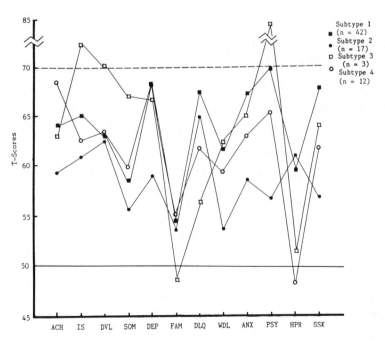

FIGURE 10.4. Plot of *T*-score means for each subtype: personality measures.

TABLE 10.8. Frequency of Behavior Problems and Activity Levels for
Each Subtype

	Subtype			
Variable	1	2	3	4
Activity Rating Scale				
"Not at all"	14.62	15.80	15.00	17.50
"Sometimes true"	9.10	8.57	8.00	8.80
"Often true"	6.95	6.97	8.80	3.67
Behavior Problem Checklist				
"Not at all"	34.73	38.90	38.20	40.77
"Sometimes true"	18.38	16.70	15.80	14.43
"Often true"	12.03	10.00	10.20	9.03

With respect to the external validation procedures, only a small number of variables actually differentiated significantly among the subtypes. However, this may result from the rather restricted ranges of WRAT standard scores employed. That is, use of a highly selected sample of arithmetic-disabled children virtually "stacks the deck" against finding multiple subtypes. Nevertheless, four subtypes did emerge.

The most obvious concern regarding the present four-cluster solution is the small number of subjects found to comprise Subtype 3. Although one may, at first blush, choose to consider these individuals as outliers, enough evidence exists to suggest the contrary. First, there is the striking similarity of Subtype 3 children to children with NLD as described by Rourke (1987, 1988, 1989). The similarities hold not only for their neuropsychological abilities but also for their personality profiles. Furthermore, the small number of subjects comprising this subtype is consistent with previous estimates regarding frequency of occurrence of this subtype (Del Dotto, 1982).

For example, Del Dotto found 9% of right-handed and 14% of left-handed learning-disabled children to have WRAT Arithmetic centile scores less than 30 and Reading and Spelling centile scores greater than 30. Given the more exclusionary criteria of the present study (i.e., WRAT Reading centile greater than 40 and Arithmetic centile less than 27), it is not surprising to find the incidence of NLD children to be only 5.1%. This low incidence rate may result from several factors. The most obvious is an overemphasis on the identification and remediation of language-related learning disabilities. Children with specific arithmetic and related "nonverbal" disorders may be identified at much lower rates in the educational system. The low incidence may also be a reflection of the referral sources employed by various researchers. School-based referrals for learning disabilities would obviously reflect the ratios noted above. However, assessment of children with psychiatric disorders may yield a quite different sample. For instance, approximately 16% of consecutive referrals for neuropsychological assessment in a childens' psychiatric hospital evidenced the NLD syndrome (DeLuca, in preparation). While this incidence rate does not reflect the entire hospital population (i.e., inpatients, outpatients, and day hospital children), it may represent a lower-bound estimate of the actual number of NLD children in such a facility.

Description of Subtypes

Throughout the descriptions of the subtypes, the following definitions apply: mildly impaired refers to performances equal to or greater than 1 standard deviation (*SD*) below the mean to less than 2 *SD* below the mean; moderately impaired refers to performances equal to or greater than 2 *SD* below the mean to less than 3 *SD* below the mean; clearly or severely impaired refers to performances 3 *SD* or more below the mean.

SUBTYPE 1

Subtype 1 was comprised of 78 children, the largest of the four subtypes (69 males and 9 females). These children evidenced the second-largest WISC Verbal IQ–Performance IQ split, favoring PIQ. Mean centile scores on the WRAT were as follows: Reading, 60; Spelling, 35; Arithmetic, 14.

Although sound–symbol matching (i.e., Speech-Sounds Perception Test) and vocabulary skills (i.e., WISC Vocabulary subtest) were age-appropriate, performances on tests of general information (i.e., WISC Information subtest), phonemically cued verbal fluency (i.e., Verbal Fluency Test), mental calculation (i.e., WISC Arithmetic subtest), and memory for sentences of gradually increasing length (i.e., Sentence Memory Test) were low average to mildly impaired. However, Subtype 1 children exhibited no difficulty in remembering series of digits in either a forward or reverse order (i.e., WISC Digit Span subtest) or in transcribing nonverbal symbols under speeded conditions (i.e., WISC Coding subtest). Subtype 1 children may experience difficulty on auditory–verbal tasks requiring concentration and memory as the material increases in complexity.

These children had no difficulty on tasks requiring the perception of visual detail (i.e., WISC Picture Completion subtest), the appreciation of cause–effect relationships presented pictorially (i.e., WISC Picture Arrangement subtest), and visual–spatial organization and synthesis (i.e.,

WISC Block Design subtest). However, tasks involving some forms of visual–spatial sequencing (e.g., the completion of visual–spatial arrays on the basis of numerical cues or short-term memory for sequences; Trail Making Test, Part A and Target Test, respectively) were more problematic for them.

Subtype 1 children evidenced average performances on the combined individual trials of a nonverbal problem-solving task (i.e., Tactual Performance Test); this task involves psychomotor coordination and the ability to benefit from tactile input and kinesthetic feedback. However, performance on a third trial of this test using both hands together was more problematic for them. Also, performance on a test of finger localization was mildly to moderately impaired; performance on a measure of finger dysgraphesthesia was mildly impaired.

Simple motor speed (i.e., Finger-Tapping Test), speeded eye–hand coordination (i.e., Grooved Pegboard Test), and kinetic motor steadiness skills were within normal limits. In fact, this subtype evidenced the best overall performances of all four subtypes on tests of finger-tapping speed and kinetic motor steadiness.

Their performances on a task requiring conceptual flexibility, symbolic shifting, verbal mediation, and the ability to keep more than one idea in mind simultaneously (i.e., Trail Making Test, Part B) were somewhat poor. They had no difficulty on a complex nonverbal test involving concept formation, the ability to benefit from immediate positive and negative informational feedback, hypothesis testing, deductive reasoning, and problem-solving skills (i.e., Halstead Category Test).

With respect to personality functioning, Subtype 1 evidenced the highest (i.e., most pathological) ratings of all four subtypes on the following PIC scales: Depression, Deliquency, Anxiety, Social Skills, and Adjustment. Furthermore, their rating on the PIC Psychosis scale was the second highest of all four subtypes. What follows are the sorts of behaviors expected for children with such profiles as described by Wirt et al. (1977). These children were characterized by difficulties in social interaction and comprehension. Evidence of inappropriate affect, cognitive disorientation, social withdrawal, and depression were noted. Delinquent traits such as a disregard for limits, limited tolerance for frustration, sadness, hostility, limited social participation, and disrespect for authority were often present as well.

Although the frequency of ratings on the Activity Rating Scale was moderate relative to the other subtypes, this group evidenced the highest frequency of problem behviors on the Behavior Problem Checklist.

It may be the case that the latter behaviors represent a method of coping, albeit in an ineffective fashion, with increased levels of anxiety and depression associated with limited social interaction. Moreover, neuropsychological deficiencies in tactile perception, in conceptual flexibility, and in concentration and short-term memory may serve to exacerbate existing socioemotional difficulties. That is, these children may experience difficulty in "getting a feel for things" (in a figurative sense), in discarding a particular mind set when it is appropriate to do so, or in remembering what is said to them. As a result, these children may often be viewed as "oppositional" or noncompliant.

Although no other subtype of learning-disabled children has been reported to evidence similar patterns of neuropsychological skills, Subtype 1 does exhibit a personality profile similar to that of a subtype of learning-disabled children (Group 2; Serious Internalized Psychopathology) described by Porter and Rourke (1985). For instance, both groups evidenced a mean WISC VIQ that was approximately 7 to 8 points lower than their mean PIQ. In addition, WRAT Reading performances were generally better than were Spelling and Arithmetic performances in both instances. However, the most interesting similarity between these two groups is the fact that the PIC profiles are virtually identical (see Figure 10.5).

SUBTYPE 2

This subtype was composed of 33 children (29 males and 4 females). WISC Verbal and Performance IQs were virtually equivalent. They obtained the following WRAT centile scores: Reading, 84; Spelling, 56; Arithmetic, 16.

Subtype 2 evidenced intact rote verbal (i.e., WISC Information and Vocabulary subtests) and sound–symbol matching skills (i.e., Speech-Sounds Perception Test) within the context of somewhat poorer performances on tests of phonemically cued verbal fluency (i.e., Verbal Fluency Test) and short-term memory for sentences of gradually increasing length (i.e., Sentence Memory Test). They had no difficulty in remembering series of digits in either forward or reverse orders, in transcribing nonverbal symbols, or in mental calculation (i.e., WISC Digit Span, Coding, and Arithmetic subtests, respectively).

Visual–spatial skills, such as perception of visual detail, appreciation of cause–effect relationships, and organization and synthesis (i.e., WISC Picture Completion, Picture Arrangement, and Block Design subtests, respectively), were within normal limits. In contrast, these children performed in a low-average to mildly impaired fashion on tests requiring visual–spatial sequencing skills (e.g., the completion of a visual–spatial array on the basis of numerical cues and short-term memory for sequences; Trail Making Test, Part A and Target Test, respectively).

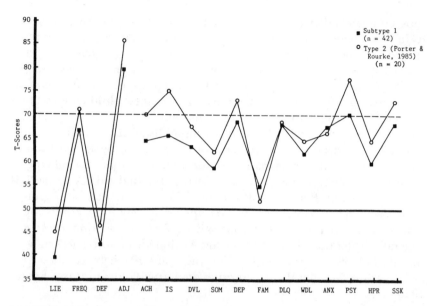

FIGURE 10.5. Comparison of PIC profiles for Porter and Rourke's Type 2 emotionally disturbed group and Subtype 1.

Tactile–perceptual skills including finger localization, fingertip number writing, and complex "hands-on" learning (i.e., Tactual Performance Test) were uniformly impaired. With the exception of a low-average level of performance on a test of speeded eye–hand coordination (i.e., Grooved Pegboard Test), performances on other motor and psychomotor tasks (i.e., simple motor speed and kinetic motor steadiness) were unremarkable.

Conceptual flexibility, symbolic shifting, planning, and verbal mediation skills were mildly to moderately impaired (i.e., Trail Making Test, Part B). In fact, Subtype 2 children evidenced the poorest level of performance of all subtypes on the latter test. Nonverbal problem-solving and concept-formation skills (i.e., Halstead Category Test) were within normal limits.

With respect to ratings on the PIC, Subtype 2 children evidenced the highest ratings of all four groups on the Delinquency and Hyperactivity scales. According to Wirt et al. (1977), the following sorts of behavior are expected for children with such profiles. These children were found to evidence a disregard for limits, low tolerance for frustration, impulsive and hostile behaviors, limited social participation, restlessness, emotional lability, and a disrespect for authority. This group evidenced moderate to high levels of activity and frequencies of problem behaviors on the Activity Rating Scale and the Behavior Problem Checklist, respectively.

It may be the case that the socioemotional problems exhibited by Subtype 2 children are, to a considerable extent, a reflection of their neuropsychological deficiencies. That is, difficulties with respect to their capacity to benefit and coordinate "hands-on" experience in addition to problems in planning, judgment, conceptual flexibility, verbal expression, and attentional deployment skills may foster "delinquent" or resistant behaviors. For example, ineffective planning and poor judgment skills may lead some of these children into conflict with respect to rules and expectations established at home and at school. Some of these children may, in fact, experience substantial difficulties in planning and in preparing for assignments at school or for chores at home. In other instances, some of these children may exhibit "delinquent" behaviors as the results of poor judgment. Such children are likely to be followers rather than leaders. Moreover, they are more likely to be the ones who get caught or apprehended when carrying out antisocial behavior because of their deficiencies in planning and judgment. These children may also be prone to physical aggression when provoked verbally because of their difficulty in dealing with such situations in a verbal fashion.

Breen and Barkley (1983) describe a group of hyperactive children who exhibit PIC profiles that are similar, in some respects, to those of Subtype 2. Both groups evidenced differences with regard to the degree of family unrest and a tendency to withdraw from unpleasant situations. According to the PIC scale descriptions provided by Wirt et al. (1977), both Subtype 2 and Breen and Barkley's hyperactive group evidenced a relative propensity to exhibit the following: a disregard for limits, irritability, low tolerance for frustration, impulsivity, restlessness, insensitivity in the context of interpersonal exchange, poor interpersonal skills, emotional lability, and "discipline" problems (see Figure 10.6). In addition, Porter and Rourke's (1985) Subtype 4 also displays a similar profile on the PIC.

Subtype 2 also exhibits many of the characteristics hypothesized as Subtype C (see Introduction). The latter include aspects of the DOF syndrome, consisting of problems in sequencing, planning, verbal expression, visuomotor and psychomotor abilities, and impulse-control skills.

SUBTYPE 3

This subtype consisted of eight children (four males and four females), the smallest number of all four groups. They also evidenced the youngest

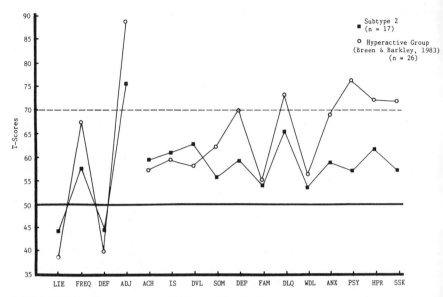

FIGURE 10.6. Comparison of PIC profiles for Breen and Barkley's hyperactive group and Subtype 2.

mean age (i.e., 10.7 years). This was the only subtype exhibiting a lower WISC Performance IQ relative to Verbal IQ. WRAT Reading and Spelling performances were above the 85th centile. Although Subtype 3 evidenced the highest WRAT Arithmetic centile score of all four groups (i.e., 18), none of the subtypes was significantly different on this variable.

With the exception of their performance on a measure of short-term memory for sentences (i.e., Sentence Memory Test), auditory–verbal skills (i.e., WISC Information and Vocabulary subtests, Verbal Fluency Test, and Speech-Sounds Perception Test) were at least age-appropriate. In fact, Subtype 3 evidenced the highest performances of all four subtypes on measures of general information, verbal fluency, and sound–symbol matching skills. Mental calculation skills and the ability to transcribe nonverbal symbols were somewhat poor (i.e., WISC Arithmetic and Coding subtests, respectively). However, Subtype 3 children exhibited a high average level of performance (the best of all four groups) on a test requiring short-term memory for series of digits (i.e., WISC Digit Span subtest).

Simple visual–spatial skills (e.g., perception of visual detail and visual–spatial sequencing; WISC Picture Completion subtest, Trail Making Test, Part A) were within normal limits. However, levels of performance on tests involving more complex visual–spatial–organizational skills (e.g., appreciation of cause–effect relationships, short-term memory for sequences, and visual–spatial organization and synthesis (WISC Picture Arrangement subtest, Target Test, and WISC Block Design subtest, respectively) were the poorest of all four subtypes.

With the exception of a mild to moderate impairment on a test of finger agnosia, performances on tests of tactile–perceptual functioning (i.e., fingertip number writing and complex "hands-on" learning) were age-appropriate. Levels of performance on some tests of motor skills (i.e., simple motor speed, kinetic motor steadiness, and speeded eye–hand coordination) were the most impaired of all four subtypes. Conceptual flexibility skills (i.e., Trail Making Test, Part B) were mildly impaired in the context of age-appropriate nonverbal problem-solving and concept-formation skills (i.e., Halstead Category Test).

On the PIC, Subtype 3 children evidenced the highest ratings of all four subtypes on the Frequency, Intellectual Screening, Development, Somatic, and Psychosis scales. The Adjustment scale was also significantly elevated (i.e., a *T*-score greater than 70; Wirt et al., 1977). What follows are the sorts of behaviors expected for children with such profiles as described by Wirt et al. (1977). These children are characterized by poor motor coordination and school performance, frequent somatic complaints, social withdrawal, limited social skills, delayed pragmatic skills, depressive symptoms, inappropriate affect, and cognitive disorientation. PIC ratings were highest on scales associated with internalized psychopathology.

This group evidenced the highest level of activity and a moderate to high level of problem behavior on the Activity Rating Scale and the Behavior Problem Checklist, respectively.

This subtype appears quite similar, in many respects, to the hypothesized Subtype A or the NLD group described by Rourke (1987, 1988, 1989). Both the NLD group and Subtype 3 children exhibit (1) average to above-average reading and spelling skills within the context of poor arithmetic calculation skills, (2) haptic-perceptual and psychomotor problems, and (3) well-developed sound–symbol matching and rote verbal skills. Although some of the Subtype 3 children in the present study did not evidence poor nonverbal problem-solving skills, their levels of performance on measures of visual–spatial skills were the lowest of all four subtypes. Moreover, both groups evidenced their highest ratings on PIC scales reflecting internalized psychopathology (i.e., Depression, Withdrawal, Anxiety, Psychosis, and Social Skills). In fact, Subtype 3 children exhibited, in general, higher ratings on these scales than did the NLD children reported by Strang and Rourke (1985b) (see Figure 10.7).

One possible explanation for the discrepancies noted between Subtype 3 and NLD children may be the younger ages of the former. In this

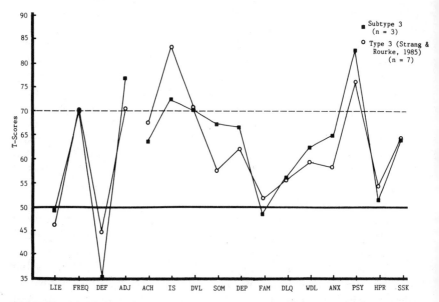

FIGURE 10.7. Comparison of PIC profiles for Strang and Rourke's Type 3 and Subtype 3.

connection, it should be pointed out that Ozols and Rourke (1988) found the neuropsychological manifestations of the NLD syndrome to be less prominent in younger as compared to older children.

SUBTYPE 4

This group consisted of 37 children (36 males and 1 female). They comprised the second largest and the oldest (i.e., 12.25 years) of all four subtypes. Subtype 4 children also evidenced the largest WISC VIQ–PIQ split (96 and 106, respectively). WRAT Reading centile scores were within normal limits; Spelling and Arithmetic performances were the lowest of all four subtypes.

Although vocabulary and sound–symbol matching skills (i.e., WISC Vocabulary subtest and Speech-Sounds Perception Test, respectively) were age-appropriate, performances on tests of general information (i.e., WISC Information subtest), verbal fluency, and short-term memory for sentences (i.e., Sentence Memory subtest) were mildly impaired. These children performed in a normal manner on tests requiring short-term memory for series of digits (i.e., WISC Digit Span subtest) and the transcription of nonverbal symbols under speeded conditions (i.e., WISC coding subtest). Mental calculation skills (i.e., WISC Arithmetic subtest) were the poorest of all four subtypes. Subtype 4 children also had difficulties on tests of visual–spatial sequencing (i.e., completing a visual–spatial array on the basis of numerical cues and short-term memory for sequences; Trail Making Test, Part A and the Target Test, respectively). However, they had no difficulty on tasks involving the perception of visual detail, the appreciation of cause–effect relationships presented pictorially, or visual–spatial organization and synthesis (i.e., WISC Picture Completion, Picture Arrangement, and Block Design subtests, respectively). In fact, their levels of performance on the latter tests were the highest of all four subtypes.

Although they exhibited adequate performance on a test of nonverbal problem solving involving "hands-on" learning (i.e., Tactual Performance Test), tactile–perceptual skills (i.e., finger localization and fingertip number writing) were mildly to moderately impaired. Motor and psychomotor skills were within normal limits. In fact, their performance on a test of speeded eye–hand coordination (i.e., Grooved Pegboard Test) was the highest of all four subtypes.

Planning, symbolic shifting, and the ability to maintain more than one idea in mind simultaneously (i.e., Trail Making Test, Part B) were problematic for these children. Performances on a test of nonverbal problem-solving and concept-formation skills (i.e., Halstead Category Test) was the highest of all four groups.

These children exhibted the highest ratings of all four subtypes on the PIC Achievement and Depression scales. Ratings on the Adjustment, Delinquency, and Psychosis scales were also somewhat elevated. According to Wirt et al. (1977), the following behaviors are expected for children with such profiles. These children exhibited poor levels of academic achievement and significant depressive symptoms. Subtype 4 children were characterized, to some degree by a disregard for limits, low tolerance for frustration, hostility in interpersonal situations, limited social participation, poor social skills and pragmatic skills, and inappropriate affect. Impulsive behavior, poor concentration and study skills, and difficulty in completing assignments are also found to be typical of such youngsters. On the Activity Rating Scale and the Behavior Problem Checklist, this group evidenced the lowest level of activity and frequency of problem behaviors of all four subtypes, respectively.

In short, Subtype 4 children evidenced difficulties in verbal expression, in the retrieval and manipulation of visual–symbolic material, in planning, and in symbolic shifting. It may be the case that these children experience difficulty when required to recall or revisualize the visual–symbolic aspects of verbal material in spelling to dictation. Problems in completing complex arithmetic calculations may also result. For instance, difficulties in accessing the appropriate answer to a multiplication problem from a stored "table" of mathematical facts may occur. On the other hand, some of these children may have deficiencies in visualizing and in manipulating visual–symbolic number images during mental calculation.

The difficulties in organization and expression experienced by some of these children may account for their poor school performance in general and for their difficulty in completing assignments in particular. Poor study habits, concentration, and expressive skills would also be consistent with the neuropsychological deficiencies that they exhibit. In fact, organizational and expressive difficulties may pervade many areas of functioning, including general level of activity and social interaction. If such be the case, the resistance to the requests of adults, social isolation, daydreaming, and the generally "depressed" appearance of these children could be viewed in a different perspective. It may very well prove to be the case that the socioemotional status of these children is largely the result of underlying neuropsychological deficiencies and not solely of external or environmental factors.

This group of children appears to evidence patterns of neuropsychological skills and personality functioning that are similar, at least in some respects, to those of the hypothesized Subtype B or the DOF children characterized by Levine et al. (1981). Both the DOF and Subtype 4 children evidenced intact reading skills within the context of rather poor spelling and arithmetic performances. In addition, consistent with the suggestion that DOF emerges in middle to late childhood, the average age of Subtype 4 children was the highest of all four groups in this study. Verbal expression, fine motor coordination, finger localization, attentional deployment, and retrieval memory difficulties are characteristic of both groups of children. Moreover, both groups exhibit poor work habits, a difficulty or a reluctance to complete assignments, organizational problems, and poor study skills. Comparisons of measures of writing and the organization of information from multiple sources were not possible.

Subtype 4 or DOF children may constitute another NLD subtype. DOF children, whose deficiencies emerge in later childhood and adolescence, exhibit intact auditory–verbal and psycholinguistic skills. Their disorders are "nonverbal" in the sense that skills involved in the coordination and expression of receptive and central processing skills are implicated. That is, skills involving retrieval, organization, expression, directed attention, and motor output were impaired. Receptive skills (e.g., sound blending, sound–symbol matching, perception of visual detail, visual–spatial organization and synthesis) were age-appropriate, as were nonverbal problem-solving skills.

Summary and Implications

In summary, four different groups of learning-disabled children with poor arithmetic and intact reading skills were identified. Both similarities and differences were noted among the patterns of academic, neuropsychological, and personality functioning of these subtypes. While it was obvious that the neuropsychological abilities of Subtypes 1 and 2 were quite similar, their ratings on measures of personality functioning were quite different. In addition, Subtype 3 children exhibited relationships among academic, neuropsychological, and personality functioning that would be predicted on the basis of the NLD model. Most striking, however, were the differences noted in the academic, neuropsychological, and personality functioning of Subtypes 3 and 4. Whereas Subtype 3 children exhibited above-average reading and spelling skills within the context of poor arithmetic, Subtype 4 children exhibited average reading skills and rather deficient spelling and arithmetic skills. On this basis, one must question the generalizability of the findings of studies that do not control for level of spelling performance in children with poor arithmetic and intact reading skills.

The results of the present study have provided support for the investigation of learning disabilities in an integrated, holistic fashion. Piecemeal approaches that serve to compartmentalize areas of adaptive functioning (i.e., academic, neuropsychological, and personality) in artificial and unrealistic manners may no longer be adequate or useful. Although it was clear that some subtypes evidenced similar neuropsychological profiles, several subtypes still differed in terms of their personality functioning. In other cases, subtypes differed on both dimensions. It is clear that the type of multidimensional approach to the study of brain–behavior/adaptive relationships adopted in this investigation is necessary if such complex interrelationships in learning-disabled children are to be understood.

Implications for Intervention

The clarification and differentiation of the quality and patterns of academic, neuropsychological, and personality dysfunctions associated with learning difficulties have some straightforward remedial management implications. On one hand, the delineation of various subtypes of learning-disabled children provides a basic foundation from which one should be able to develop effective remedial strategies. On the other hand, one must be cognizant of the fact that the existence of homogeneous subtypes does not necessarily imply that all the children within a particular group are identical. Rourke (1985, p. 12) suggested that other factors (e.g., early or current environmental influences, reinforcement patterns) may serve to alter the outcome of treatment programs. Although children within a particular subtype may exhibit similar patterns of adaptive strengths and weaknesses, Rourke (1985) contended that, ultimately, prognoses (predictions) and treatments must account for common subtypal properties within the context of individual (unique historical) characteristics. In this sense, subtype analysis provides an intermediate classification system between two extremes. That is, the extreme of classifying all individuals as simply learning-disabled and the classification of each individual learning-disabled child as a unique subtype.

As mentioned above, specific remedial strategies developed to account for individual differences in patterns of academic, neuropsychological, and personality functioning are critical components of an effective treatment regimen. In fact, the generation of a specialized remedial program is one of the primary goals of a treatment-oriented approach to neuropsychological assessment (Rourke et al., 1986).

The following provides a brief overview of some of the remedial strategies that appear appropriate for each of the four subtypes of children identified in the present study.

For Subtype 1 children, it is unlikely that remedial assistance will be effective until their emotional problems are dealt with in an effective manner. That is, it is highly probable that their emotional difficulties serve to impede the development and utilization of many of the age-appropriate abilities they exhibit. Given their intact nonverbal problem-solving skills, both behavioral and insight-oriented approaches may be useful. It appears probable that some form of family intervention would be appropriate for many of these children.

Subtype 2 children would likely benefit from practice in talking, reciting, and taking part in social discourse. Emphasis should be placed on the encouragement and reinforcement of verbal and emotional expression. Use of some type of metacognitive strategies, such as the *Think Aloud* program (Bash & Camp, 1985), could be employed in order to decrease impulsiveness and to improve planning and self-directed behavior. For example, teaching these children to memorize step-by-step verbal recipes that can be used to "talk themselves through" a task may be productive. Once these verbal mediation skills are developed to a sufficient degree, these skills can be utilized to monitor, organize, and plan their behavior more effectively. These exercises may serve to increase concentration, attention, self-monitoring, and self-reflective skills. A behavior modification program would likely prove to be effective with respect to their socioemotional difficulties.

Subtype 3 children are likely to benefit most from some form of behavioral management program as opposed to insight-oriented psychotherapy. That is, Subtype 3 children may have difficulty in gaining insight into their own and others' behaviors, in understanding the subtle nuances of interpersonal exchange, and in understanding novel, complex, and abstract informational input. Social skills should be taught in a direct fashion, and they should be provided with exercises in reality-based role playing. The emphasis on and encouragement of social involvement and the extinguishing of extraneous verbal output would be most helpful. In reading, it may be beneficial to stress comprehension of the material. Problem-solving and study skills should be taught in a direct fashion. These children may need extra time to adjust to novel and/or complex information. In this respect, it may be useful to teach such children in a systematic, step-by-step manner utilizing a parts-to-whole approach to learning. A more detailed outline of remedial strategies for NLD children has been provided by Rourke (1989).

With Subtype 4 children, verbal and emotional (including prosodic and gestural) expression should be encouraged and reinforced. A behavioral management program may be more effective than insight-oriented psychotherapy, at least in the initial stages of treatment, in order to address socioemotional problems (e.g., flat affect, depressed appearance, decreased social involvement). A morphographic approach to spelling that stresses the creative and problem-solving aspects of words may be useful. In addition, the use of drill, repetition, and other verbal mnenonic devices may be beneficial with respect to memory (retrieval) difficulties. A programmed and/or computer-based approach to mathematics may be most effective. These children will likely require additional time to complete written work. Moreover, the amount of required written output should be lessened. In this respect, a tape recorder to take notes or typewritten handouts could be employed to advantage.

The above recommendations for intervention are offered as a heuristic framework. Consideration of them may help to form a preliminary, general framework within which treatment can be initiated. Assessing the validity of the framework's hypotheses in the individual case would constitute a type of "external validity" for the treatment program. More generally, studies along the lines suggested by Lyon (1985) and Lyon and Flynn (Chapter 11, this volume) are necessary for the more rigorous assessment of the validity of these intervention plans.

Acknowledgments

The authors wish to thank Drs. Kenneth Adams, Jack Fletcher, Douglas Shore, and Noel Williams for their advice during the initial phase of this project. The editorial efforts of Marilyn Chedour and Mary L. Stewart are also greatly appreciated.

References

Adams, K. M. (1985). Theoretical, methodological, and statistical issues. In B. P. Rourke (Ed.), *Neuropsychology of learning disabilities: Essentials of subtype analysis* (pp. 17–39). New York: Guilford Press.

Aldenderfer, M. S., & Blashfield, R. K. (1984). *Cluster analysis*. Beverly Hills: Sage Publications.

Badian, N. A. (1983). Dyscalculia and nonverbal disorders of learning. In H. R. Myklebust (Ed.), *Progress in learning disabilities* (Vol. 5, pp. 235–264). New York: Grune & Stratton.

Badian, N. A., & Ghublikian, M. (1983). The personal–social characteristics of children with poor mathematical computation skills. *Journal of Learning Disabilities, 16,* 154–157.

Bash, M. A., & Camp, B. W. (1985). *Think Aloud: Increasing social and cognitive skills—a problem-solving program for children.* Champaign, IL: Research Press.

Blashfield, R. K., & Morey, L. (1980). A comparison of four clustering methods using MMPI Monte Carlo data. *Applied Psychological Measurement, 4,* 57–64.

Breen, M. J., & Barkley, R. A. (1983). The Personality Inventory for Children (PIC): Its clinical utility with hyperactive children. *Journal of Pediatric Psychology, 8,* 359–366.

Del Dotto, J. E. (1982). *Differential subtypes of sinistral learning disabled children: A neuropsychological, taxonomic approach.* Unpublished doctoral dissertation, University of Windsor, Windsor, Ontario.

DeLuca, J. W. (in preparation). *Interface between clinical neuropsychology and child psychopathology: Assessment and classification issues.*

DeLuca, J. W., Adams, K. M., & Rourke, B. P. (in press). Two-stage cluster analysis: Methodological and statistical issues.

DeLuca, J. W., Del Dotto, J. E., & Rourke, B. P. (1987). Subtypes of arithmetic disabled children: A neuropsychological, taxonomic approach. *Journal of Clinical and Experimental Neuropsychology, 9,* 26. (Abstract)

Edelbrock, C. (1979). Mixture model tests of hierarchical clustering algorithms: The problem of classifying everybody. *Multivariate Behavioral Research, 14,* 367–384.

Edelbrock, C., & McLaughlin, B. (1980). Hierarchical cluster analysis using interclass correlation: A mixture model study. *Multivariate Behavioral Research, 15,* 299–318.

Everitt, B. (1974). *Cluster analysis.* London: Heinemann Educational Books.

Fisk, J. L., & Rourke, B. P. (1979). Identification of subtypes of learning-disabled children at three age levels: A neuropsychological, multivariate approach. *Journal of Clinical Neuropsychology, 1,* 289–310.

Francis, D. J., Fletcher, J. M., & Rourke, B. P. (1988). Discriminant validity of lateral sensorimotor tests in children. *Journal of Clinical and Experimental Neuropsychology, 10,* 779–799.

Jastak, J. F., & Jastak, S. R. (1978). *The Wide Range Achievement Test.* Wilmington, DE: Jastak Associates.

Knights, R. M. (1970). Smoothed normative data on tests for evaluating brain damage in children. Ottawa: Carleton University.

Knights, R. M., & Moule, A. D. (1967). Normative and reliability data on finger and foot tapping in children. Perceptual and Motor Skills, 25, 717–720.

Knights, R. M., & Moule, A. D. (1968). Normative data on the motor steadiness battery for children. Perceptual and Motor Skills, 26, 643–650.

Knights, R. M., & Norwood, J. A. (1980). Revised smoothed normative data on the neuro-psychological test battery for children. Ottawa: Carleton University.

Lachar, D., & Gdowski, C. L. (1979). Actuarial assessment of children and adolescent personality: An interpretive guide for the Personality Inventory for Children. Los Angeles: Western Psychological Services.

Levine, M. D. (1984). Cumulative neurodevelopmental debts: Their impact on productivity in late middle childhood. In M. D. Levine & P. Satz (Eds.), Middle childhood: Development and dysfunction (pp. 227–243). Baltimore: University Park Press.

Levine, M. D., Oberklaid, F., & Meltzer, L. (1981). Developmental output failure: A study of low productivity in school-aged children. Pediatrics, 67, 18–25.

Lyon, G. R. (1985). Educational validation studies of learning disability subtypes. In B. P. Rourke (Ed.), Neuropsychology of learning disabilities: Essentials of subtype analysis (pp. 228–253). New York: Guilford Press.

McLeod, T. M., & Crump, W. D. (1978). The relationship of visuospatial skills and verbal ability to learning disabilities in mathematics. Journal of Learning Disabilities, 11, 237–241.

Mezzich, J. E. (1978). Evaluating clustering methods for psychiatric diagnosis. Biological Psychiatry, 13, 265–281.

Milligan, G. W. (1980). An examination of the effect of six types of error perturbation on fifteen clustering alogrithms. Psychometrika, 45, 325–342.

Milligan, G. W., & Cooper, M. C. (1987). Methodology review: Clustering methods. Applied Psychological Measurement, 11, 329–354.

Morey, L. C., Blashfield, R. K., & Skinner, H. A. (1983). A comparison of cluster analysis techniques within a sequential validation framework. Multivariate Behavioral Research, 18, 309–329.

Morris, R., Blashfield, R., & Satz, P. (1981). Neuropsychology and cluster analysis: Problems and pitfalls. Journal of Clinical Neuropsychology, 3, 79–99.

Ozols, E. J., & Rourke, B. P. (1985). Dimensions of social sensitivity in two types of learning-disabled children. In B. P. Rourke (Ed.), Neuropsychology of learning disabilities: Essentials of subtype analysis (pp. 281–301). New York: Guilford Press.

Ozols, E. J., & Rourke, B. P. (1988). Characteristics of young learning-disabled children classified according to patterns of academic achievement: Auditory–perceptual and visual–perceptual abilities. Journal of Clinical Child Psychology, 17, 44–52.

Porter, J. E., & Rourke, B. P. (1985). Socio-emotional functioning of learning disabled children: A subtypal analysis of personality patterns. In B. P. Rourke (Ed.), Neuropsychology of learning disabilities: Essentials of subtype analysis (pp. 257–280). New York: Guilford Press.

Quay, H. C., & Peterson, D. R. (1979). Manual for the Behavior Problem Checklist. Available from author.

Reitan, R. M. (1966). A research program on the effects of brain lesions in human beings. In N. R. Ellis (Ed.), International review of research in mental retardation (Vol. 1, pp. 153–218). New York: Academic Press.

Reitan, R. M. (1974). Psychological effects of cerebral lesions in children of early school age. In R. M. Reitan & L. A. Davison (Eds.), Clinical neuropsychology: Current status and applications (pp. 53–90). Washington: Winston.

Rourke, B. P. (1982). Central processing deficiencies in children: Toward a developmental neuropsychological model. *Journal of Clinical Neuropsychology, 4,* 1–18.

Rourke, B. P. (Ed.). (1985). *Neuropsychology of learning disabilities: Essentials of subtype analysis.* New York: Guilford Press.

Rourke, B. P. (1987). Syndrome of nonverbal learning disabilities: The final common pathway of white-matter disease/dysfunction? *Clinical Neuropsychologist, 1,* 209–234.

Rourke, B. P. (1988). Socioemotional disturbances of learning-disabled children. *Journal of Consulting and Clinical Psychology, 56,* 801–810.

Rourke, B. P. (1989). *Nonverbal learning disabilities: The syndrome and the model.* New York: Guilford Press.

Rourke, B. P., Bakker, D. J., Fisk, J. L., & Strang, J. D. (1983). *Child neuropsychology.* New York: Guilford Press.

Rourke, B. P., & Finlayson, M. A. J. (1978). Neuropsychological significance of variations in patterns of academic performance: Verbal and visual–spatial abilities. *Journal of Abnormal Child Psychology, 6,* 121–133.

Rourke, B. P., Fisk, J. L., & Strang, J. D. (1986). *Neuropsychological assessment of children: A treatment-oriented approach.* New York: Guilford Press.

Rourke, B. P., & Strang, J. D. (1978). Neuropsychological significance of variations in patterns of academic performance: Motor, psychomotor, and tactile-perceptual abilities. *Journal of Pediatric Psychology, 3,* 62–66.

Rourke, B. P., Young, G. C., & Leenaars, A. A. (1989). A childhood learning disability that predisposes those afflicted to adolescent and adult depression and suicide risk. *Journal of Learning Disabilities, 22,* 169–187.

Rourke, B. P., Young, G. C., Strang, J. D., & Russell, D. L. (1986). Adult outcomes of central processing deficiencies in childhood. In I. Grant & K. M. Adams (Eds.), *Neuropsychological assessment in psychiatric disorders: Clinical methods and empirical findings* (pp. 244–267). New York: Oxford University Press.

SAS Institute Inc. (1985). *SAS user's guide: Statistics, version 5 edition.* Cary, NC: SAS Institute Inc.

Satz, P., & Morris, R. (1981). Learning disability subtypes: A review. In F. Pirozzollo & M. Wittrock (Eds.), *Neuropsychological and cognitive processes in reading* (pp. 109–141). New York: Academic Press.

Siegel, L. S., & Feldman, W. (1983). Nondyslexic children with combined writing and arithmetic disabilities. *Clinical Pediatrics, 22,* 241–244.

Siegel, L. S., & Linder, B. A. (1984). Short-term memory processes in children with reading and arithmetic learning disabilities. *Developmental Psychology, 20,* 200–207.

Strang, J. D., & Rourke, B. P. (1983). Concept-formation/nonverbal reasoning abilities of children who exhibit specific problems with arithmetic. *Journal of Clinical Child Psychology, 12,* 33–39.

Strang, J. D., & Rourke, B. P. (1985a). Arithmetic disability subtypes: The neuropsychological significance of specific arithmetic impairment in childhood. In B. P. Rourke (Ed.), *Neuropsychology of learning disabilities: Essentials of subtype analysis* (pp. 167–186). New York: Guilford Press.

Strang, J. D., & Rourke, B. P. (1985b). Adaptive behavior of children who exhibit specific arithmetic disabilities and associated neuropsychological abilities and deficits. In B. P. Rourke (Ed.), *Neuropsychology of learning disabilities: Essentials of subtype analysis* (pp. 302–330). New York: Guilford Press.

Webster, R. E. (1979). Visual and aural short-term memory capacity deficits in mathematics disabled students. *Journal of Educational Research, 72,* 277–283.

Webster, R. E. (1980). Short-term memory in mathematics-proficient and mathematics disabled students as a function of input-modality/output-modality pairings. *Journal of Special Education, 14*, 67–78.

Wechsler, D. (1949). *Wechsler Intelligence Scale for Children*. New York: Psychological Corporation.

Werry, J. S. (1968). Developmental hyperactivity. *Pediatric Clinics of North America, 15*, 581–599.

Wirt, R. D., Lachar, D., Klinedinst, J. K., & Seat, P. D. (1977). *Multidimensional description of child personality: A manual for the Personality Inventory for Children*. Los Angeles: Western Psychological Services.

Wishart, D. (1978). *CLUSTAN user manual: Version 1C, release 2* (3rd ed.). Edinburgh, Scotland: Edinburgh University Program Library Unit.

Subtype $\times$ Treatment Interaction Studies

CHAPTER 11

Educational Validation Studies with Subtypes of Learning-Disabled Readers

G. Reid Lyon and Jane M. Flynn

A complicated task facing researchers, clinicians, and teachers is to identify and understand the instructional factors and decisions that must be considered when teaching learning-disabled (LD) individuals. By current definition, the learning disabled do not process information in a manner that allows them to comprehend, remember, and generalize concepts relevant to the development of reading, oral language, writing, mathematics, and/or social skills. Within this context, the value of treatment (e.g., educational remediation) is central to the concept of LD. From a clinical standpoint, it is our view that the descriptive and predictive validity of the LD diagnosis depends on the facility by which it generates testable hypotheses about instructional methodologies that have the highest probability of success with a given LD individual (Lyon, 1985a; Lyon & Moats, 1988; Lyon, Moats, & Flynn, 1988).

However, the complexity of studying instructional methods and outcomes with LD students is increased by factors related to the heterogeneous nature of the LD population, the multivariate and dynamic problem-solving demands inherent within the instructional decision-making process, and the methodological requirements necessary to identify valid interactions between "subtypes" of LD individuals and different forms of educational treatment. Each of these factors is considered here.

Population Heterogeneity and Treatment Effectiveness

It is well documented that individuals diagnosed as LD do not constitute a homogeneous group (Lyon & Watson, 1981; Rourke, 1985; Satz & Morris, 1981). In fact, current definitions of learning disabilities specify that LD consists of several major subgroups identified on the basis of different handicapping conditions (e.g., oral language disorders, basic reading and reading comprehension disorders, arithmetic calculation and reasoning disorders, written language disorders). Recent classification research has also indicated that a number of these major diagnostic subgroups are themselves composed of homogeneous subtypes, each of which can be distinguished from one another by a particular array of information-processing, neuropsychological, and/or academic achievement characteristics. Space does not permit extensive discussion of these findings, but interested readers are referred to Fletcher and Morris (1986), Hooper and Willis (1989), and Rourke (1985) for extensive coverage of current LD subtype research findings.

The important point to note is that meaningful conclusions regarding treatment efficacy and outcomes for the learning disabled cannot be made until population heterogeneity is recognized, accounted for in an internally and externally valid fashion, and incorporated into LD subtype × treatment method designs. This point may take on added relevance when one considers that, even when samples of LD individuals are identified and grouped according to stringent selection criteria (e.g., similar academic achievement deficits, IQ above 100, middle to upper-middle socioeconomic status, and control for exposure to different curricula), there still exists substantial heterogeneity with respect to the development and manifestation of skills that are correlated with specific forms of academic underachievement. Thus, even within "well-defined" samples of LD individuals, there continues to exist substantial heterogeneity, indicating that not all LD children learn poorly for the same reasons; consequently, they do not respond equally well to the same teaching tactics or methodologies (see Lyon, 1985b).

Some advances have been made in accounting for both LD population and sample heterogeneity via the application of empirical, clinical, and rational classification methodologies to identify subtypes. However, our understanding of specific relationships between LD subtype characteristics and treatment responsiveness remains tentative because of a number of practical and logistical factors. We now turn to a discussion of some of these factors.

Factors That Impede the Educational Validation of LD Subtypes

Even when the heterogeneity of LD samples has been accounted for via the formation of typologies that contain individuals of like characteristics, understanding how and why each subtype responds to different treatments is difficult for a variety of logistical and pedagogical reasons. For example, it is often the case that individuals who have participated in subtype identification studies are not available for subsequent treatment investigations. In other cases, parents and teachers are sometimes reluctant to have their children receive a form of instruction with which they may disagree or instruction that reduces time spent in other classes or school activities.

It also must be recognized that educational treatment outcomes are difficult to quantify accurately, priamrily because remediation may not produce immediate changes in cognitive and academic functioning. Moreover, the degree of relationship between subtype, instructional treatment method, and outcome is difficult to interpret because of limitations in accoutning for and measuring departures from treatment fidelity, teacher preparation and style, classroom climate, and the LD student's previous and concurrent instructional experiences (Lyon & Moats, 1988). Investigators planning to carry out educational validation studies with LD subtypes must not only consider the practical and logistical design factors addressed here, but they should also become acquainted with the theoretical and methodological features that exemplify quality aptitude (e.g., subtype) X treatment (e.g., teaching method) research.

Educational Validation of LD Subtypes: Theoretical and Methodological Considerations

In addition to the practical constraints cited earlier, another significant difficulty encountered when conducting educational validity studies of LD subtypes is satisfying the theoretical and methodological demands of classification research in general and aptitude X treatment experiments in particular. A necessary first step in such investigations is to delineate, in an *a priori* fashion, the scope, purpose, and theoretical basis for the subtype identification and educational validation study. From this context, theory-driven hypotheses can be formulated. These hypotheses, in turn, should lead to tentative descriptions of anticipated subtypes and specification of how predicted subtypes will respond to treatment.

Once theory-driven hypotheses have been developed to specify the possible range and nature of the subtype solution, both classification and external educational validation variables must be selected (see Lyon & Flynn, 1990, for a discussion of issues related to variable selection). Variables designated as classification variables are chosen to assess the critical attributes of the predicted subtypes. The educational validation variables (outcome measures) should be selected to assess multiple dimensions of change even within specific content domains (e.g., reading). This is necessary because subtype × teaching method interactions may exist for some behaviors (e.g., reading accuracy) but not for others (e.g., reading speed). Variable selection is a complex process and should be guided by informed theoretical, psychometric, content, and developmental perspectives. As a general guideline for subtype validation studies, variables should be selected on the basis of the following:

1. Their theoretical coherence and ability to permit unconfounded and fine-grained analysis of hypothesized subtypal attributes and outcomes.
2. Their relationship to known paths of development within the content domain being studied (e.g., reading). This insures that the measurement of a subtypal attribute or validation domain is appropriate to the developmental level of the individuals in the sample.
3. Evidence that the variables constitute valid measurements of the classification (subtype) attributes and the educational validation treatments and outcomes.
4. Evidence that the variables possess adequate reliability.
5. Evidence that the classification and educational validation variables accomplish nonredundant assessments of subtypal attributes and treatment outcomes.

It is also useful to note that difference scores (e.g., scores reflecting change between pre- and posttest conditions) are frequently reported to be unreliable and thus limited in their usefulness in detecting treatment effects. Interested readers are referred to Cronbach and Snow (1977) for a discussion of this issue and recommendations for the selection of appropriate treatment-dependent variables.

The actual statistical procedures that can be used to detect subtype × teaching method interactions are complex and beyond the scope of this chapter. Although a brief overview of the recommended methodology is provided here, the reader is referred to Cronbach and Snow (1977) for more complete coverage. In general, studies designed to predict treatment response on the basis of subtype characteristics require regression analysis (Cronbach, 1977) and/or ANOVA designs (Bracht, 1970). In the case of the regression design, subjects are measured on a set of aptitude measures and then randomly assigned to one of two or more treatment (teaching) methods. Following completion of the teaching condition, the aptitude scores are used to predict the treatment outcome scores obtained by members of each group. The regression lines are then examined for parallelism and plotted to determine whether they interact within the effective range of the aptitude (subtype) measures.

In the ANOVA design, subjects are administered aptitude measures (e.g., neuropsychological tasks) and then assigned, according to their scores, to one of several levels of the aptitude (subtype) factor in a factorial analysis of variance. (Keep in mind that subtypes may be formed through multivariate empirical classification procedures, clinical assignment via visual inspection of the data, or application of rational grouping procedures.) Bracht (1970) has recommended that, following the teaching intervention(s), an ANOVA be computed to assess possible disordinal interactions among levels of the aptitude (subtype) factor and levels of the treatment (teaching method) factor. A disordinal interaction exists if the analyses of simple effects are significant *and* the mean cell differences have different algebraic signs.

When carrying out subtype × teaching method research, careful consideration has to be given to determining the number of subjects per aptitude × treatment condition needed to achieve a given level of power for the interaction. In the main, a relatively large sample size is recommended for this type of research. With both the regression and ANOVA designs, subjects should be equated on preintervention achievement and preintervention regression between achievement and aptitude *or* must be randomly assigned to the different teaching conditions if the results of the data analysis are to be interpretable. Obviously, the matching of subjects on preintervention achievement variables and the random assignment of subjects to teaching conditions would require a large sample size. This is particularly true if subjects from several identified subtypes are being randomly assigned to several teaching conditions.

No doubt, the complexity of conducting well-designed educational validation studies of LD subtypes has limited the number of investigations completed to date and has also reduced the quality of the few that have been published. Nevertheless, it may be useful to provide an overview of three research programs that are currently pursuing subtype remediation research. In doing so, our goal is to describe the current "state of the art" with an eye toward making improvements in future educational validation studies. The reader should note that Bakker's subtype validation studies are not reviewed in this chapter since he accomplishes this task in Chapter 7 (Bakker, Licht, & van Strien, this volume).

Selected Educational Validation Studies of LD Subtypes

To date, a few research programs have reported preliminary data that suggest that LD subtypes respond differently to various forms of treatment (remediation). Although the studies reported here have all been carried out with LD readers, the studies differ with respect to theoretical orientation, assessment tasks used to characterize subtypes, and classification methodologies employed to identify subtypes.

For example, Lyon and his associates have identified several LD subtypes by applying empirical multivariate quantitative methods to information-processing task scores obtained by large samples of LD readers. External educational validation studies have then involved attempts to teach the disabled readers and to identify subtype × teaching method interactions. In contrast, Lovett and her colleagues (Lovett, Ramsby, & Barron, 1988) and Flynn and her group (Flynn & Deering, 1989) have concentrated on clinically identifying dyslexic subtypes on the basis of their reading and spelling patterns and then assigning subjects to different treatment conditions.

The three research groups have presented pilot data showing that children who display varied subtype attribute patterns respond in different ways to instructional formats. Each of these research programs is reviewed in greater detail in this section. Emphasis is placed on describing the theoretical orientation that serves as the context for variable selection, the types of treatment procedures used, and the clinical relationship between tasks and interventions. Attention is also given to the methodological shortcomings associated with each program of research.

The Lyon Research Program

Lyon and his associates (Lyon, 1983, 1985a, 1985b; Lyon, Stewart, & Freedman, 1982; Lyon & Watson, 1981) have questioned the appropriateness of a single-deficit classification model for reading disability and have hypothesized that LD readers (dyslexics) constitute a population that is composed of a number of subtypes, each of which is defined by its own particular array of linguistic, perceptual, and reading characteristics. The theoretical background underlying Lyon's research can be viewed as a logical extension of Luria's (1966, 1973) clinical neuropsychological theory and Benson and Geschwind's (1975) multiple-syndrome model of alexia. For example, Lyon (1983) proposed that reading development is a complex process that requires the concerted participation of cognitive, linguistic, and perceptual subskills. As such, deficiencies in any one subskill can limit the acquisition of fluent decoding and/or reading comprehesion abilities.

SUBTYPE VALIDATION STUDIES WITH OLDER LD READERS

Within this theoretical context, an initial series of studies was conducted (Lyon, Rietta, Watson, Porch, & Rhodes, 1981; Lyon & Watson, 1981) in which a battery of tasks designed to assess linguistic and perceptual skills related to reading development was administered to 100 LD readers and 50 nomal readers matched for age (11–12 years) and IQ ($M = 104$). The data were submitted to a series of cluster analyses to test the hypothesis that subtypes could be identified. Six distinct subtypes were delineated and characterized by significantly different patterns of linguistic and perceptual deficits. The six-subtype solution remained stable across internal validation studies employing different variable subsets and clustering algorithms. Further, 94% of subjects were recovered into similar subtypes in a cross-validation study using a new subject sample (Lyon, 1983). A brief description of each of the subtypes' information-processing characteristics is provided here, followed by an overview of the intervention program. Readers are referred to cited references for specific details.

Children who were assigned empirically to Subtype 1 ($n = 10$) exhibited significant deficits in language comprehension, the ability to blend phonemes, visual–motor integration, visual–spatial skills, and visual memory skills, with strengths in naming and auditory discrimination skills. Analysis of the reading and spelling errors made by members of Subtype 1 indicated significant deficits in the development of both sight-word vocabulary and word-attack skills.

Children in Subtype 2 ($n = 12$) also exhibited a pattern of mixed deficits, but in a milder form than that observed in Subtype 1. Specifically, significant problems in language comprehension, auditory memory span, and visual–motor integration were observed and may have been related to the reading problems of these subjects. No deficits were seen in these youngsters' performance on naming, auditory discrimination, sound-blending, visual–spatial, and visual memory tasks. Subtype 2 members produced mixed orthographic and phonetic errors when reading, but to a much milder degree than did Subtype 1 children.

Members of Subtype 3 ($n = 12$) manifested selective deficits in language comprehension and sound blending, with corresponding strengths in all other linguistic and visual–perceptual skills measured. The oral reading errors made by Subtype 3 youngsters were primarily phonetic in nature, as would be expected from their diagnostic profile.

Children in Subtype 4 ($n = 32$) displayed significant deficiencies on a visual–motor integration task and average performance on all other measures. These youngsters presented with an assorted sample of oral reading errors, though most errors were made when they attempted to read phonetically irregular words.

Subtype 5 ($n = 12$) members displayed significant deficits in language comprehension, auditory memory span, and sound blending, with corresponding strengths in all measured visual–perceptual and visual-motor skills. These characteristics appeared related to the severity of their oral reading and written spelling errors. The major academic characteristic that distinguished Subtype 5 youngsters from the other children was their consistently poor application of word-attack (phonetic) skills to the reading and spelling process.

The pattern of scores obtained by members of Subtype 6 ($n = 16$) indicated a normal diagnostic profile. These results were unexpected. It is quite possible that these children were reading poorly for reasons that were not detected by the assessment battery.

Following this subtype identification study, an external validation investigation (Lyon, 1983) was carried out to determine whether subtypes would respond differently to reading instruction. However, because of the relatively small sample size, an aptitude × treatment study designed according to the criteria discussed earlier could not be conducted. Therefore, it was decided to explore the possibility that the six subtypes might respond differently to one teaching condition. Since the children for this exploratory study had to be matched for preintervention achievement levels and other relevant variables (age, IQ, sex, socioeconomic status), the initial subject pool available from the subtype identification study was reduced to 30. Thus, random assignment of children from each of the six subtypes to several teaching conditions was not feasible.

In light of these logistical difficulties, five subjects were selected from each of the six subtypes. They were matched on their ability to read single words, age, IQ, race, and sex. All 30 subjects were white males ranging in age from 12.3 years to 12.7 years and in Full Scale IQ from 103.5 to 105. Preintervention grade equivalents on the Reading Recognition subtest of the Peabody Individual Achievement Test (PIAT; Dunn & Markwardt, 1970) ranged from 3.0 to 3.3, with centile ranks ranging from 4 to 8. It was not possible to control for the amount and type of previous reading instruction experienced by the children, their present curriculum, and the amount of time spent in classrooms for LD youngsters. Thus, the results obtained from this study must be evaluated in light of these confounding features.

The teaching method selected for the study was a synthetic phonics program (Traub & Bloom, 1975). This program was chosen because of its sequenced format, its coverage of major phonics concepts, and its familiarity to the teachers in training who were providing the instruction. All subjects were provided 1 hour of reading instruction per week (in addition to their special and regular classroom instruction) for 26 weeks.

Following the 26 hours of phonics instruction, the 30 children were posttested with the PIAT Reading Recognition subtest, and gain scores employing centile ranks were computed. A one-way analysis of variance indicated significant differences among the six subtypes for gain scores achieved from preintervention to posttesting. An analysis of subtype gain scores and subsequent pairwise comparisons indicated that members of Subtype 6 made the most progress (mean centile rank gain = 18.0), followed by members of Subtype 4 (mean centile rank gain = 8.2). On the other hand, Subtypes 1, 2, 3, and 5 made minimal gains and were also not significantly different from one another in terms of the gains achieved. Subtypes 6 and 4 were both significantly different from one another and from all other subtypes with respect to their improvement in the oral reading of single words.

The data obtained in this subtype remediation study indicate that, for some subtypes, a synthetic phonics teaching intervention appeared to enhance significantly the ability to read single words accurately. Clearly, members of Subtypes 6 and 4 demonstrated robust improvements in their decoding capabilities. Whether or not the absence of auditory–verbal deficits in these two subtypes was associated with their good response to instruction cannot be answered clearly at this time, but one could hypothesize that this might be the case. This hypothesis is made more tenable by the observation that those subtypes with the most severe linguistic and memory-span deficits made either minimal gains (i.e., Subtypes 2 and 3) or no gains (i.e., Subtypes 1 and 5) in the ability to pronounce single words accurately and fluently.

SUBTYPE VALIDATION STUDIES WITH YOUNGER LD READERS

In a related program of research carried out with younger disabled readers (*M* age = 8.1 years) (Lyon, 1985b; Lyon et al., 1982), five LD subtypes were identified and validated internally and externally by using different variable subtests, clustering algorithms, and subtype × teaching method interaction studies. Again, a brief description of each of the subtypes' information-processing characteristics is provided, followed by an overview of the external validation intervention program.

Children assigned to Subtype 1 (*n* = 18) manifested significant deficits in visual perception, visual–spatial analysis and reasoning, and visual–motor integration. Visual memory was also below average, but not significantly so. All measured linguistic and verbal expressive skills were within the average range. The reading errors made by members of Subtype 1 appeared to be related to their diagnostic profile. Frequent mispronunciations resulting from confusion of orthographically similar words were noted, as were reading errors involving medial vowels and vowel combinations.

Children in Subtype 2 (*n* = 10) displayed selective deficits in morphosyntactic skills, sound blending, language comprehension, auditory memory span, auditory discrimination, and naming ability, with corresponding strengths in all measured visual–perceptual skills. These deficits across linguistic and verbal memory-span domains appeared to impede seriously their ability to decode single words and to apply decoding principles to the pronunciation of nonsense words.

Members of Subtype 3 ($n = 12$) scored in the normal range on all diagnostic measures and, thus, can be compared with subjects in the subtype identified by Lyon and Watson (1981) that scored significantly below normal on reading tasks without concomitant low performance on the diagnostic test battery. It is possible that members of Subtype 3 read inefficiently for social or affective reasons rather than because of inherent oral language or perceptual deficiencies. It is also quite possible that the diagnostic battery employed did not assess effectively all skills relevant to the developmental reading process. As was the case with Lyon and Watson's (1981) Subtype 6 (normal diagnostic profile), members of Subtype 3 scored higher than all other subgroups on the reading measures. These youngsters did have relatively more difficulties in comprehending reading passages than in the other measured reading skills. No systematic patterns of errors could be identified from analysis of their performance on word recognition and word attack measures.

Children in Subtype 4 ($n = 15$) displayed significant deficiencies in sound blending, language comprehension, auditory memory span, naming ability, and some aspects of visual perception. The difficulties manifested by Subtype 4 members in remembering, analyzing, synthesizing, and correctly sequencing verbal information appeared to have a significant effect on their ability to decode phonetically regular real and nonsense words.

Members of Subtype 5 ($n = 9$) manifested significant mixed deficits in morphosyntactic skills, sound blending, visual perception, visual-motor integration, visual–spatial analysis, and visual memory. These youngsters committed primarily orthographic errors when reading single words (both real and nonsense), possibly reflecting the influence of deficiencies in visual–verbal analysis and memory.

Following the subtype identification phase with the younger disabled readers, Lyon (1985b) carried out a pilot remediation study. Similar to the Lyon (1983) subtype remediation study, a relatively small sample size and other logistical difficulties (funding, sample migration) prohibited any attempts to assign members randomly from each of the five identified subtypes to a variety of teaching approaches. However, rather than teaching all subtype members with the same method, as was done in the first intervention study, one subtype (Subtype 2) was divided, with half of the members receiving reading instruction via a synthetic phonics approach and the other half receiving instruction through a combined whole-word and analytic phonics method.

Although this approach represents a significant departure from the experimental design necessary for an aptitude (subtype) × treatment (teaching method) interaction study, Lyon attempted to gain preliminary information about how children who are similar to one another diagnostically would respond to different teaching methods. Subtype 2 ($n = 10$) was chosen as the target subtype for this pilot study because all of its members displayed both significant linguistic deficits (auditory discrimination, auditory comprehension, auditory memory span) and verbal expressive deficits (retrieval, syntax, sequencing) within the context of robust visual perceptual–motor–memory strengths. Because all of the Subtype 2 members manifested significant difficulties reading single words and connected language, the opportunity existed to determine how two different reading approaches affected these skills in the presence of a number of linguistic subskill impairments.

For this pilot study, five children were randomly assigned to a synthetic phonics approach (Traub & Bloom, 1975), whereas the remaining five were placed randomly in a combined sight-word, contextual analysis, structural analysis, and analytic phonics group. Preintervention assessment using the Woodcock Reading Mastery Word Identification subtest (Woodcock, 1973) indicated that the five children in each remediation group were reading between the 8th and 10th centile ranks for age. The mean centile ranks for the two groups were not significantly different (Mann–Whitney $Z > .05$) prior to the initiation of the remediation programs.

Both remediation groups received approximately 30 hours of individualized instruction (3 hours a week for 10 weeks). Unfortunately, it was not possible to control for the type of previous exposure to reading instruction or for the type of ongoing regular and special class instruction the children were receiving in their typical school day. Thus, as in the Lyon (1983) study, any conclusions drawn from the results of this study must be interpreted in light of these confounding factors.

The synthetic phonics remediation group was taught via the scope and sequence presented in the Traub and Bloom (1975) reading program. A brief description of the instructional format for this approach was presented earlier. The combined remediation group learned to label whole words (three nouns, three verbs) rapidly by first pairing the words with pictures, then recognizing the names of the words (by a pointing response), and then finally reading the words in isolation. Following the development of rapid reading ability for these six words, function words (the, is, was, are) were introduced and taught. Following stable reading of these words, short sentences using combinations of the sight and function words were constructed and read in order to introduce the concept of contextual analysis and to develop metalinguistic awareness of reading as a meaningful language skill. Following contextual reading drills, the combined group received instruction in structural analysis and the reading and comprehension of the morphosyntactical markers -ed, -s, and -ing. These morphemes were written as anagrams and introduced into context so that the children could readily grasp their effect on syntax and meaning. Finally, analytic phonics drills were initiated to develop letter-sound correspondences with the context of whole words. Specifically, phonetically regular words that could be read rapidly by sight were presented, and children were first asked to recognize a particular letter-sound correspondence ("Point to the letter that makes the /a/ sound.") and then to provide a recall response ("What sound(s) does this letter make?"). As children became more adept at recalling grapheme-phoneme relations, drills in auditory analysis and blending were initiated.

Following the 30 hours of remediation, children in both groups were posttested with an alternate form of the Woodcock Reading Mastery Word Identification subtest. Significant differences were found between the two remediation groups with respect to postintervention reading centile rank scores (Mann–Whitney $A < .003$). Children within the combined remediation group gained, on the average, 11 centile rank points, whereas members of the synthetic phonics group gained approximately 1 centile rank point.

There is little doubt that Subtype 2 members responded significantly differently to two forms of reading instruction. Apparently, the auditory receptive and auditory expressive language deficits that characterized each member of Subtype 2 impeded response to a reading instructional method that required learning letter–sound correspondences in isolation followed by blending and contextual reading components. A tentative hypothesis might be that Subtype 2 children did not have the linguistic subskills necessary for success with this approach but could deploy their relatively robust visual–perceptual and memory skills more effectively with whole words, as seen within the combined remediation. A more tenable hypothesis is that whole-word reading placed far less linguistic demands on these readers than did alphabetic approaches that require a phonological awareness of (1) sound structure and acoustic boundaries and (2) the relationship of these units to letter sequences. Thus, whereas Subtype 2 members learned to read whole words in structured, isolated context, their ability to generalize phonological concepts to read new words remained limited.

In general, the data derived from this series of subtype identification and remediation studies support a model of dyslexia that presumes that a number of diverse information-processing deficits can have specific reading disability as a common correlate. Although the results from these basic research endeavors are interesting, the findings have limited clinical utility for a number of reasons. First, the kinds of subtypes identified and their descriptions are limited by the range and quality of the classification tasks that provided the data for cluster analysis. For example, the tasks selected for use in Lyon's assessment batteries did not provide adequate fine-grained coverage of some linguistic factors (particularly phonology) implicated in the developmental reading process. Second, the specific nature of the relationship between subtype assessment characteristics and response to reading instruction is difficult to determine because the assessment tasks are indirect measures of associated symptomatology. Third, it is not well understood whether the correlated information-processing deficits constitute necessary and/or sufficient conditions for reading disability. Fourth, methodological limitations in sample size and the number and type of dependent reading measures preclude adequate interpretations and confident generalization of the subtype × teaching method interaction studies. Finally, even though particular teaching (treatment) approaches had differential effects for some subtypes, it is difficult to determine if the effects should be attributed to subtype characteristics, the instructional program, the interaction between the two, the teacher, the time spent in remediation, or previous or concomitant educational experiences.

The Lovett Research Program

A subtype × teaching method study by Lovett et al. (1988) exemplifies a classification system that used direct measures of reading behaviors to identify subtypes of reading-disabled children who fail at crucial stages of reading acquisition. Lovett and her colleagues hypothesized that some readers (accuracy-disabled) fail at the initial stage of reading development, which involves the ability to recognize accurately and decode single words. Others (rate-disabled), although accurate decoders, demonstrate a deficiency at a later stage of reading characterized by the development of speed and fluency. Differential response to treatment was predicted on the basis of pretreatment reading and language characteristics of children assigned to either an accuracy-disabled or a rate-disabled subtype.

From a clinic-referred sample of 8- to 13-year-old children, Lovett selected 112 disabled readers based on multiple measures of accuracy and speed of single-word recognition and contextual reading. Accuracy-disabled readers were identified on the basis of substandard performance on four out of five tests of untimed word recognition. Rate-disabled children were classified on similar criteria for reading speed in the presence of average decoding accuracy. The groups did not differ significantly in age or IQ. However, accuracy-disabled children were significantly different from rate-disabled subjects on pretreatment language characteristics (i.e., receptive vocabulary, naming opposites, and syntax).

Because it is generally desirable to classify children based on nonredundant measurements (see Lyon & Flynn, 1990), a word about Lovett's use of multiple measurements to assess single constructs is in order. Because standardized reading tests vary significantly in the number, regularity, and complexity of words used as stimuli (Lovett et al., 1988; Voeller & Armus, 1988), Lovett used multiple measures of critical reading skills in order to avoid a classification artifact based on the idiosyncratic content of single instruments.

Following identification, children from each subtype received 40 hours of remediation with random assignment to one of two treatments or a control condition. A decoding skills program (DS) emphasized acquisition of single-word recognition for both regular and exception words of high frequency. The second treatment condition (OWLS) emphasized reading in context, listening and reading comprehension, vocabulary development, syntactical elaboration, and written compositions. Finally, a control condition taught classroom survival skills (CSS) with no direct instruction in reading or exposure to print.

Pre- and posttests measured several dimensions of reading skill. The dependent variables included an experimental test of phonetically regular and exception words, standardized tests of word recognition singly and in context, and language measures. Given the theoretical framework of the study, these measures appear to constitute ecologically valid measurements of subtypal attributes and treatment conditions. Unfortunately, reliability data were not reported. This information would have been additionally helpful in interpreting the results of the experimental word recognition test, which does appear to have adequate content validity from both a classification and treatment standpoint.

Data were analyzed using a series of ANOVAs. For instance, analysis of the experimental word task included a five-way analysis of variance with nesting of subjects according to sample (rate-disabled, accuracy-disabled) and treatment program (DS, OWLS, CSS). Repeated measures factors consisted of word type (regular, exception), word frequency class (high, medium, low), and time of test (pretest, posttest). Posttest cell means were adjusted for pretest performance differences.

Results of the experimental word recognition test were interesting with respect to subtype × teaching method interactions. For example, rate-disabled readers in both the DS and OWLS conditions made significant gains on nonphonetic words but not on phonetically regular words as compared to their control peers in CSS. On the other hand, accuracy-disabled readers demonstrated posttest gains for both regular and non-phonetic words, with greater gains made on nonphonetic words in the DS condition. This latter finding was unexpected, given the presumed additional processing demands for remembering sight words as opposed to words that conform to sound–symbol patterns. Lovett et al. (1988) speculated that this finding reflected the fact that more time was spent teaching individual nonphonetic words, while phonetically regular words were presented in word patterns. An alternate explanation could be that nonphonetic words represented more salient entities than phonetically regular words presented in pattern drills and were thus more readily mastered. The ambiguity inherent in this interpretation illustrates the complexity of accounting for educational outcomes even in well-controlled treatments with relatively precise dependent variables.

The standardized test results also illustrate the difficulty of measuring change given a relatively brief treatment period. Both accuracy-disabled and rate-disabled readers in DS and OWLS demonstrated significantly greater performance on the Wide Range Achievement Test—Revised (Jastak & Wilkinson, 1984) compared to children in CSS. However, inspection of the posttest raw data reveals that superior posttest performance involved raw score differences of only one or two words. Because CSS children received no reading instruction, this statistically significant finding does not appear to be clinically useful in choosing a treatment program.

Despite the difficulties noted, the Lovett et al. (1988) subtype $\times$ teaching method study is important for a number of reasons. First, the classification system was based on direct observation of reading behaviors within a developmental framework. Second, multiple measures were used to classify children, thus avoiding classification artifacts associated with sizable differences in word type found in different standardized tests. Third, a large number of disabled readers, well matched on IQ and age, were assigned to clearly defined reading treatments and a nonreading control condition. Fourth, project teachers implemented all three treatments, thus controlling for teacher differences. The distinctiveness and fidelity of each treatment were also well documented through random observation and coding of student and teacher activities by two raters with resultant good interrater reliability. Finally, the dependent measures included theory-based experimental tasks as well as standardized tests of reading skills in order to assess educational outcomes adequately.

The Flynn Research Program

A similar classification and educational validation pilot study of longer duration was conducted by Flynn (see Flynn & Deering, 1989; Lyon et al.,

1988). Similar to the Lovett et al. (1988) study, direct measures of reading and spelling behaviors were chosen to classify children and to generate hypotheses about instructional methodologies that have a predicted probability of success with identified subtypes.

Assessment tasks were chosen to represent key subskills in an interactive reading model conceptualized to include lower-level processes (alphabetic, logographic, orthographic word recognition skills) and higher-level processes (syntax, semantics, experiential knowledge, executive monitoring skills). Ecological assessment of intact, deficient, and compensatory reading strategies included oral reading samples to classify errors and the Boder Tests of Reading–Spelling Behaviors (Boder & Jarrico, 1982). Thus, test content was directly related to the tasks that children face on a daily basis and led to testable hypotheses regarding subtype responses to specified instructional methodologies.

Children who demonstrated significant difficulties with sound–symbol relationships, the decoding and spelling of single words, and contextual reading were classified as dysphonetic. These children are clinically similar to Lovett's accuracy-disabled readers. Dyseidetic (rate-disabled) children demonstrated normal decoding abilities on phonetically regular words and produced good phonetic equivalents in their misspellings, but they had difficulty recognizing nonphonetic words and read slowly.

Using these criteria, Flynn identified 27 first, second, and third grade children. Because of limited sample size, matching on IQ, age, and other variables generally related to achievement was not possible. The two groups did not differ significantly with respect to receptive vocabulary, age, parents' educational level, and school history. This pilot study was conducted during the school day, and therefore random assignment to treatment was difficult because of classroom scheduling conflicts. Nevertheless, children's assignments to treatment were randomized as much as possible across ages and subtypes. As in the Lovett et al. (1988) study, no attempt was made to control for concomitant reading instruction in the regular classroom or at home. The children participated in reading remediation for 33 weeks, three times a week for 45 minutes per session during the first year of the study and for four sessions per week during the second year. Differences in teacher preparation and style were accounted for by assigning teachers to different remediation groups at midyear.

It was hypothesized that dysphoneic (accuracy-disabled) readers would respond to a program that controlled the phonetic complexity of English orthography through use of the Initial Teaching Alphabet (ITA). In addition, phonetic principles were presented analytically to children in this subtype through a language experience approach. Conversely, dyseidetic (rate-disabled) children were hypothesized to have intact auditory–linguistic reading skills and were predicted to respond best to a synthetic phonics program. The Distar Reading Program (Engelmann & Bruner, 1984) was chosen as the synthetic phonics program. Children in the two treatment groups did not differ significantly on age, verbal IQ, or pretreatment reading level. The final sample of children available for posttesting in these two treatment programs consisted of 12 dysphonetic readers and 5 dyseidetic readers. Educational validation variables chosen to measure the critical dimensions of reading accuracy and fluency included tests of single-word recognition, contextual reading, and spelling. As with the Lovett et al. (1988) study, these measures appear to have content validity for both the classification system and hypothesized responses to instruction.

Results obtained from the contextual reading measures are reported here to illustrate principles relevant to our discussion of educational validation research. First, different scores were compiled to provide a summary of average gain by subtype (dysphonetic, dyseidetic) within each treatment (ITA, Distar). Given the small number of subjects per cell and the unreliability of difference scores (Cronbach & Snow, 1977), tests of significance were not computed. Rather, graphing and visual inspection of the data were used to refine and generate hypotheses for future studies with a larger sample.

Visual inspection of average gains on measures of contextual reading suggested that, as hypothesized, dysphonetic (accuracy-disabled) children made greater gains via the language experience, analytic phonics program using the ITA than in Distar. Unexpectedly, dyseidetics in ITA also made greater gains than in the Distar condition.

Despite difficulties in sample size and assignment to treatments, the Flynn study does provide additional support for the use of direct measurements of reading and spelling behaviors in the identification of subtypes and in conducting ecologically relevant educational validation studies. Two findings may be especially important in designing future studies. First, the variability of results within each treatment condition and subtype demonstrates the inadequacy of a design that implies a simple match between reading subtype and optimal treatment program. Further, second-year data derived from the Flynn study suggest that longitudinal investigations are needed in order to measure adequately the critical dimension of reading fluency. Specifically, while only three of the eight children (38%) in the ITA condition could read fluently at grade level by the end of the first year of remediation, 9 out of 15 ITA-instructed children (60%) were fluent readers by the end of the second year.

This overview of the Lovett and Flynn studies may be helpful in designing future educational validation research. For instance, all subtypes in both investigations made the most progress in analytic phonics programs (Lovett's DS and Flynn's ITA) and in language experience approaches that emphasized reading- and writing-connected discourse (Lovett's OWLS and Flynn's ITA). This finding suggests that subtype differentiation is unnecessary if broadly based treatment conditions are implemented. However, apart from developmental considerations that make both accuracy and fluency data important in identifying poor readers, subtyping may be important in explaining individual outcomes. That is, similar treatment outcomes may have occurred through subtle differences in teacher–child interactions within a program. This could be especially true in the language experience approaches (OWLS and ITA) but could have also occurred in the analytic phonics (DS) treatment as teachers adjusted rate and manner of presentation to each child's attentional, motivational, processing, and prior knowledge characteristics.

The possibility that these subtle adaptations were made by teachers points out the need for more dynamic aptitude × treatment interaction studies. The contamination of age ranges and concomitant and/or prior interventions in both the Lovett and Flynn studies further suggest the need for longitudinal investigations that begin in preschool and follow the children for a sufficient period of time to measure reading mastery adequately. The challenge of these and other language-based intervention studies will be to allow the teacher freedom to vary the approach and methodology while accounting for teacher–child–content–context variables that result in specific educational outcomes.

Conclusions

Identifying subtype × treatment method interactions may be one useful procedure to establish the external validity of a particular subtype solution. Findings derived from educational validation studies also serve to establish the predictive and clinical validity of a classification system. It is important to note, however, that educational validations are extraordinarily complex and difficult to conduct, primarily because of the dynamic nature of the teaching process. Proficient teachers and clinicians constantly attempt to manipulate and control learner, task, and setting (e.g., classroom) variables. Within this context, expert teachers continuously modify representations of concepts for different students, monitor and adjust the number of conceptual elements being presented, routinely induce strategies for learning, motivate students to persist in difficult-to-learn tasks, and perform all of these instructional elements simultaneously or in rapid succession to produce learning (Lyon & Moats, 1988).

Because of this complexity, our initial attempts at predicting treatment options on the basis of subtype characteristics fall far short of the educational task confronting us. Ultimately, the best classification (subtyping) for educational purposes may result from documenting how children at risk for educational failure respond to specific instructional methodologies. Students' responses to different representations and strategies, etc. may be used as attribute variables that would allow for assignment to a particular subtype. As one example, it could be hypothesized that children with general and/or nonspecific reading delays on first grade entrance would respond equally well to any intervention methodology, whereas children at risk for failure in accuracy or fluency stages of reading would require longer periods of intervention and more specific instructional methodologies. Likewise, children who respond to reading approaches that provide explicit representations and explanations of phonological codes may differ substantially from students who benefit more from global orthographic representations. What is clear is that the appropriate use of subtyping methodology in educational settings will require creative research methodologies that are as dynamic, fluid, and flexible as is the teaching process itself.

Acknowledgments

The preparation of this chapter was made possible by a Research Scientist grant to G. Reid Lyon from the Gundersen Medical Foundation, LaCrosse, WI, and by a grant to Jane M. Flynn from the Initial Teaching Alphabet Foundation, Roslyn Heights, NY. The authors wish to thank Tanya Prindle and Mary Vaassen for critical comments on drafts of this chapter.

References

Benson, D. F., & Geschwind, N. (1975). The alexias. In D. J. Vinkis & G. W. Bruyn (Eds.), *Handbook of clinical neurology* (Vol. 4, pp. 325–350.). New York: American Elsevier.

Boder, E., & Jarrico, S. (1982). *The Boder Test of Reading-Spelling Patterns: A diagnostic screening text for subtypes of reading disability.* New York: Grune & Stratton.

Bracht, G. H. (1970). Experimental factors related to aptitude treatment interactions. *Review of Educational Research, 40,* 627–645.

Cronbach, L. J. (1977). How can instruction be adapted to individual differences? In R. M. Gagne (Ed.), *Learning and individual differences,* (pp. 79–90). Columbus, OH: Charles E. Merrill.

Cronbach, L. J., & Snow, R. E. (1977). *Aptitudes and instructional methods.* New York: Irvington.

Dunn, L. M., & Markwardt, F. D. (1970). *Manual, Peabody Individual Achievement Test.* Circle Pines, MN: American Guidance Service.

Engelmann, S., & Bruner, E (1984). *Distar Reading.* Chicago: Science Research Associates.

Fletcher, J. M., & Morris, R. (1986). Classification of disabled learners: Beyond exclusionary definitions. In S. J. Ceci (Ed.), *Handbook of cognitive, social, and neuropsychological aspects of learning disabilities* (Vol. 1, pp. 55–80). Hillsdale, NJ: Lawrence Erlbaum.

Flynn, J. M., & Deering, W. M. (1989). Subtypes of dyslexia: Investigation of Boder's system using quantitative neurophysiology. *Developmental Medicine and Child Neurology, 31,* 215–223.

Hooper, S. R., & Willis, W. G. (1989). *Learning disability subtyping: Neuropsychological foundations, conceptual models, and issues in clinical differentiation.* New York: Springer-Verlag.

Jastak, S., & Wilkinson, G. (1984). *The Wide Range Achievement Test—Revised.* Wilmington, DE: Jastak Associates.

Lovett, M. W., Ransby, M. J., & Barron, R. W. (1988). Treatment, subtype, and word type effects in dyslexic children's response to remediation. *Brain and Language, 34,* 328–349.

Luria, A. R. (1966). *Higher cortical functions in man.* New York: Basic Books.

Luria, A. R. (1973). *The working brain: An introduction to neuropsychology.* New York: Basic Books.

Lyon, G. R. (1983). Subgroups of learning disabled readers: Clinical and empirical identification. In H. R. Myklebust (Ed..), *Progress in learning disabilities.* (Vol. 5, pp. 103–134). New York: Grune & Stratton.

Lyon, G. R. (1985a). Educational validation of learning disability subtypes. In B. P. Rourke (Ed.), *Neuropsychology of learning disabilities: Essential of subtype analysis* (pp. 228–256). New York: Guilford Press.

Lyon, G. R. (1985b). Identification and remediation of learning disability subtypes: Preliminary findings. *Learning Disabilities Focus, 1,* 21–35.

Lyon, G. R., & Flynn, J. M. (1990). Assessing subtypes of learning abilities. In H. L. Swanson (Ed.), *Handbook on the assessment of learning disabilities: Theory, research, and practice* (pp. 59–74). San Diego: College-Hill Press.

Lyon, G. R., & Moats, L. C. (1988). Critical issues in the instruction of the learning disabled. *Journal of Consulting and Clinical Psychology, 56,* 830–835.

Lyon, G. R., Moats, L. C., & Flynn, J. M. (1988). From assessment to treatment: Linkages to interventions with children. In M. Tramontana & S. Hooper (Eds.), *Issues in child neuropsychology: From assessment to treatment* (pp. 113–142). New York: Plenum Press.

Lyon, G. R., Rietta, S., Watson, B., Porch, B., & Rhodes, J. (1981). Selected linguistic and perceptual abilities of empirically derived subgroups of learning disabled readers. *Journal of School Psychology, 19,* 152–166.

Lyon, G. R., Stewart, N., & Freedman, D. (1982). Neuropsychological characteristics of empirically derived subgroups of learning disabled readers. *Journal of Clinical Neuropsychology, 4,* 343–365.

Lyon, G. R., & Watson, B. (1981). Empirically derived subgroups of learning disabled readers: Diagnostic characteristics. *Journal of Learning Disabilities, 14,* 256–261.

Rourke, B. P. (1985). *Neuropsychology of learning disabilities: Essentials of subtype analysis.* New York: Guilford Press.

Satz, P., & Morris, R. (1981). Learning disability subtypes: A review. In F. H. Pirozzolo & M. C. Wittrock (Eds.), *Neuropsychological and cognitive processes in reading* (pp. 109–141). New York: Academic Press.

Traub, M., & Bloom, F. (1975). *Recipe for reading.* Cambridge, MA: Educators Publishing Service.

Voeller, K. S., & Armus, J. (1988, November). *Analysis of word characteristics in specific reading tests, based on information-processing models: Implications for evaluating dyslexics.* Paper presented at the 37th Annual Orton Dyslexia Society conference, Tampa, FL.

Woodcock, R. (1973). *Woodcock Reading Mastery Test.* Circle Pines, MN: American Guidance Service.

CHAPTER 12

From Theory to Practice with Subtypes of Reading Disabilities

Christina A. M. Fiedorowicz and Ronald L. Trites

The development of effective intervention programs for the reading disabled is an issue of considerable significance. Follow-up studies have indicated that the learning problems and their sequelae persist into adulthood (Bruck, 1985; Schonhaut & Satz, 1983; Spreen, 1982; Trites & Fiedorowicz, 1976). The reasons for the poor outcome are unclear. Are the reading disabilities intractable, or are they amenable to intervention? What constitutes effective intervention? These are important questions that educators and researchers alike need to pursue, not only to develop a better understanding of the disorder and its management from a scientific perspective but also because the consequences of the reading disabilities have serious long-term practical effects academically, vocationally, socioeconomically, and emotionally.

A review of the literature has indicated that in general, the traditional methods of remediation of reading disabilities are largely ineffective (Balow, 1965; Bateman, 1977; Benton, 1978; Buerger, 1968; Fiedorowicz & Trites, 1987; Guthrie, 1978; Johnson, 1978; Vernon, 1971; Zigmond, 1978). Some researchers have interpreted this poor outcome as indicative of an intractable disorder (Balow, 1965; Buerger, 1968) or at least one that is "highly resistant to instruction" (Vernon, 1971). However, many others consider the interventions *per se* to be inadequate, or the methods of evaluating the effectiveness of treatment to be flawed (Arter & Jenkins, 1979; Doehring, Trites, Patel, & Fiedorowicz, 1981; Hewison, 1982; Johnson, 1978; Torgeson, 1979; Wong, 1979).

The interpretation of an intractable disorder appears to be a premature overgeneralization, and a pessimistic one at that. Before such a conclusion can be drawn, it is necessary to determine that the interventions employed for the reading disabled incorporate exemplary teaching strategies and that methodological issues are adequately addressed in the investigation of the efficacy of the remedial techniques.

In this chapter, one intervention approach with demonstrated effectiveness is presented. This approach, called the Autoskill Component Reading Subskills (CRS) Program, was developed in accordance with several current theoretical issues related to reading disabilities.

The major theoretical principles integrated in the program include the identification, through computerized testing, of different subtypes of reading difficulties and then the remediation of the deficits with differential training subprograms specific to each type of reading difficulty. Another important feature of the program involves the automaticity theory, the basis of which is the idea that component skills for reading letters, syllables, and words must be overlearned to a level of rapid automatic responding so that higher levels of reading, such as comprehension, can be attained. A combination of task-analytic and process-oriented approaches has been incorporated to identify component skills of reading word recognition and profiles of reading subskills so that training can proceed in a sequential format to remediate weaknesses in the reading subskill profile. Behavioral principles have also been integrated in the program to enhance learning through immediate positive reinforcement of correct responses and presentation of correct answers when errors have been made. Graphing of all results to monitor progress is provided on an ongoing basis along with an extensive automated record-keeping system for rapid access to all testing and training data.

The importance of these theoretical perspectives is summarized, followed by research studies evaluating the efficacy of this approach.

Relevance of the Subtype Concept

One possible factor complicating the understanding of reading disabilities is that, traditionally, research investigations were based on the assumption that all reading-disabled persons belonged to a homogeneous group. The focus of research was on finding a single cause for a unitary form of reading disability and finding a single treatment intervention. This model resulted in the reporting of a vast array of symptoms and etiological factors associated with the disorder and little understanding of the underlying disability. However, each reading-disabled person does not share all of the characteristics, deficits, and strengths of other reading-disabled persons. This single-syndrome paradigm was criticized as too simplistic in that it ignored the complexities of reading as a multidimensional process.

An alternative multiple-syndrome paradigm that allows for subtypes of reading disabilities was suggested as a more appropriate model (Applebee, 1971; Doehring, 1978; Doehring & Hoshko, 1977; Doehring et al.,

1981; Satz & Morris, 1981; Wiener & Cromer, 1967). Further, it was hypothethized that, if distinct homogeneous subtypes could be determined, remedial intervention specific to the individual subtype could result in a better outcome (Aaron, Grantham, & Campbell, 1982; Boder, 1973; Doehring et al., 1981; Fiedorowicz, 1986; Fiedorowicz & Trites, 1987; Petrauskas & Rourke, 1979; Satz & Morris, 1981).

Doehring (1976) devised a battery of reading subskill tests based on a task analysis of reading word recognition. Individual letters, pronounceable nonsense syllables, and one-syllable words were presented by four different procedures: visual matching-to-sample, auditory–visual matching-to-sample, oral reading (reading aloud), and visual scanning. Normative data for the test battery were obtained on a sample of average prereaders and readers in kindergarten through grade 11. The tests were administered to a sample of 34 reading-disabled subjects aged 8 to 17 years, and three subtypes were determined: Type O, oral reading deficit subtype; Type A, intermodal-associative subtype; and Type S, sequential relations deficit subtype.

All of the students performed more poorly on all of the tasks relative to average or normal readers, and the deficits of the reading disability subtypes showed three specific patterns of performance. The subjects categorized as Type O, the oral reading subtype, were characterized by poor oral reading of words and syllables with performance on visual and auditory–visual matching-to-sample tasks relatively good. The predominant impairment of Type A was in auditory–visual matching of letters, syllables, and words, and it was considered that the main difficulty of readers of this type was in intermodal association. Type S readers, or the sequential deficit subtype, could match single letters well but were notably poor in matching syllables and words, and therefore it was hypothesized that their main difficulty was in sequencing (Doehring & Hoshko, 1977). The same three subtypes were identified in a second sample of 88 reading-disabled subjects aged 8 to 27 (71% of the subjects were aged 8 to 14), thus replicating the initial findings (Doehring et al., 1981).

The method of classification for both studies was the Q-technique of factor analysis (Nunnally, 1967; Overall & Klett, 1972). Cluster analysis and discriminant function analysis were used to illustrate the stability of the subtypes, and several analyses of subsamples yielded consistent results. In addition, comparisons of average readers and children with other types of learning problems, and with external criteria such as teacher evaluations, also demonstrated the stability of the subtypes (Doehring, Hoshko, & Bryans, 1979; Doehring et al., 1981). The same subtypes were identified in two other subsequent studies of 15 reading-disabled boys aged 8 to 14 (Fiedorowicz, 1986) and 74 reading-disabled boys and girls aged 8 to 19 (Fiedorowicz & Trites, 1987).

The neuropsychological and linguistic profiles of each subtype were evaluated in the study involving the 88 reading-disabled subjects. The neuropsychological characteristics were determined based on a variety of cognitive, sensory, and motor measures (Trites, 1977). Each subtype exhibited differential profiles (Doehring et al., 1981; Fiedorowicz, Trites, & Doehring, 1980). Type O appeared to be the least impaired subtype, and although there were a few mild asymmetries on the tests of motor and sensory function, performance levels were above the clinical average, and there was no evidence of cerebral dysfunction. Type A was the most impaired group, and the profile was interpreted as consistent with left hemisphere dysfunction. The predominant deficit of Type S appeared to be spatial in nature, with evidence of cerebral dysfunction in the posterior regions of the brain, possibly with greater right hemisphere involvement.

The analysis of the linguistic profiles was based on an extensive battery of language tests (Doehring et al. 1981). The pattern of language deficit for the sample as a whole suggested that the predominant difficulty was on tests of low levels of language skill such as phonemic segmentation, blending, serial naming, and morphophonemic knowledge, whereas tests involving higher levels of semantic knowledge were near normal. No consistent clear-cut differential patterns were found for each subtype with the following exceptions: Type O was associated with a short-term verbal memory deficit and word retrieval deficit, and Type A and Type S were associated with poor serial naming and difficulty following instructions.

Further study of both the neuropsychological and linguistic characteristics is necessary before definite statements can be made about these aspects of the Type O, A, and S subtypes. However, there is strong evidence to suggest that these reading subtype profiles are viable in view of the replicability across different samples and stability across different types of analyses. It was, therefore, considered that the three reading disability subtypes were appropriate to form the basis of a treatment program with differential training corresponding to each of the specific subtypes.

Rationale for Rapid Automatic Responding in Reading

LaBerge and Samuels (1974) developed a theoretical model of information processing in reading in which words in print are transformed into meaning through a series of processing stages of visual, phonological, episodic, and semantic systems. It was hypothesized that if each stage or component process required attention, the capacity of attention would be overloaded. Therefore, automatic processing must occur in order to execute such a complex skill.

Automaticity at the level of recognition of letters, syllables, and words would allow a greater amount of attention to be available for higher-level aspects of reading, such as comprehension. It was suggested that the method of achieving automatic responding or fluent reading was through overlearning, practice, repetition, or drill. Fluent reading was defined as consisting of two components, including accuracy of word recognition and reading speed.

The issue of establishing accuracy before training reading speed has been discussed extensively (Carver & Hoffman, 1981; Chall, 1979; Chomsky, 1978; Perfetti & Lesgold, 1979; Samuels, 1979). At the time of the development of the training procedures incorporated in the Autoskill CRS Program, several authors had pointed to the importance of automaticity in reading (Fisher, 1979, LaBerge, 1979; LaBerge, Peterson, & Norden, 1977; Lesgold & Resnick, 1981; Perfetti & Lesgold, 1979; Sternberg & Wagner, 1982), and investigations had been carried out in which the theory of automaticity had been applied (Carver & Hoffman, 1981; Chomsky, 1978; Gonzales & Elijah, 1975: LaBerge 1973; LaBerge & Samuels, 1973; Samuels, 1979; Terry, 1974). Although there were positive findings in the training studies, there were methodological problems (Fiedorowicz, 1983; Fiedorowicz & Trites, 1987), and of central importance, the automaticity model had not been applied to subtypes of reading disabilities.

The use of computerized training was implemented in this context, since computer technology lends itself readily to the concept of automaticity. Computerized programs provided a fast and efficient method for measuring latency of response, delivering immediate reinforcement, keeping detailed records, and, of particular importance, presenting the training stimuli in a rapid fashion. All of these features were considered crucial in a method emphasizing skill and practice (Carver & Hoffman, 1981; Perfetti & Lesgold, 1979).

A Combined Process-Oriented/Task-Analytic Approach

Arter and Jenkins (1979) have critically evaluated a common treatment model used in special education, the Differential Diagnosis–Prescriptive Teaching (DD-PT) model. DD-PT involves the assessment of various psycholinguistic and perceptual–motor abilities that are presumed to be necessary for the acquisition of basic academic skills. Then, based on the pattern of strengths and weaknesses, treatment programs are prescribed. The asumption of this process-oriented approach is that the disability is the result of deficiencies in one or more of the basic psychological processes required for learning (Estes, 1974; Werner, 1973). The general psychological processes examined have included various auditory, visual, cross-sensory perceptual, and psycholinguistic abilities (Arter and Jenkins, 1979). Instruction is then matched to the individual learning needs (Kirk, 1972). This approach has been described as the "majority position within the field of learning disabilities over the past 20 to 30 years" (Haring & Bateman, 1977).

Arter and Jenkins (1979) criticized this approach as failing to validate several assumptions inherent in the DD-PT model. Their overall conclusions included the following: poor reliability and validity of the DD-PT tests used in measuring psychological processes, poor success rate in training the underlying psychological process, poor success rate in improvement in academic skills following training in the underlying psychological process, and that modality–instruction matching failed to improve achievement. Although their review cast doubt on the validity of the DD-PT model, they suggested that their results do not mean that this approach is theoretically untenable but rather, that the current instructional programs and tests are not successful.

Torgeson (1979) also criticized the effectiveness of treatments based on process-oriented theories. He raised questions similar to Arter and Jenkins regarding whether or not psychological processes necessary for learning could, in fact, be identified and measured. He concluded that although specifically defined subprocesses can be trained so that performance on a given task is improved, generalization to other academic skills is poor. He contrasted the process-oriented approach with the task-analytic approach.

There are no inferences about processing problems with the task-analytic model. Rather, the assumption is that poor performance on tests of a prerequisite skill is secondary to a lack of practicing the skill (Smead, 1977). A major advantage of this approach is that information directly relevant to instruction in academic skills is provided. On the other hand, task analysis does not consider individual differences in cognitive functioning, whereas process-oriented theories recognize sources of variance other than practice. Torgeson, therefore, suggested an integration of both approaches beginning with an analysis of the academic task into component skills and then a development of tests to assess the processes required to learn the skills. This view is supported by others (Doehring et al., 1981, Wong, 1979).

In the Autoskill CRS Program an integration of the task-analytic and process-oriented models is incorporated into the training procedures. There are three different procedures involved in the training in the Autoskill CRS Program: oral reading, auditory–visual matching-to-sample, and visual matching-to-sample. Each of the training procedures involves the training of component reading skills, which were identified through a task-analytic process. The task analysis used to identify the component reading skills is a feature in keeping with the task-analytic model.

Performance levels on the three different procedures can be defined in terms of either strengths or weaknesses in component reading subskills, and training can proceed according to either the strengths or the weaknesses. This feature is similar to the process-oriented model in that individual characteristics can be treated differentially. However, a major alteration from the typical process-oriented procedure is that the differential profiles are based on component reading skills and not general psychological processes, which is what the process-orientated procedure usually involves.

Irrespective of which of the three procedures is used, the training consists of improving rapid automatic responding through practice. This feature is in keeping with both the task-analytic approach and the theory of automatic information processing, since both approaches emphasize drill and repetition to a level of rapid automatic responding.

A Component Reading Subskills Approach

Research Study I

The first major study (Fiedorowicz, 1983, 1986) investigating the effectiveness of the training procedures that are incorporated into the Autoskill CRS Program was carried out in the Renfrew County Board of Education, Ontario, during the 1981–1982 academic year. The study included 16 boys referred by school personnel, each of whom met rigorous criteria of reading disability.

It has been generally acknowledged that the term reading disability refers to those children who fail to acquire normal reading proficiency despite average intelligence, sociocultural opportunity, conventional instruction, and freedom from gross sensory, emotional, or neurological handicap (Benton, 1975, 1978; Critchley, 1970; Rourke, 1978). It has also been generally acknowledged that such a definition is problematic, since it is one of exclusion and describes a residual syndrome (Benton, 1978; Rutter, 1978).

Recently, some investigators have emphasized a less restrictive approach (Doehring et al., 1981; Ross, 1976; Rutter, 1978; Satz & Morris, 1981). A redefinition following a more inclusive concept that recognizes variants such as children with neurological, intellectual, social, emotional, or educational handicaps has been suggested as an alternative. The basic argument of those who support this position is that children diagnosed as reading disabled should not be distinguished from other failing readers along the dimensions included in the definition, specifically academic, neurological, and emotional characteristics. They differ significantly from other failing readers on all of the dimensions specified in the current definition (Satz & Morris, 1981). However, Benton (1978) cautions that, following this tack, there is a risk of becoming so diffuse as to be no longer clinically or theoretically relevant. Some limiting descriptions of the condition are necessary for a meaningful basis of comparison in research. For this reason, stringent criteria for inclusion in the first evaluation study were applied.

The average age of the sample was 11 years, with a range of 8 to 13 years. All subjects were at least 1.5 grade levels behind in word recognition reading skills, with an average of a 2.3-grade-level delay as measured by the Wide Range Achievement Test (WRAT; Jastak & Jastak, 1976). The average reading word recognition grade level was 3.7. All subjects had at least average intelligence (as defined by a score of 90 on the Verbal IQ, Performance IQ, and Full Scale IQ scales on the Wechsler Intelligence Scale for Children—Revised [WISC-R; Wechsler, 1974]). None of the children had emotional or behavioral problems according to the Conners Teacher Symptom Questionnaire (Conners, 1969) completed by the teacher and according to the Beitchman Self-Report Psychiatric Questionnaire (Beitchman & Raman, 1981) completed by the student. None had visual or auditory impairment as indicated through eye and audiometric examinations carried out by the Public Health Nurse, and there was no evidence of overt neurological dysfunction based on clinical history interviews and health records. All children were white, middle-class (Blishen & McRoberts, 1976) boys.

Following an assessment of component reading subskills, the subjects were classified into subtypes. There were five subjects in each of the Type O, Type A, and Type S subtypes. An additional subject participated in the pre- and posttesting but not the training. There were no significant subtype differences on any of the selection variables as determined by an analysis of variance.

Type O subjects were trained on the oral reading procedure, Type A subjects on the auditory–visual matching-to-sample procedure, and Type S subjects on the visual matching-to-sample procedure. The training stimuli, presented according to the respective procedures, included single letters, cv–vc syllables, and cvc, cvvc, and cvcc syllables and words (c = consonant, v = vowel). Each subject received half-hour sessions, 4 to 5 days per week, for a total of 21.5 hours over 11 weeks.

Eight subjects, randomly selected, were trained during the first half of the academic year on Schedule 1, and seven subjects during the second half of the year on Schedule 2. Schedule 1 consisted of pretest, training,

posttest, no training, posttest. Schedule 2 consisted of pretest, no training, pretest, training, and posttest, with an approximate interval of 2.5 to
3 months for the training and no-training periods. This design allowed
the subjects on Schedule 2 to serve as an untrained control group (waiting
list) and for follow-up data to be obtained with subjects on Schedule 1.

The assessment battery administered at all pre- and posttraining periods consisted of measurements of accuracy and latency of response to
trained stimuli on trained and untrained procedures and to untrained
stimuli on trained and untrained procedures. In addition, a variety of
reading achievement measures of word recognition and connected text were
also administered to measure the transfer-of-training effect to the reading
task in general. The Student Problem Individual Reading Evaluation
(SPIRE; Alpert & Kravitz, 1971) was used as measure of reading word
recognition. The Gallistel–Ellis Test of Coding Skills (G-E; Gallistel &
Ellis, 1974) was used as a measure of phonetic knowledge. The SPIRE was
also used as a measure of paragraph reading fluency, retention, and comprehension. The Qualitative Analysis of Silent and Oral Reading
(QASOR; Aulls, 1981) was used to assess the reading of cloze passages.

A series of repeated-measures ANOVAs was applied. The rationale
for the statistical analysis as well as the details of the analyses have been
reported elsewhere (Fiedorowicz, 1983, 1986) and only the main findings
are summarized here.

1. Significant improvement specific to subtype classification and
corresponding training procedures was obtained for trained stimuli presented according to training procedures in comparisons of trained versus
untrained subjects and for the total sample as well. Further, there was a
significant transfer-of-training effect as measured by the reading tests.

2. The subjects trained during the first part of the study showed
marked improvement in the component reading skills, reading word
recognition, and phonetic knowledge in comparison to the subjects who
received no training during that same period. When the subjects were
pooled following training of all subjects, all subjects showed marked
improvement in these same areas.

3. Accuracy and speed of response were significantly improved on the
oral reading and auditory–visual matching-to-sample procedures, and
speed of response was significantly improved on the visual matching-to-
sample procedure. Accuracy did not improve on the visual matching-to-
sample procedure; this is probably because accuracy levels at pretesting
were very high, with little potential for improvement.

4. There was a grade-level-equivalent improvement of slightly more
than 1 grade level on the SPIRE word recognition and a 17% improvement in phonetic knowledge of words on the G-E test. These gains, over
2½ months of training, were an important and positive outcome of this

study, since reading-disabled children typically do not achieve 1 grade level in reading over the course of 1 full academic year.

5. There was a significant transfer of training to reading text with the total sample analysis but not with the trained versus untrained comparisons. This finding was disappointing in that, based on the automaticity model, it was predicted that the significant transfer in training effects of component reading subskills should improve paragraph-reading fluency and comprehension. An explanation for the inconsistent transfer to paragraph reading and comprehension may be related to the small sample size in the trained versus untrained comparisons. Alternatively, it may be that it is unrealistic to expect that such a short period of training would be sufficient to remediate the component skill deficits entirely, and therefore a longer period of training would be necessary, especially in view of the inclusion of moderate and severe reading-disabled subjects (some had projected grade delays of up to 4.9 grade levels). Further, it may be that specific training in paragraph-reading fluency is important to enhance the process.

6. The analyses of the follow-up results indicated that the students who were trained during the first part of the study, posttested immediately following training, and then posttested in a follow-up after a 4 month interval maintained their gains.

7. Analyses of the specific subtype results indicated that training the deficient component reading skills according to subtype significantly improved the skills trained, and the effects on the component skills were differential to the specific subtype. Type O and A subjects were significantly more accurate on their respective training procedures at posttest, and Type S subjects were significantly faster on their training procedure. However, there were no significant differences among the subtypes in the gains made on the independent reading tests. This may be reflecting a problem with the small sample size or the short training period. Alternatively, it may be an indication that, once the predominant deficit, which is different for each subtype, is remediated, the rate of gain in reading words then progresses at a consistent rate regardless of subtype.

LIMITATIONS OF STUDY I

Overall, the results of this initial evaluation were encouraging, and it was concluded that training in deficient component reading subskills, according to differential subtype training procedures, was a viable approach to enhancing reading skills. However, there were limitations in this first study, both with regard to methodology and to the expected outcome in paragraph reading. It was apparent that there were important issues to explore further in a more extensive investigation.

Several features of the testing and training procedures were altered and expanded and became part of the Autoskill CRS Program. It was also considered important to study a larger sample of reading-disabled children, both male and female, over a longer period of training. Alternative control groups needed to be incorporated into the design. In addition, training procedures were implemented by teachers to determine how readily the program could be administered in the schools and other educational settings on an ongoing basis.

All of these issues were incorporated in the second study evaluating the effectiveness of the training procedures.

Research Study II

In the second study (Fiedorowicz & Trites, 1987)), five school boards of education in the Eastern Region of Ontario participated. Altogether, 26 schools, 35 teachers, and 115 reading-disabled students (all of whom met rigorous criteria for reading disability as defined in the first study) were involved. There were 26 Type O, 22 Type A, and 26 Type S subjects selected for the Autoskill-trained group and 17 subjects for the untrained control group. The average age of the sample was 11.2 years, with a range 7.3 to 14.6 years. There were 57 males and 16 females. The average projected reading grade delay (word recognition) utilizing the Wide Range Achievement Test—Revised (WRAT-R; Jastak & Wilkinson, 1984) was 3.0 grades (range of 1.2 to 6.2 grades). The mean Verbal IQ was 93.0 (range of 80 to 118); the mean Performance IQ was 101.3 (range of 80 to 130); and the mean Full Scale IQ was 96.3 (range of 85 to 123). The WISC-R was administered (Wechsler, 1974). There were no significant differences among the subtypes on any of the variables (age, projected reading grade delay, VIQ, PIQ, or FSIQ).

There were 24 reading-disabled subjects selected for the alternate computer-trained control group. These were matched with a subsample of the Autoskill-trained subjects for age (M age = 11.0; range 9 to 14 years), sex (14 males, 10 females), and projected reading grade delay (3.0 grades). None of these subjects had major visual, hearing, neurological, or emotional/behavioral conditions.

The Autoskill-trained subjects were trained on the Autoskill CRS Program between October and May of the academic year 1985 to 1986 for half-hour sessions, three times per week, for a total of 56.4 hours. Each subtype was trained differentially according to their subtype classification, with Type O trained on oral reading, Type A on auditory–visual matching-to-sample, and Type S on visual matching-to-sample procedures. The training stimuli included single letters, cv–vc syllables, cvc, cvvc, cvcv, ccvc, and cvcc syllables, and words. In addition, two-word and three-word phrases, sentences and paragraphs were also included. The untrained control group subjects were pre- and posttested at the same time of the academic year as were the Autoskill-trained groups, but in the interim period the untrained control group proceeded normally within the school system. The purpose of the untrained control group was to define a sample of reading-disabled subjects and follow their progress in whatever programming the School Boards typically provided for them.

The alternative computer-trained control group subjects were provided with computer-assisted programs concerned with some aspects of language arts development for three half-hour sessions per week for a total of 30 hours. They were compared with the matched subsample of Autoskill–trained subjects trained for 30 hours. The purpose of this control group was predominantly to control for the effect of working on computer-assisted programs related to language arts development. The programs were selected following consultation with specialists within each School Board, and the teachers were permitted to use their choice of programs for language arts.

The pre- and posttest assessment battery included the Autoskill CRS Program Test Battery to evaluate component reading subskills, the WRAT-R (Jastak & Wilkinson, 1984) to assess reading word recognition, the G-E to assess phonetic knowledge, the SPIRE to assess paragraph-reading fluency, retention, and comprehension, as well as the QASOR, a measure of reading of cloze paragraphs. (The alternate computer-trained control subjects did not receive the Autsoskill CRS Program Test Battery or the QASOR, but they received all of the other tests.)

The main findings of this study are summarized below. The full descriptions and results of the statistical analyses have been published elsewhere (Fiedorowicz & Trites, 1987).

1. In the comparisons of the Autoskill-trained group and the untrained control group, the Autoskill-trained group exhibited significant improvement on component reading subskills, reading word recognition, phonetic knowledge of letters and syllables, and paragraph-reading accuracy, speed, retention, and comprehension; they also exhibited better graphic representation and meaning of inserted words in cloze passages.

2. These same results were obtained in an analysis of a subsample of Autoskill-trained subjects matched for Full Scale IQ, age, sex, and projected reading grade delay in word recognition with the untrained control subjects.

3. Analyses of specific subtype comparisons to the untrained control group indicated that each subtype made significant gains in contrast to the untrained control group. The only significant subtype difference among the three subtypes was exhibited on a measure of comprehension

of silently read paragraphs. In this instance, Type S subjects showed greater improvement than did Type O and Type A subjects.

4. In the comparisons of the alternate computer-trained control group and the matched Autoskill-trained subsample, the Autoskill-trained subsample exhibited significant improvement on measures of reading word recognition as well as speed and accuracy of paragraph reading.

5. Other findings in this study, based on statistical analyses, indicated that there were no sex differences in outcome; there were no differences in outcome of students trained by teachers in comparison to those trained by research assistants (all teachers underwent extensive training in the procedures and were provided with year-long supervision and support); and there were no differences among the five School Boards involved throughout the region.

Overall, the results of this investigation indicated significant gains for the reading-disabled students trained on the Autoskill CRS Program. Not only were the findings of the first study replicated, but there were further benefits of training, most important of which was the transfer of training to paragraph-reading fluency and comprehension.

The ultimate goal of any remedial training program for the reading disabled is to improve general reading skills, including word recognition, but particularly reading of connected text. The Autoskill-trained groups improved not only reading word recognition skills but also reading and comprehending paragraphs at a level corresponding to their word recognition skills as well as at their projected grade levels (i.e., the level at which they should be able to read based on their chronological age expectation). This was evident on measures involving passages read aloud and silently in addition to cloze passages. Each subtype was significantly improved at posttest in comparison to pretest; in addition, all were improved at posttest relative to the untrained control group.

FOLLOW-UP

The issue of whether the improvements in reading skills are maintained beyond the intervention phase is important in evaluating the effectiveness of treatment. In the first evaluation study, it was demonstrated that the gains were maintained after a 4 month interval, but there was no assessment as to whether the reading skills continued to improve after training was discontinued. The results of a 1-year follow-up with the subjects in the second study are not yet fully analyzed. However, the preliminary findings indicated that, for most of the Autoskill-trained subjects, the gains were maintained. Furthermore, several of the subjects continued to make progress at a rate faster than would be expected on age level gains alone. It appears that the subjects who made the greatest improvements during the training period were the same subjects who continued to make a rapid rate of progress thereafter.

LIMITATIONS OF STUDY II

The results of these studies lend support to the effectiveness of applying the subtype concept in the treatment of reading disabilities. Component reading subtypes of reading disabilities were identified and trained according to differential procedures that were matched to the respective subtype profiles. In both studies, the selection of training procedures was based on the predominant deficit of the subtype profile, with good results. However, the effectiveness of training according to other aspects of the subtype profiles has not been investigated. Studies involving systematic training according to the strength in the profile, or random assignment of the training procedures, would be of value in determining which training strategies are most effective.

Another question that arises in all treatment studies is the long-term benefits of training. Follow-up investigations of the students in these studies over longer periods of time would be important to determine whether or not the benefits extend beyond the 4-month period.

The applicability of the subtype concept to other types of reading failure, not typically included in the exclusionary definition of reading disability, is another concern that is addressed below.

Beyond the Exclusionary Definition

In all of the studies associated with the development of a component reading subskills approach over the last 13 years, the subjects met rigorous criteria associated with the exclusionary definition of reading disabilities. This is in keeping with the methodology employed in a majority of research studies of reading disabilities, particularly within the field of neuropsychology. In the education system, students who are not progressing in reading skill acquisition and require special intervention to assist them in developing reading skills are identified in a variety of ways. Typically, less stringent criteria are applied in the identification process. The students may be experiencing reading difficulties for a number of reasons, and the predominant concern is that the students are not achieving in reading at a level in keeping with their age- and grade-level peers. In the selection of remedial reading programs for these students, the question arises whether a program developed for specific reading-disabled students that has demonstrated effectiveness with this particular population can be an effective and efficient method of remediation for a more inclusive group of reading difficulties. Is the approach of identifying component reading profiles with corresponding training procedures effective for other types of reading failure? In particular, are the strategies integrated in the Autoskill CRS Program effective for this application? Several sites across Canada and the United States have implemented the program with varied reading-deficient groups. The main findings are reflected in the reports of five different sites described below.

Although the following field site reports may be criticized as lacking in several aspects as research studies, the teachers and their administrators should be acknowledged for their efforts to obtain some objective criteria for evaluating the usefulness and benefits of a new remedial reading program within their respective sites. Pre- and posttesting on standardized reading measures, particularly when a comparison group is included, is an important first step in an evaluation process. Relevant observations have been made that lend support to the subtype approach to treatment of more inclusive reading problems.

Santa Fe Public School District

Chapter 1 students (from low-income families) with identified reading difficulties below the 25th centile of reading on New Mexico state-wide norms were involved. In a preliminary pilot study, 86 students from one school described as "being most in need," since they were below the first centile on the state-wide norms, were tested and trained on the Autoskill CRS Program. The schedule of training was half-hour sessions, three times per week, for 8 weeks. They were pre- and posttested on the Metropolitan Reading Diagnostic Test (MAT6) in the area of comprehension. A comparison control group of students involved in the usual program was also assessed. The results indicated significant gains for the Autoskill group (Gutierrez & Reed, 1988).

During the academic year 1987 to 1988, nine schools were involved in the project, involving 450 Chapter 1 students with reading difficulties. They received half-hour sessions, three times a week, throughout the year. Again, significant gains on the Metropolitan Reading Diagnostic Test in comprehension were attained relative to controls and relative to all past state-wide norms for similar grade-level classes. The average gain for the 450 predominantly Hispanic students across grades 1 to 8 was 14.8 normal curve equivalents, with a range of 6.9 to 27.3 (Gutierrez & Reed, 1988). Based on the success of this project, the Autoskill CRS Program will be implemented state-wide for Chapter 1 students in New Mexico, and a more extensive evaluation is anticipated in the future.

Salinas Union High School District

Officials at the Alisal High School in Salinas, California, evaluated the effectiveness of the Autoskill CRS Program with a high school population with reading difficulties; these students were predominantly of Hispanic origin and low socioeconomic status. There were 62 students who received training during the academic year 1986 to 1987, and 50 students (another sample) during the 1987 to 1988 school year. Approximately half of the students in each group were underachieving in reading skills, since they had limited English language skills and were enrolled as ESL students (English as a second language). The pre- and posttest standardized reading measure was the Woodcock Reading Mastery Tests (Woodcock, 1973). The students received half-hour training sessions for a total of 17 hours. Results for each group indicated an approximate 2.4-grade-equivalent gain. No control groups were included (Griffin, 1988).

Dade County Jail

A pilot investigation involving 60 juveniles who were incarcerated at the Dade County Jail, Miami, Florida, was carried out to determine the effectiveness of the Autoskill CRS Program with a group of high-school-aged juveniles who were not only several years below age-expected reading levels but who were drop-outs and described as having no interest in a school learning environment. Pre- and posttest results on the Metropolitan Achievement Test Form JS, Levels Advanced 1 and 2, indicated significant gains following 90 days on the program. Students on average gained 1.82 grades in reading comprehension with slightly over 20 hours of training. The project was considered a "huge success" not only because of the gain in reading levels but also because the interest in learning and the behavior of the participants were judged to be improved (Buckhalt & Burton, 1988).

Humber Community College

Seventeen students enrolled at Humber College, Toronto, Ontario, were involved in assessing the benefits of the Autoskill CRS Program with a community college adult population. The students were below a grade 8 level in reading word recognition skills and were enrolled in the Academic Preparation Program at the College as part of their language upgrading to assist them in their course of studies of technical–vocational programs. They received training during five 35-minute sessions per week for approximately 27 hours. The pre- and posttest standardized reading measures included the WRAT-R and the Woodcock. The results indicated an improvement in component reading subskills for both accuracy and latency along with a 4.7-grade-level improvement in reading word recognition and a 1.2-grade-level gain in reading comprehension. No comparison groups were evaluated (Muller, 1988).

Salvation Army Literacy Program

Fifty-three illiterate adults (mean age 34 years, range 23 to 60) are currently enrolled in the Salvation Army Literacy Program, Ottawa, Ontario, on the Autoskill CRS Program. Approximately half of the students have limited or no English reading skills, since they are learning English as a second language. The remaining students represent a cross section of illiteracy problems, including early school drop-out, reading disabilities, low socioeconomic status, and lack of application and motivation as well as recovering from alcoholism and drug addiction.

The Literacy Program has only been in operation for a short period, but 22 of the students have recently undergone the first 8-week semester posttest evaluation. There was an improvement in accuracy and latency of the component reading subskills as measured by the Autoskill CRS Program Test Battery, and reading word recognition skills have improved by 5.5 grade-level equivalents, with a range of 2 to 8 as measured by the WRAT-R. These 22 students were trained for an average of 49 hours. Reading comprehension scores are not yet available, nor are measures of self-esteeem. However, case study reports indicated that self-concept and self-confidence have improved according to self-reports and teacher observations, and students reported reading books for pleasure outside of the training environment (Burry & Goddard, 1989). The more extensive 12-month evaluation report will be of interest.

Discussion

Implications for the Subtype Concept

The concept of subtypes of reading disabilities developed out of an attempt to obtain a better understanding of reading dysfunction. The three profiles were based on component reading subskills that were derived by a task-analytic process and that were, theoretically, skills important to be acquired for effective word recognition. The Type O, A, and S subtypes were originally determined by a statistical procedure that contributed to greater objectivity in their identification. The same subtypes were replicated with different samples across different studies and were stable following different statistical analyses of classification, alternative concurrent validity methods, and different subsamples. On this basis, it is concluded that although these three subtypes are not definitive or exclusive, they are pertinent and viable.

In addition to providing a greater systematic understanding of a heterogeneous group of reading disabilities, the subtype concept also extends to treatment. It had been hypothesized that, if methods of teaching reading are developed in accordance with the subtype classification, this specificity of matching training strategies with the differential subtypes of reading disabilities may produce a better outcome. This supposition appeared to be logical and viable, and the results of the first two research studies evaluating the effectiveness of a component reading subskills approach offered strong supporting evidence. The groups trained according to subtype classification in the first study were significantly improved in comparison to the untrained group (waiting list control). In the second study, the students trained according to subtype were significantly improved in comparison to the untrained group, which received typical intervention by the school, as well as in comparison to the alternate computer-trained group, which received computer-assisted remedial work on other language arts programs.

The application of the program in the field evaluations also lends credence to the subtype concept. Although the samples consisted of students with more inclusive reading difficulties, the subjects were identified according to their differential performance on component reading subskills and trained on procedures specific to the differential profiles with good results. The evaluation techniques were lacking in rigorously controlled methodology and analyses, but the Santa Fe results particularly offer support in that the performance of the students trained according to subtype was considerably better than traditional methods of teaching as indicated by state-wide normative testing. The field site reports also illustrate the viability of applying the component reading subtypes approach to treatment of adolescents and adults.

Implications for Automaticity and Task-Analytic Models

Training according to the task-analytic model progresses in a sequential order from the beginning stages of single-letter names and sounds and progresses in a hierarchic fashion, training deficient component skill areas in both accuracy and latency. Most traditional remedial programs focus on accuracy only. The role of improved speed of accurate reading is also of considerable importance. Theoretically, according to the automaticity model of information processing, component skills for reading letters, syllables, and words must be overlearned to a level of rapid automatic responding to attain higher-level comprehension in reading.

The results of the first two research studies evaluating the effectiveness of the training procedures seem to indicate that the improvement of both accuracy and latency in all component reading subskills to the level of overlearning and automaticity requires extended training. In the first study, after 21.5 hours of training, group results indicated significant gains in component reading subskills, reading word recognition, and phonetic knowledge. After 56.4 hours of training in the second study, in addition to significant gains in component reading subskills, phonetic knowledge, and reading word recognition, there were also significant gains in paragraph-reading fluency, retention, comprehension, and cloze. The longer period of training to attain better levels of accuracy and latency over a greater number of component reading subskill areas appears to have a greater benefit of performance of reading and understanding paragraphs. Much of this additional improvement is secondary to transfer-of-training effects and not to a direct effect of training on paragraphs, since many of the students did not progress through the program to the point of paragraph training by the end-of-year posttesting.

The field evaluation results are consistent with these findings. The initial gains with a shorter training period appear to be in reading word recognition, with minimal paragraph-reading gain (Humber College), with significant paragraph-reading gain being observed over a longer duration of training (Santa Fe, Salinas). The specific number of hours is no doubt just a rough gauge, but the duration of training may be related to the automaticity model. One hypothesis is that there is a process of improvement that occurs in stages. As a greater proficiency in the component reading subskill areas is attained, there is an initial transfer-of-training effect to phonetic knowledge and word recognition. Then, with increased proficiency over time, there is a transfer effect to paragraph-reading comprehension. If this interpretation is accurate, these results lend credence to the automaticity model.

However, it appears that some modifications in the model are necessary. In an analysis of the progress of each individual student in Study II, the majority did very well as reflected in the group means; however, some of the students made poor progress, and some did exceptionally well. On the basis of reading word recognition alone, 36% of the sample made up to 1 grade level gain, 21% gained up to 2 grade levels, and a further 16% gained up to 4 grade levels. The students who made the most gains progressed further along in the program to practice paragraph-reading fluency. Therefore, it may be the case that training in component reading skills does transfer to paragraph-reading fluency and comprehension, but the process is enhanced if the training progresses to include not only all of the accuracy and latency of component subskill areas but paragraphs as well.

Individual Differences

The reasons for some students progressing through the program more quickly than others are unclear, as are the follow-up findings that some students continue to make considerable improvement once training is discontinued. Further investigation is necessary to consider such factors as the subtype and severity of the disability. The results of the field evaluations seem to indicate that greater progress is made in shorter periods of time with the more inclusive sample of students who experience reading failure for reasons such as low socioeconomic factors, ESL, former school drop-outs, and others. A slower rate of gain was attained by the students who met the more rigorous definition of reading disabilities.

The results of the students with poor progress also raise important research questions. For 6% of the Autoskill-trained group in Study II, there was no gain on standardized reading tests. In evaluating the progress of the individual students in this 6% group, it was found that these students also failed to improve in accuracy and latency of component reading subskills. Before it can be concluded that they represent a subsample of "highly resistant" or intractible reading disabilities, alternative teaching strategies would need to be implemented. Certainly, identifying the characteristics of this subsample, along with a means of differentiating them from those with greater probability of succeeding, would be a most beneficial addition to the program.

Conclusion

In summary, although there are several questions requiring further exploration through research, some conclusions can be made. The primary conclusion is that the three subtypes of reading disabilities, Type O, Type A, and Type S, are viable and meaningful subtypes. The Autoskill CRS Program appears to be a highly effective training approach for these specific reading disabilities. This component reading skills-subtyping approach also appears to be an effective program for a more inclusive group of reading difficulties. Short-term follow-up indicated that the benefits of training are maintained, and, for many of the students, the gains continued after the training period. The long-term benefits and outcome still need to be evaluated. The success of this approach is attributed to the integration of several current theoretical issues that have been incorporated into the diagnostic process and training strategies. The subtype concept is an integral aspect of both.

Acknowledgments

The research for Study I was supported by a grant from the Toronto Hospital for Sick Children Foundation, Toronto, Canada, and a scholarship from the Natural Science and Engineering Research Council, Ottawa, Canada. Awards received for this research include the Outstanding Dissertation Award Finalist, International Reading Association, May 1985, and the First Annual Outstanding Dissertation Award Winner, Orton Dyslexia Society, November 1985. The research for Study II was supported by funding from the Ministry of Education, Computers in Education Branch and Research Branch, Toronto, Ontario. Awards received for this research include the Ottawa Council for Exceptional Children Award, September 1988, and the Canadian Council for Exceptional Children, Sam Rabinovitch Evaluation for Research Award, October 1988. The authors wish to gratefully acknowledge these awards and the financial support.

References

Aaron, P. G., Grantham, S. L., & Campbell, N. (1982). Differential treatment of reading disability of diverse etiologies. In R. N. Malatesha & R. G. Aaron (Eds.), *Reading disorders: Varieties and treatments* (pp. 449–452). New York: Academic Press.

Alpert, M., & Kravitz, A. (1971). *SPIRE I and SPIRE II.* New York: New Dimensions in Education Inc.

Applebee, A. N. (1971). Research in reading retardation: Two critical problems. *Journal of Child Psychology and Psychiatry, 12,* 91–113.

Arter, J. A., & Jenkins, J. R. (1979). Differential diagnosis–prescription teaching: A critical appraisal. *Review of Education Research, 49,* 517–555.

Aulls, M. (1981). *Qualitative analysis of silent and oral reading.* Unpublished test, McGill University, Montreal.

Balow, B. (1965). The long-term effect of remedial reading instruction. *The Reading Teacher, 18,* 581–586.

Bateman, B. (1977). Teaching reading to learning disabled children and other hard-to-reach children. In L. B. Resnick & P. A. Weaver (Eds.), *Theory and practice of early reading* (Vol. 1, pp. 227–259). Hillsdale, NJ: Lawrence Erlbaum.

Beitchman, J. M., & Raman, S. (1981). *Clinical applications and diagnostic validity of a new children's self report psychiatric rating scale.* Unpublished manuscript.

Benton, A. L. (1975). Developmental dyslexia: Neurological aspects. *Advances in Neurology, 7,* 1–47.

Benton, A. L. (1978). Some conclusions about dyslexia. In A. L. Benton & D. Pearl (Eds.), *Dyslexia: An appraisal of current knowledge* (pp. 453–476). New York: Oxford University Press.

Blishen, B. R., & McRoberts, H. A. (1976). A revised socioeconomic index for occupations in Canada. *Canadian Review of Sociology and Anthropology, 13,* 71-79.

Boder, E. (1973). Developmental dyslexia: A diagnostic approach based on three atypical reading-spelling patterns. *Developmental Medicine and Child Neurology, 15,* 663-687.

Bruck, M. (1985). The adult functioning of children with specific learning disabilities: A follow-up study. In I. E. Sigel (Ed.), *Advances in applied developmental psychology* (Vol. 1, pp. 91-129). Norwood, NJ: Ablex.

Buckhalt, R. W., & Burton, Z. T. (1988, May). *Evaluation of the computer learning program in reading.* Education report to the Dade County School Board, Miami, FL.

Buerger, T. A. (1968). A follow-up of remedial reading instruction. *The Reading Teacher, 21,* 329-334.

Burry, J., & Goddard, L. (1989, May). *The Salvation Army & Booth Centre Literacy Program report.* Interim evaluation report for the Secretary of State Canada, Ottawa, Ontario.

Carver, R. P., & Hoffman, J. V. (1981). The effect of practice through repeated reading on gain in reading ability using a computer-based instructional system. *Reading Research Quarterly, 16*(3), 374-390.

Chall, J. S. (1979). The great debate: Ten years later, with a modest proposal for reading stages. In L. B. Resnick & P. A. Weaver (Eds.), *Theory and practice of early reading* (Vol. 1, pp. 29-55). Hillsdale, NJ: Lawrence Erlbaum.

Chomsky, C. (1978). When you still can't read in third grade: After decoding, what? In S. J. Samuels (Ed.), *What research has to say about reading instruction* (pp. 13-30). Newark, DE: International Reading Association.

Conners, C. K. (1969). A teacher rating scale for use in drug studies with children. *American Journal of Psychiatry, 126,* 884-888.

Critchley, M. (1970). *The dyslexic child.* Springfield, IL: Charles C. Thomas.

Doehring, D. G. (1976). The acquisition of rapid reading responses. *Monographs of the Society of Research in Child Development, 41*(2).

Doehring, D. G. (1978). The tangled web of behavioral research on developmental dyslexia. In A. L. Benton & D. Pearl (Eds.), *Dyslexia: An appraisal of current knowledge* (pp. 123-135). New York: Oxford University Press.

Doehring, D. G., & Hoshko, I. M. (1977). Classification of reading problems by the Q-technique of factor analysis. *Cortex, 13,* 281-294.

Doehring, D. G., Hoshko, I. M., & Bryans, B. N. (1979). Statistical classification of children with reading problems. *Journal of Clinical Neuropsychology, 1,* 5-16.

Doehring, D. G., Trites, R. L., Patel, P., & Fiedorowicz, C. (1981). *Reading disabilities: The interaction of reading, language and neuropsychological deficits.* New York: Academic Press.

Estes, W. K. (1974). Learning theory and intelligence. *American Psychologist, 29,* 740-749.

Fiedorowicz, C. (1983). *Component reading skills training of three subtypes of reading disability.* Unpublished doctoral dissertation, McGill University, Montreal.

Fiedorowicz, C. (1986). Training of component reading skills. *Annals of Dyslexia, 36,* 318-334.

Fiedorowicz, C., & Trites, R. (1987). *An evaluation of the effectiveness of computer-assisted component reading subskills training.* Toronto: Queen's Printer for Ontario.

Fiedorowicz, C., Trites, R. L., & Doehring, D. (1980, February). *Neuropsychological correlates of three subtypes of dyslexia.* Paper presented at the eighth annual meeting of the International Neuropsychology Society, San Francisco.

Fisher, D. F. (1979). Dysfunctions in reading disability: There's more than meets the eye. In L. B. Resnick & P. A. Weaver (Eds.), *Theory and practice of early reading* (Vol. 1, pp. 109-135). Hillsdale, NJ: Lawrence Erlbaum.

Gallistel, E., & Ellis, K. (1974). *Manual: Gallistel–Ellis Test of Coding Skills.* Hamden, CT: Montage Press.

Gonzales, P. G., & Elijah, D. V. (1975). Rereading: Effect on error patterns and performance levels on the IRI. *The Reading Teacher, 28,* 647–652.

Griffin, J. (1988, October). *Compensatory Education Program: Alisal High School.* Education report of Salinas Union High School District, Salinas, CA.

Guthrie, J. T. (1978). Principles of instruction: A critique of Johnson's "remedial approaches to dyslexia." In A. L. Benton & D. Pearl (Eds.), *Dyslexia: An appraisal of current knowledge* (pp. 423–433). New York: Oxford University Press.

Gutierrez, G., & Reed, J. (1988, September). *An exemplary approach for children at risk.* Education report, Santa Fe Public Schools, Santa Fe, New Mexico.

Haring, N. G., & Bateman, B. (1977). *Teaching the learning disabled child.* Englewood Cliffs, NJ: Prentice-Hall.

Hewison, J. (1982). The current status of remedial intervention for children with reading problems. *Developmental Medicine and Child Neurology, 24,* 183–186.

Jastak, J., & Jastak, S. (1976). *Wide Range Achievement Test.* Wilmington, DE: C. L. Story.

Jastak, S., & Wilkinson, G. S. (1984). *Wide Range Achievement Test—Revised.* Wilmington, DE: C. L. Story.

Johnson, J. L. (1978). Remedial approaches to dyslexia. In A. L. Benton & D. Pearl (Eds.), *Dyslexia: An appraisal of current knowledge* (pp. 397–421). New York: Oxford University Press.

Kirk, S. (1972). *Education of exceptional children.* Boston: Houghton-Mifflin.

LaBerge, D. (1973). Attention and the measurement of perceptual learning. *Memory and Cognition, 1,* 268–276.

LaBerge, D. (1979). The perception of units in beginning reading. In L. B. Resnick & P. A. Weaver (Eds.), *Theory and practice of early reading* (Vol. 3, pp. 31–51). Hillsdale, NJ: Lawrence Erlbaum.

LaBerge, D., Peterson, R. J., & Norden, M. (1977). Exploring the limits of cueing. In B. S. Dornic (Ed.), *Attention & performance VI* (pp. 285–306). Hillsdale, NJ: Lawrence Erlbaum.

LaBerge, D., & Samuels, S. J. (1973). *On the automaticity of naming artificial letters* (Technical Report No. 7, Minnesota Reading Research Project). Minneapolis: University of Minnesota.

LaBerge, D., & Samuels, S. J. (1974). Toward a theory of automatic information processing. *Cognitive Psychology, 6,* 293–323.

Lesgold, A. M., & Resnick, L. B. (1981). *How reading difficulties develop: Perspectives from a longitudinal study.* Pittsburgh: Learning Research and Development Centre.

Muller, P. (1988, November). *Autoskill computer-based reading software evaluation.* Humber College project report to Ontario Ministry of Skills Development, Toronto, Ontario.

Nunnally, J. C. (1967). *Psychometric theory.* New York: McGraw-Hill.

Overall, J., & Klett, J. (1972). *Applied multivariate analysis.* New York: McGraw-Hill.

Perfetti, C. A., & Lesgold, A. M. (1979). Coding and comprehension in skilled reading and implications for reading instruction. In L. B. Resnick & P. A. Weaver (Eds.), *Theory and practice of early reading* (Vol. 1, pp. 57–84). Hillsdale, NJ: Lawrence Erlbaum.

Petrauskas, R. J., & Rourke, B. P. (1979). Identification of subtypes of retarded readers: A neuropsychological, multivariate approach. *Journal of Clinical Neuropsychology, 1,* 17–37.

Ross, A. (1976). *Psychological aspects of learning disability and reading disorders.* New York: McGraw-Hill.

Rourke, B. (1978). Neuropsychological research in reading retardation: A review. In A.

Benton & D. Pearl (Eds.), *Dyslexia: An appraisal of current knowledge* (pp. 139–171). New York: Oxford University Press.

Rutter, M. (1978). Prevalence and types of dyslexia. In A. Benton & D. Pearl (Eds.), *Dyslexia: An appraisal of current knowledge* (pp. 3–28). New York: Oxford University Press.

Samuels, S. J. (1979). The method of repeated readings. *The Reading Teacher,* January, 403–408.

Satz, P., & Morris, R. (1981). Learning disability subtypes: A review. In F. J. Pirozzolo & M. C. Wittrock (Eds.), *Neuropsychological and cognitive processes in reading* (pp. 109–141). New York: Academic Press.

Schonhaut, S., & Satz, P. (1983). Prognosis for children with learning disabilities: A review of follow-up studies. In M. Rutter (Ed.), *Developmental neuropsychiatry* (pp. 542–563). New York: Guilford Press.

Smead, V. S. (1977). Ability training and task analysis in diagnostic–prescriptive teaching. *Journal of Special Education, 11,* 114–125.

Spreen, D. (1982). Adult outcome of reading disorders. In R. N. Malatesha & P. G. Aaron (Eds.), *Reading disorders: Varieties and treatments* (pp. 473–492). New York: Academic Press.

Sternberg, R. J., & Wagner, R. R. (1982). Automatization failure in learning disabilities. *Topics in Learning and Learning Disabilities, 2,* 1–11.

Terry, P. (1974). *The effect of orthographic transformations upon speed and accuracy of semantic categorization.* Unpublished doctoral dissertation, University of Minnesota.

Torgeson, J. K. (1979). What shall we do with psychological processes: *Journal of Learning Disabilities, 12,* 514–521.

Trites, R. L. (1977). *Neuropsychological test manual.* Montreal: Ronalds Federated.

Trites, R., & Fiedorowicz, C. (1976). Follow-up study of children with specific (or primary) reading disability. In R. M. Knights & D. J. Bakker (Eds.), *The neuropsychology of learning disorders: Theoretical approaches* (pp. 41–50). Baltimore: University Park Press.

Vernon, M. D. (1971). *Reading and its difficulties.* Cambridge, England: Cambridge University Press.

Wechsler, D. (1974). *Manual: Wechsler Intelligence Scale for Children—Revised.* New York: Psychological Corporation.

Werner, H. (1973). Process and achievement—a basic problem of education and developmental psychology. *Harvard Educational Review, 7,* 353–368.

Wiener, M., & Cromer, W. (1967). Reading and reading difficulty: A conceptual analysis. *Harvard Educational Review, 37,* 620–643.

Wong, B. (1979). The role of theory in learning disabilities research. Part 1: An analysis of problems. *Journal of Learning Disabilities, 12,* 585–595.

Woodcock, R. W. (1973). *Woodcock Reading Mastery Tests.* Arile Pines, MN: American Guidance Service.

Zigmond, N. (1978). Remediation of dyslexia: A discussion. In A. L. Benton & D. Pearl (Eds.), *Dyslexia: An appraisal of current knowledge* (pp. 435–448). New York: Oxford University Press.

Developmental Dimensions

Cross-Sectional and Longitudinal Studies

CHAPTER 13

Construct Validation of the Nonverbal Learning Disabilities Syndrome and Model

Joseph E. Casey and Byron P. Rourke

In the last resort, all diagnostic concepts stand or fall by the strength of the prognostic and therapeutic implications they embody.—R. E. Kendell (1975)

The purpose of this chapter is to describe one integrated approach to the determination of the validity of the nonverbal learning disabilities (NLD) syndrome and model as proposed by Rourke (1989). The methods by which this is to be accomplished are threefold: first, to consider briefly the validity of the NLD syndrome and model within the context of a framework proposed by Skinner (1981); second, to present in some detail the results of two developmental studies recently completed in our laboratory that bear on the issue of the external validity of the NLD syndrome; and third, to apply the results derived from the above exercises to summarize the strengths and weaknesses of the NLD model. It was thought that the latter considerations would point to areas wherein future research would likely prove contributory to the broadening of our understanding of the characteristics, dynamics, and clinical utility of the syndrome and the model.

Construct Validation and the NLD Syndrome

Skinner (1981) describes his three-component framework as a "meta-theory of classification which has heuristic value for the evaluation of particular classification systems" (p. 69). Thus, it appears to be well suited to an analysis of the NLD syndrome and model. The first component of the framework, that of theory formulation, involves the specification of the classification theory. It includes a description of the variables on which the typology is based and the relationship of the typology to various external variables (e.g., outcome). The internal validation component is concerned with issues relating to the typology's reliability, homogeneity, and coverage. Finally, the external validation component involves the typology's generalizability to other populations and its predictive, descriptive, and clinical validity.

This framework is especially appealing because it provides a logical structure by which to consider systematically the types of validity that a classificatory system or typology possesses. In addition, this system emphasizes the continuing interplay between theory development and empirical analyses. This emphasis appears to be important when one's aims are to achieve a reliable separation of individuals into homogeneous groups (an actuarial endeavor) and to understand the relationship of the derived typology to etiological, prognostic, and treatment considerations (a theoretical endeavor aimed at explaining underlying processes).

Although it was originally conceived with psychiatric classifications in mind, the applicability of this framework to the evaluation of learning disabilities subtyping research has already been demonstrated (Fletcher, 1985). In this work, Fletcher focused on the external validation component of Skinner's framework to evaluate classification systems based on patterns of academic strengths and weaknesses and on central processing deficiencies. However, rather than considering typology systems from a broad perspective, our attention is directed to the validity of one particular subtype of learning disability, that which has been termed "nonverbal learning disabilities" (Myklebust, 1975).

Theory Formulation Component

According to Skinner, an adequate articulation of the classification theory should include a precise definition of each type and a specification of how the types are related, an explication of the development and etiology of the type, an indication of the population for which the classification applies, and a description of appropriate treatment interventions and prognosis. The theory formulation need not be particularly elaborate. More important is the theory's functional utility—regardless of whether the theory is concerned with an entire classification system or with a single subtype—which, in part, is measured by its ability to generate testable hypotheses. As Skinner states, a "classification should be viewed as a scientific theory that is open to empirical falsification" (p. 69). To what extent does the NLD syndrome meet the conditions of Skinner's theory formulation component? Does it possess, by virtue of its specifications, the quality of falsifiability? Before attempting to answer these questions, we first consider each of the conditions individually as they relate to the syndrome and model.

The identification of the NLD syndrome and the formulation of the model emerged, in part, from research that began some 20 years ago in our laboratory as a general approach to the neuropsychology of learning disabilities. Early studies examined the neuropsychological and academic manifestations of learning-disabled (LD) children classified according to VIQ–PIQ discrepancies on the Wechsler Intelligence Scale for Children (WISC; Rourke, Dietrich, & Young, 1973; Rourke & Telegdy, 1971; Rourke, Young, & Flewelling, 1971). Subsequent studies were conducted to determine the neuropsychological and socioemotional correlates of LD children classified according to their performance on academic achievement tests of reading (word recognition), spelling, and arithmetic (Rourke & Finlayson, 1978; Rourke & Strang, 1978; Strang & Rourke, 1983). Together, these studies (1) led to the identification of the NLD syndrome, (2) delineated its neuropsychological relationship to other LD types (e.g., reading disabilities), and (3) provided the foundations for the development of the NLD model.

The elaboration of the model, which was advanced for the purposes of explaining the manifestations and dynamics of the NLD syndrome, was accomplished through the incorporation of neuropsychological theory and research, Piaget's theory of cognitive development (especially as it relates to the sensorimotor stage), and the Goldberg and Costa (1981) model. Furthermore, the theoretical and empirical information derived from these three domains of knowledge was employed to a large extent for the explication of the developmental changes that have been observed in children classified as NLD.

Rourke (1989) recently presented in detail the neuropsychological, academic, and socioemotional features that characterize the NLD syndrome in children. These have been summarized as follows (Rourke, 1987):

1. Bilateral tactile–perceptual deficits, usually more marked on the left side of the body.

2. Bilateral psychomotor coordination deficiencies, often more marked on the left side of the body.

3. Outstanding deficiencies in visual–spatial–organizational abilities.

4. Marked deficits in nonverbal problem solving, concept formation, hypothesis testing, and the capacity to benefit from positive and negative informational feedback in novel or otherwise complex situations. Included are significant difficulties in dealing with cause–effect relationships and marked deficiencies in the appreciation of incongruities (e.g., age-appropriate sensitivity to humor).

5. Very well developed rote verbal capacities, including extremely well developed rote verbal memory skills.

6. Extreme difficulty in adapting to novel and otherwise complex situations. An overreliance on prosaic, rote (and, in consequence, inappropriate) behaviors in such situations.

7. Outstanding relative deficiencies in mechanical arithmetic as compared to proficiencies in reading (word recognition) and spelling.

8. Much verbosity of a repetitive, straightforward, rote nature. Content disorders of language characterized by very poor psycholinguistic pragmatics (e.g., "cocktail party" speech). Misspellings that are almost exclusively of the phonetically accurate variety. Little or no speech prosody. Reliance on language as a principal means for social relating, information gathering, and relief from anxiety.

9. Significant deficits in social perception, social judgment, and social interaction skills. A marked tendency toward social withdrawal and even social isolation as age increases. Such children are very much at risk for the development of socioemotional disturbances, especially "internalized" forms of psychopathology.

It is clear from this description that the defining features of the syndrome rely exclusively on clinical and psychometric variables. Although not a condition of the diagnosis, a possible underlying biological determinant (i.e., etiology) has been proposed. The principal theoretical tenet of the model is that damage or dysfunction of cerebral white matter is responsible for the manifestations of the syndrome. This inference was formulated on the basis of observations that children with known white matter involvement, such as in cases of closed head injury, agenesis of the corpus callosum, and brain excision encompassing portions of the right cerebral hemisphere, to name just a few, demonstrated features that were remarkably similar to those observed in the NLD child, who typically presented with outstanding deficiencies in arithmetic. In addition, the model further stipulates that a positive relationship obtains between the amount of cerebral white matter involved and the probability that the NLD syndrome will be in evidence. Finally, important developmental dimensions that bear on the manifestations and severity of symptoms have been articulated.

The model also includes statements regarding prognosis and intervention that are based primarily on the proposed dynamics of neuropsychological strengths and weaknesses. Thus, in terms of outcome, the model predicts that there will be a relative stability over time (i.e., age-appropriate development) in some verbal, reading (word recognition), spelling, and simple motor skills. In contrast, relative declines are predicted in visual–spatial–organizational, mechanical arithmetic, and complex psychomotor skills. In terms of socioemotional functioning, it is predicted that there will be an increase in psychopathology of the internalized variety. Intervention methods for dealing with the deficiencies exhibited by such children have been well described (Strang & Rourke, 1985; Rourke, 1989). In general, they have been designed to enlist NLD children's neuropsychological strengths to compensate for their deficiencies.

From even this very brief description, it should be clear that the NLD syndrome and model satisfy most, if not all, of the conditions considered by Skinner to be fundamental to any sound classification theory. Moreover, the manner in which the syndrome is defined and the model articulated render the NLD typology open to empirical investigation, statistical hypothesis testing, and, hence, falsification.

Internal Validation Component

Essentially, internal validation is concerned with the reliability of the typology. The typology is said to be reliable to the extent that it is not dependent on a certain method or statistical technique for its derivation and can be replicated in new samples (Fletcher & Satz, 1985; Skinner, 1981). Determining reliability in this manner is important because, as Kendell (1975) points out, "it establishes the ceiling for validity; the lower it is, the lower validity necessarily becomes" (p. 39). Considerations for evaluating the internal validity of the NLD typology would include (1) the reliability of the syndrome's manifestations (e.g., interrater reliability), (2) the degree of similarity among the individuals so classified (i.e., its homogeneity), (3) the number of individuals successfully classified (i.e., coverage), and (4) the replicability of the syndrome across techniques and samples (Skinner, 1981).

Within Skinner's framework, internal validity is likely the weakest component of the NLD model. Some of the aforementioned considerations have been addressed in the literature in relation to the Wide Range Achievement Test (WRAT) typology, for example, the typology's replicability (see Fletcher, 1985, for a discussion of these studies). However, whereas these studies provide evidence suggestive of the model's internal validity, this support cannot be viewed as direct because the groups employed in these studies were formulated on the basis of WRAT patterns and not the features of the NLD syndrome as defined by Rourke (1989). Other than these studies, little research has been conducted that has any bearing on the internal validation component.

Although not constituting direct attempts at determining the reliability of the NLD syndrome, many of the features that comprise the syndrome have been reported in several independent studies examining both children (Voeller, 1986) and predominantly adults (Abramson & Katz, 1989; Tranel, Hall, Olson, & Tranel, 1987; Weintraub & Mesulam, 1983). The constellation of features described in these studies has been labeled variously as follows: right hemisphere developmental learning disability (Tranel et al., 1987); right hemisphere deficit syndrome (Voeller, 1986); and developmental learning disabilities of the right hemisphere (Weintraub & Mesulam, 1983). Although they were not collected with a view to doing so, the results of these studies can be construed as evidencing support for the internal validity of the NLD syndrome.

External Validation Component

If it can be demonstrated that a typology is externally valid, then by necessity it is also reliable. However, despite the obvious importance of external validation in the clinical sciences, this component has been the most neglected in classification research (Skinner, 1981). As outlined by Skinner, the external validity of a typology is supported to the extent that it can demonstrate generalizability to other populations, clinical meaningfulness, convergent and discriminant validity, and prognostic usefulness (predictive validity).

Although the NLD syndrome was originally isolated in children who presented with outstanding academic difficulties in arithmetic, it has been found that many children suffering from certain other conditions also exhibit neuropsychological profiles that are remarkably similar. These include children with moderate to severe head injuries (e.g., Fletcher & Levin, 1988), children with hydrocephalus (e.g., Rourke, Bakker, Fisk, & Strang, 1983, pp. 290–297), survivors of acute lymphocytic leukemia and other forms of childhood cancer who had received very large doses of X-irradiation over a prolonged period of time (e.g., Fletcher & Copeland, 1988), children with congenital absence or partial agenesis of the corpus callosum (e.g., Casey, Del Dotto, & Rourke, 1990; Rourke, 1987), and children with significant tissue removal from the right cerebral hemisphere (e.g., Rourke et al., 1983, pp. 230–238). These findings have provided strong evidence for the generalizability of the NLD syndrome to populations other than those who present with the developmental manifestations of the syndrome.

One of the appealing aspects of the NLD typology is its clinical meaningfulness. If the specification of the defining features of a typology is vague or otherwise unclear, or if its relevance to clinical practice is remote, as would be the case if it were unable to predict outcome, then it is unlikely that the typology will receive acceptance by clinicians (Skinner, 1981). The previous discussion regarding the relatively precise specification of the syndrome, coupled with the evidence to be discussed shortly concerning its predictive validity, suggests that the NLD typology is "user friendly."

Finally, there is the matter of the convergent and discriminant validity of the NLD syndrome. In short, because of the relative recency of the complete formulation of the model (Rourke, 1989), this type of evidence relating to validity is limited to those studies that have examined the WRAT typology.

Apart from the exceptions to follow, studies that attempt to evaluate the predictive validity of the NLD syndrome have yet to appear in the literature. Such research could take many forms. For example, a therapeutic trial could be conducted in which the response to treatment would be predicted based on the pattern of neuropsychological strengths and weaknesses that charcterize the syndrome. Another approach might be to employ a subtype X task interaction design whereby the pattern of neuropsychological strengths and weaknesses would be utilized to predict performances on tasks not used to define the syndrome. Outcome studies that attempt to predict the future course of events given a particular syndrome provide powerful and, perhaps, the most important demonstrations of validity (Kendell, 1989). The two studies described in the second section of this chapter are examples of investigations that have been conducted for the purpose of evaluating the external validity of the NLD syndrome.

Study 1

The first investigation (Casey & Rourke, 1990) was designed to examine whether the academic and neuropsychological features of the NLD syndrome would change in a predictable manner within the childhood years. Rourke, Young, Strang, and Russell (1986) found that adults who demonstrated a configurational pattern of neuropsychological abilities and deficits similar to that observed in NLD children exhibited more pronounced deficiencies in neuropsychological and socioemotional functioning than their younger counterparts. Based on these findings and the results of case studies of children who manifest the NLD syndrome (e.g., Rourke et al., 1983, pp. 247–253), it was expected that there would be a relative stability or accelerated growth (i.e., age-appropriate or better development) in rote verbal skills, reading (word recognition), spelling, and simple motor and tactile–perceptual abilities and skills. In contrast, it was expected that there would be a relative decline (i.e., a failure to make age-appropriate gains) in visual–spatial–organizational abilities, mechanical arithmetic skills, and complex psychomotor and tactile–perceptual abilities. Several specific hypotheses were formulated concerning developmental changes expected on the measures employed in this study. These are presented following a discussion of the methodology.

Subjects

The subjects for study were selected in accordance with the neuropsychological and academic features of the NLD syndrome. For the purpose of initial selection from a computerized data base, each child had to evidence at least the following (specific variable findings and their relationship to appropriate age-dependent norms are in parentheses):

1. *Bilateral tactile perceptual deficits* (performance on measures of finger agnosia, graphesthesia, or stereognosis was 1 *SD* or more below the norm with either hand).
2. *Bilateral psychomotor deficiencies* (performance on the Grooved Pegboard Test was 1 *SD* or more below the norm with either hand).
3. *Visuospatial/organizational deficiencies* (performance on the Target Test was 1 *SD* or more below the norm, and VIQ > PIQ by 10 or more points).
4. *Good verbal capacities* (VIQ > 79 and performance on either the Speech-Sounds Perception Test or the Auditory Closure Test was neither less than, nor equal to, 1 *SD* below the norm).
5. *Mechanical arithmetic deficiencies* (performances on the WRAT Reading and Spelling subtests exceeded that of the WRAT Arithmetic subtest by 10 or more standard score points).

These liberal criteria were not interpreted as constituting the defining features of the syndrome. Rather, they were employed in order to identify all *potential* subjects. Once these were selected, their neuropsychological reports were reviewed, and only those children who were considered to exhibit the neuropsychological and academic features of the NLD syndrome were included.

Criteria relating to nonverbal problem-solving and concept-formation abilities in the younger children as well as those relating to difficulties in adapting to novel or otherwise complex situations were not employed in the selection process because it was not always possible to determine precisely that the child was experiencing such difficulties. In those cases where a child was tested more than once, if any one of the assessment protocols met the criteria for the NLD syndrome, then all the protocols for that child were included in the analyses; obviously, not doing so might have the effect of diminishing group differences by excluding the protocols of children seen at a younger age when, according to the model, some of the deficiencies may not be as conspicuous. Clinical and psychometric data reflecting socioemotional functioning were not considered in the selection of the subjects, as these were employed as outcome variables for the second study (Rourke & Casey, 1990).

Based on the aforementioned criteria and conditions, a total of 29 subjects were selected retrospectively from approximately 5,000 children who had received an extensive battery of neuropsychological tests primarily for purposes of evaluating a possible learning disability and/or perceptual problem for which it was thought that brain impairment might be a contributing factor. Two of the subjects had well-documented acquired lesions. One had sustained a severe head injury at the age of 13 years that eventuated in excision of portions of the right temporal and parietal lobes. The other had sustained a left temporoparietal depressed skull fracture at birth. At the age of 2 months this child developed hydrocephalus that was treated by a lumbar subarachnoid–peritoneal anastomosis; at 6 years of age, a ventricular–caval shunt was inserted. Two subjects had congenital brain abnormalities. One had hydrocephalus for which he was shunted within the first year of life; a second had agenesis of the corpus callosum. There were 14 boys and 15 girls. Twenty-five of the subjects were right-handed; four were left-handed.

Procedures

Twenty-one subjects had undergone neuropsychological assessment once, seven were tested twice, and one was tested three times. Because of the relative scarcity of such cases and the exploratory nature of this study, all of the resulting 38 protocols were utilized in the descriptive statistics. The protocols were separated into two groups: The "Young" group ($n = 7$) comprised those protocols of children tested at the ages of 7 and 8 years of age (inclusive); the "Old" group ($n = 31$) comprised those protocols of children tested at the ages of 9 through 14 years (inclusive). Age-adjusted scores were employed in order to make comparisons between groups and among tests possible. Data are reported in standard-score ($M = 100$, $SD = 15$) or T-score ($M = 50$, $SD = 10$) formats. T-score conversions for the neuropsychological measures were based on the normative data of Knights and Norwood (1980).

The following measures were employed: all of the subtests of the WISC except Mazes (Wechsler, 1949); the WRAT (Jastak & Jastak, 1965); the Peabody Picture Vocabulary Test (PPVT; Dunn, 1965); the Reitan-Indiana Neuropsychological Test Battery for Children (Young children; Reitan & Davison, 1974); the Halstead Neuropsychological Test Battery for Children (Old children; Reitan & Davison, 1974); Maze Coordination, Static Steadiness (Holes Test), and Grooved Pegboard tests from the Kløve–Matthews Motor Steadiness Battery (Kløve, 1963); tests of tactile imperception and suppression, Finger Agnosia, Finger-Tip Writing, and Astereognosis from the Reitan–Kløve Sensory–Perceptual Examination (Reitan & Davison, 1974); and the Underlining Test (Rourke & Gates, 1980). All tests were administered in a standardized manner by technicians trained extensively in the administration of these tests and procedures.

Hypotheses

INTELLIGENCE AND ACADEMIC ACHIEVEMENT

It was expected that (1) the PPVT IQ and WISC VIQ would not differ between Young and Old children, (2) the PIQ for Young children would exceed that of the Old children, and (3) the WISC VIQ–PIQ discrepancy (favoring the VIQ) would be larger for Old than Young children. On measures of academic achievement (Reading, Spelling, and Arithmetic subtests of the WRAT), it was expected that (1) Reading and Spelling standard scores would be higher for Old than for Young children, (2) Arithmetic standard scores would be higher for Young than for Old children, and (3) the difference between Reading and Spelling on the one hand and Arithmetic on the other (favoring Reading and Spelling) would be larger for Old than for Young children.

MOTOR, PSYCHOMOTOR, AND TACTILE–PERCEPTUAL ABILITIES

It was expected that, the more complex and novel the motor or tactile-perceptual task, (1) the poorer would be the performance of both groups relative to age-based norms, and (2) the poorer would be the age-corrected performance of the Old children as compared to the Young ones. For motor tasks, the hierarchical order of simplicity to complexity and rote to novel was considered as follows: Grip Strength, Finger-Tapping Speed, Holes Test (static steadiness), Mazes Test (kinetic steadiness), and Grooved Pegboard Test. Name-writing speed does not fit well within this hierarchy. It was assumed that name writing is a novel task for the younger child and becomes a well-practiced and relatively fluid task for the older one. As such, it was expected that name-writing speed would be quicker (relative to age-based norms) for the Old than for the Young children.

Similarly, tests of Finger Agnosia, Finger-Tip Writing (graphesthesia), and Stereognosis were considered to be more complex than tests of imperception and suppression (single and double simultaneous stimulation; SDSS). Hence, the Old children were expected to perform more poorly than the Young children on these tactile–perceptual tasks, whereas performance on SDSS would be equivalent for the two groups.

CONCEPT-FORMATION AND PROBLEM-SOLVING ABILITIES

It was expected that the Old children would perform more poorly than the Young children on (1) the Category Test and (2) all measures of the Tactual Performance Test (namely, dominant hand, nondominant hand, both hand trials; memory and location scores). Although not easily characterized because of its multifactorial demands, the Underlining Test can be viewed as a rather novel task requiring speeded performance and, at least for some subtests, fairly complex visual perceptual skills. In keeping with the other predictions regarding the difficulty for older NLD individuals to deal with tasks that are novel, complex, and demanding of visual–perceptual abilities, it was expected that the Young children would perform better than the Old children on this task.

Results

INTELLIGENCE AND ACADEMIC ACHIEVEMENT

The results illustrated in Table 13.1 revealed that (1) the scores obtained for the Old and Yound children on the PPVT IQ and WISC VIQ were similar and within the normal range; (2) the PIQ of the Young children (low-average range) exceeded that of the Old children (borderline range); and (3) the WISC VIQ–PIQ discrepancy was larger for the Old children (21.6 points) than for the Young children (16.7 points). On academic achievement measures (1) the Old children exceeded the Young in reading and spelling; (2) the Young children exceeded the Old in arithmetic; and (3) the discrepancy between reading and spelling versus arithmetic skills (favoring the former) was greater for the Old children than for the Young.

In general, both groups performed within the average range on all of the WISC Verbal subtests and on measures of psycholinguistic and verbal memory abilities. The Young children were more proficient than the Old children on measures of verbal associations (Similarities subtest), expressive word knowledge (Vocabulary subtest), and sound-blending abilities (Auditory Closure Test); their performance on these measures was in the high-average range. In contrast to the generally similar level of performance found between the two groups on measures of verbal abilities, the performance of the Young children consistently exceeded that of the Old

TABLE 13.1. Means (Standard Deviations) for the Young and Old Groups on Measures of Intelligence and Academic Achievement

	Test protocols		
Measures	Young	Old	Change
PPVT IQ	106.4 (7.7)	107.2 (18.1)	+0.8
WISC			
VIQ	104.9 (6.1)	100.1 (10.2)	−4.8
PIQ	88.1 (7.8)	78.4 (10.7)	−9.7
FSIQ	96.7 (7.6)	88.8 (10.7)	−7.9
WRAT			
Reading[a]	110.1 (9.0)	115.7 (16.3)	+5.6
Spelling[a]	103.6 (9.1)	108.2 (15.7)	+4.6
Arithmetic[a]	91.9 (7.0)	83.3 (10.6)	−8.6

[a]Standard scores.

on measures of visual–perceptual–organizational abilities (i.e., all Performance scale subtests of the WISC and the Target Test). In general, the performance level of the Young children fell within the low-average range on the Performance subtests and in the moderately impaired range on the Target Test. The Old children generally performed in the mildly impaired range on the Performance subtests and in the moderately impaired range on the Target Test.

MOTOR, PSYCHOMOTOR, AND TACTILE-PERCEPTUAL ABILITIES

The data suggested that the predictions regarding motor and psychomotor changes in performance were at least partially supported. There was a pattern for the Old children to perform better on simple motor tasks and for the Young children to perform better on more complex psychomotor tasks. The Old children performed better than the Young on measures of grip strength and name-writing speed, similar to the Young children on a measure of static steadiness (Holes Test), and poorer than the Young children on measures of finger-tapping speed, kinetic steadiness (Mazes), and speeded eye–hand coordination (Grooved Pegboard). The hierarchy of performance superiority to inferiority of the Old versus the Young children was as follows (predicted order from 1 through 5 in parentheses): Grip Strength (1), Holes Test (3), Mazes Test (4), Finger Tapping (2), and Grooved Pegboard Test (5). With the exception of finger-tapping speed in the Old children, left-hand performance was consistently poorer than the right-hand performance for both groups on all measures.

The results of the tactile–perceptual tests were as predicted. The Old children performed better than the Young only on the measure of simple tactile perception (SDSS) and performed more poorly on the higher-order tactile–perceptual tests of Finger Agnosia, Finger-Tip Writing, and Astereognosis.

CONCEPT-FORMATION AND PROBLEM-SOLVING ABILITIES

The performance of the Young children exceeded that of the Old on the Category Test and on all measures except the both-hands trial of the Tactual Performance Test. In most instances, the performance level of the Young children was within the normal range, whereas that of the Old children was within the mildly to moderately impaired range. The notable exception to this pattern was the markedly impaired performance of both groups of children on the third (both-hands) trial of the Tactual Performance Test.

On 10 of the 14 subtests of the Underlining Test, the performance of the Young children was better than that of the Old children. Generally, the performance of the Young children was in the average to mildly impaired range, whereas that for the Old children was in the mildly to moderately impaired range.

Conclusions: Study 1

The results of the first study provided convincing evidence that the academic and cognitive/neuropsychological features of the NLD syndrome evolve in a predictable manner within the childhood years. Verbal and linguistic abilities, particularly those of a more rote nature, were found to develop in an age-appropriate fashion. The superiority of the Young children on the Similarities and Vocabulary subtests is interesting in this regard, as these subtests tend to measure more concrete and automatic verbal abilities (i.e., overlearned verbal associations and definitions of objects) at this age level as compared to the greater demand placed on abstraction and concept-formation abilities (i.e., verbal abstractions/classifications and definitions of abstract words) for the Old children. With increasing age, the children demonstrated an accelerated development in the academic skills of reading and spelling.

In contrast, there was a clear failure of NLD children to make age-appropriate gains in visual–perceptual–organizational abilities and in mechanical arithmetic skills. Within sensorimotor domains, the greater the degree of task complexity in terms of the need for intermodal integration and mediational processes (e.g., SDSS versus finger agnosia; grip strength versus speeded eye–hand coordination and dexterity), the poorer was the performance of the Old children relative to the Young. In summary, all of the above findings were consistent with the predictions derived from the dynamics of the NLD model and the results of outcome studies of adults who exhibited the features of the NLD syndrome.

Study 2

The purpose of the second investigation (Rourke & Casey, 1990) was to examine whether or not the pattern of socioemotional and behavioral disturbances typically exhibited by NLD children also changed with advancing years. As described in the study by Rourke et al. (1986), adults who exhibit the neuropsychological features of the NLD syndrome do not come to professional attention with complaints of learning difficulties. Rather, their presenting problems tend to relate to (1) social ineptitude characterized by the lack of meaningful relationships and a tendency toward withdrawal and isolation, (2) low self-esteem, and (3) chronic depression. Although obviously not conclusive give the selection bias present in the Rourke et al. (1986) study, these findings nevertheless suggest that it is the emotional difficulties that are paramount in the adult with the NLD syndrome.

Subjects and Procedures

The children selected for study constituted a subset of those employed in the first investigation (Casey & Rourke, submitted). Of the 38 assessment protocols selected for the first study, 15 included ratings from the primary caretaker (usually the mother) on the Personality Inventory for Children (Wirt, Lachar, Klinedinst, & Seat, 1977), the Werry–Weiss–Peters Activity Rating Scale (ARS; Werry & Sprague, 1970), and/or the Behavior Problem Checklist (BPC; Quay & Peterson, 1975). As in Study 1, the protocols were separated into two groups: The "Young" group comprised the protocols of 7- and 8-year-olds, and the "Old" group 9- through 14-year-olds. It will be recalled that neither the results of these measures nor clinical history data regarding socioemotional functioning were employed in the selection of subjects.

Hypotheses

Based on the dynamics of the NLD syndrome and the findings of Rourke et al. (1986), several predictions were made. On the Personality Inventory for Children (PIC), the following results were expected: (1) There would be more concern regarding academic achievement and the need for "intellectual screening" among the Old as compared to the Young children; (2) significant elevations on the Adjustment scale and on those scales that contribute to the internalized psychopathology factor (Depression, Withdrawal, Anxiety, Psychosis, Social Skills) would be in evidence for both age groups; (3) moderate but significant elevations of the F scale ("degree of concern"), and higher F scales for the Old children would obtain; (4) there would be higher scores on scales that contribute to the internalized psychopathology factor for the Old as compared to the Young children; and (5) elevations on the Hyperactivity scale would be higher for the Young than for the Old children. Consistent with the last prediction, it was expected that there would be higher scores on the ARS for the Young than for the Old children. Finally, it was expected that the Old children would obtain higher scores on the BPC than would the Young children, thus reflecting an increase in the frequency and/or severity of socioemotional disturbances.

Results

Figure 13.1 illustrates the profile configurations on the PIC for the Young and Old children. It reveals that (1) concerns over academic achievement and the need for intellectual screening were higher in the Old versus the Young children, with the elevation on the Intellectual Screening scale falling within the pathological range for the Old children; (2) significant elevations for both groups were observed on the Adjustment, Psychosis, and Social Skills scales, but not the Depression, Withdrawal, or Anxiety scales; (3) moderate but significant elevations were obtained on the F scale ("degree of concern"), with a marginally higher score evident for the Old children; (4) higher scores were evidenced by the Old children as compared to the Young on all of the scales that contribute to the internalized psychopathology factor; and (5) a lower score for the Young children was obtained on the Hyperactivity scale. For the most part, predictions regarding the PIC profiles were confirmed.

Exceptions to predictions were noted in the following instances: Neither group demonstrated significant elevations on the Withdrawal and Anxiety scales (although in both instances the Old children obtained

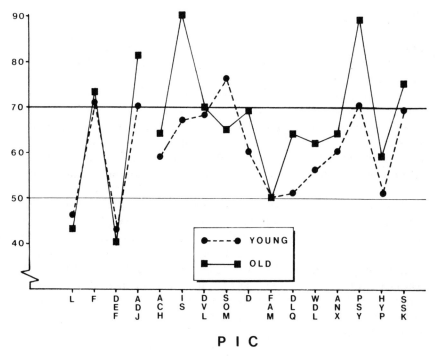

FIGURE 13.1. *T*-scores for the Young and Old groups on the Personality Inventory for Children.

higher scores); the Old group only approached the clinically significant range on the Depression scale; and marginally higher scores were obtained by the Old children on the Hyperactivity scale. Finally, there was no substantial difference between the groups on either the ARS or the BPC (Table 13.2).

Conclusions: Study 2

Generally, the results of the second investigation supported the predictions put forth. A significant degree of parental concern regarding the psychological adjustment of both the Young and Old children was present. Disturbances were primarily with respect to interpersonal relationships, withdrawal, and a tendency toward social isolation. This overall pattern is quite consistent with that observed in adults who exhibit the neuropsychological features of the NLD syndrome.

In addition to increasing concerns regarding the need for intellectual screening in the Old children—which was now in the clinically signifi-

TABLE 13.2. Means (Standard Deviations) for the Young
and Old Groups on the Activity Rating Scale and
Behavior Problem Checklist

	Test protocols	
Measures	Young	Old
ARS (32 items)		
No	9.3 (5.7)	12.0 (7.3)
A little	11.9 (3.6)	11.2 (6.0)
Very much	11.1 (6.5)	7.0 (4.8)
BPC (64 items)		
No	35.3 (7.9)	32.9 (13.0)
A little	16.3 (5.2)	18.8 (8.9)
Very much	14.4 (8.1)	11.7 (7.4)

cant range—there was also evidence of an exacerbation of the same
emotional disturbances that were found in the Young children.

However, contrary to our predictions, the Young children did not
exhibit a greater degree of hyperactivity or any other form of conduct
disorder as compared to the Old children; indeed, the reverse seemed to
hold. The Old children obtained higher scores on the Hyperactivity and
Delinquency scales of the PIC, though both remained in the clinically
nonsignificant range. However, confusing the issue somewhat is the fact
that the Young and Old children obtained similar overall ratings on the
ARS and BPC; this suggests a generally stable level of overall behavioral
disturbance. Taken together, the results of the PIC, ARS, and BPC suggest that the changes in behavioral conduct are minimal and tend to be in
the direction of increasing levels of disturbance with advancing age.

Conclusions: Studies 1 and 2

Based on the results of these two exploratory investigations, the following
tentative conclusions regarding the developmental dynamics of the NLD
syndrome can be drawn:

1. Some of the features of the NLD syndrome do evolve with advancing age during the childhood years of 7 to 14 and do so in a
   manner that is predicted by the NLD model.
2. The pattern of changes observed is such that there is a relative
   stability of verbal and auditory linguistic abilities and a relative
   decline in visual–perceptual–organizational abilities.

3. Regardless of sensory modality, as children who exhibit the features of the NLD syndrome become older, they experience greater difficulty with novel or otherwise complex tasks, especially when those tasks stress problem-solving and concept-formation abilities.
4. Such children demonstrate increasing degrees of socioemotional disturbances, particularly of the internalized variety. In contrast, externalized types of disturbances, such as hyperactivity and delinquency, remain at nonsignificant levels.

Strengths and Weaknesses of the NLD Syndrome and Model and the Implications for Future Research

In its present form, the NLD typology possesses many strengths that make it worthy of further investigative efforts. Particularly notable in this regard is the theoretical formulation of the typology. The specification of the features that comprise the syndrome is clearly articulated. Obtaining data on the vast majority of the variables in order to identify individuals who exhibit the features of the syndrome would be straightforward within the context of a complete neuropsychological evaluation. For this reason, in addition to the apparent relevance of the syndrome for predicting outcome (particularly as it relates to socioemotional adjustment), it is suggested, based on this preliminary analysis, that the NLD typology does possess clinical validity.

In addition, the model does not merely describe the research findings that have led to its formulation, but it also addresses the underlying mechanisms (both psychological and neuroanatomical) that are thought to be responsible for the syndrome's manifestations and their developmental course.

Among the model's strengths are its apparent internal consistency and amenability to empirical investigation via hypothesis testing. As such, it is open to falsification. The broad scope of the model—covering intellectual, academic, neuropsychological, socioemotional, and neuroanatomical aspects of the syndrome—together with its integration of previous research findings and established theories comprise a quality that one would expect from a reasonably thorough scientific theory (Miller, 1983). Taken together, the merits of the NLD syndrome and model suggest that it is capable of fulfilling one of its major purposes, that being to "encourage empirical examination and test of [its] elements" (Rourke, 1989).

Despite its strengths, the NLD typology is still in need of refinement. One area where additional work is required concerns issues relating to its internal validity. For example, there are no published studies that have directly evaluated the reliability of the NLD syndrome. The extent to which agreement would be obtained among diagnosticians who are given the same data protocols to classify (interrater reliability) is not yet known.

Although the domains of functional abilities and deficiencies are clearly delineated and seemingly internally consistent, the typology's level of success at correctly identifying individuals remains speculative. To some extent, this may be influenced by the weight placed on the individual features of the syndrome. Clinical experience suggests that some features are almost pathognomonic of the NLD syndrome (e.g., severely impaired performance on tasks of speeded eye–hand coordination and fine finger dexterity with the left hand), whereas others may not be as predictive (e.g., the presence of an arithmetic disability). More likely, there probably exists a subset of the features that serve best to identify individuals considered to exhibit the NLD syndrome. Obviously, these are all important issues in establishing the typology's construct validity and should be subjected to empirical investigation.

Because the NLD syndrome and model have only recently been developed, it is not surprising that its external validity remains largely unexplored. Research studies focusing on children classified according to their pattern of academic achievement, especially as they relate to the arithmetic-disabled subtype, have provided much, although indirect, support for the external validity of the NLD syndrome. A recent study by Loveland, Fletcher, and Bailey (1990) is an excellent example of the type of research that could be conducted to examine the external validity of the syndrome. In this study, a subtype × task interaction design was employed to examine the communication skills of LD children classified according to their WRAT pattern. It was found that arithmetic-disabled children encountered more difficulties with social communication that involved nonverbal presentations and enact responses as compared to a group of children who exhibited both reading and arithmetic disability. In contrast, the reading- and arithmetic-disabled children made more errors than the arithmetic-disabled children with verbal presentations and describe responses. It should be noted that these results are quite consistent with the predictions that would be derived from the NLD model.

Studies are beginning to emerge that have been designed for the explicit purpose of examining the syndrome's external validity. The two developmental studies presented herein provided examples of how the hypothesized dynamics of the syndrome can be put to the empirical test. Also, they have provided strong evidence supporting the predictive validity of the NLD typology. Other studies have been conducted recently that have sought to test the hypothesized relationship between white matter damage or dysfunction and the manifestations of the NLD syndrome (e.g., Casey et al., 1990; Del Dotto, Barkley, & Casey, 1989; Fletcher, Thompson, & Miner, 1989). The results of these studies, coupled with the findings of this preliminary analysis, suggest that the NLD syndrome (and its associated model) holds considerable promise as a valid typology and will likely generate many interesting research studies.

References

Abramson, R., & Katz, D. A. (1989). A case of developmental right hemisphere dysfunction: Implications for psychiatric diagnosis and management. *Journal of Clinical Psychiatry, 50,* 70-71.

Casey, J. E., Del Dotto, J. E., & Rourke, B. P. (1990). An empirical investigation of the NLD syndrome in a case of agenesis of the corpus callosum. *Journal of Clinical and Experimental Neuropsychology, 12,* 29.

Casey, J. E., & Rourke, B. P. (submitted) *Syndrome of nonverbal learning disabilities: Age differences in neuropsychological skills and abilities.*

Del Dotto, J. E., Barkley, G., & Casey, J. E. (1989). Neuropsychological and MRI aspects of multiple sclerosis. *The Clinical Neuropsychologist, 3,* 281.

Dunn, L. M. (1965). *Expanded manual for the Peabody Picture Vocabulary Test.* Minneapolis: American Guidance Service.

Fletcher, J. M. (1985). External validation of learning disability typologies. In B. P. Rourke (Ed.), *Neuropsychology of learning disabilities: Essentials of subtype analysis* (pp. 187-211). New York: Guilford Press.

Fletcher, J. M., & Copeland, D. R. (1988). Neurobehavioral effects of central nervous system prophylactic treatment of cancer in children. *Journal of Clinical and Experimental Neuropsychology, 10,* 495-537.

Fletcher, J. M., & Levin, H. S. (1988). Neurobehavioral effects of brain injury in children. In D. K. Routh (Ed.), *Handbook of pediatric psychology* (pp. 258-295). New York: Guilford Press.

Fletcher, J. M., & Satz, P. (1985). Cluster analysis and the search for learning disability subtypes. In B. P. Rourke (Ed.), *Neuropsychology of learning disabilities: Essentials of subtype analysis* (pp. 40-64). New York: Guilford Press.

Fletcher, J. M., Thompson, N. H., & Miner, M. E. (1989). Ability discrepancies in hydrocephalic children. *The Clinical Neuropsychologist, 3,* 282.

Goldberg, E., & Costa, L. D. (1981). Hemisphere differences in the acquisition and use of descriptive systems. *Brain and Language, 14,* 144-173.

Jastak, J. F., & Jastak, S. R. (1965). *The Wide Range Achievement Test.* Wilmington, DE: Guidance Associates.

Kendell, R. E. (1975). *The role of diagnosis in psychiatry.* Oxford: Blackwell.

Kendell, R. E. (1989). Clinical validity. *Psychological Medicine, 19,* 45-55.

Kløve, H. (1963). Clinical neuropsychology. In F. M. Forster (Ed.), *The medical clinics of North America* (pp. 1647-1658). New York: Saunders.

Knights, R. M., & Norwood, J. A. (1980). *Revised smoothed normative data on the neuropsychological test battery for children.* Ottawa, Ontario: Author, Department of Psychology, Carleton University.

Loveland, K. A., Fletcher, J. M., & Bailey, V. (1990). Verbal and nonverbal communication of events in learning disability subtypes. *Journal of Clinical and Experimental Neuropsychology, 12,* 433-447.

Miller, P. H. (1983). *Theories of developmental psychology.* New York: W. H. Freeman.

Myklebust, H. R. (1975). Nonverbal learning disabilities: Assessment and intervention. In H. R. Myklebust (Ed.), *Progress in learning disabilities* (Vol 3, pp. 85–121). New York: Grune & Stratton.

Quay, H. C., & Peterson, D. R. (1975). *Manual for the Behavior Problem Checklist.* Coral Gables, FL: Authors, University of Miami, Program in Applied Social Sciences.

Reitan, R. M., & Davison, L. A. (Eds.). (1974). *Clinical neuropsychology: Current status and applications.* Washington, DC: Winston.

Rourke, B. P. (1987). Syndrome of nonverbal learning disabilities: The final common pathway of white-matter disease/dysfunction? *The Clinical Neuropsychologist, 1,* 209–234.

Rourke, B. P. (1989). *Nonverbal learning disabilities: The syndrome and the model.* New York: Guilford Press.

Rourke, B. P., Bakker, D. J., Fisk, J. L., & Strang, J. D. (1983). *Child Neuropsychology: An introduction to theory, research, and clinical practice.* New York: Guilford Press.

Rourke, B. P., & Casey, J. E. (1990). *Syndrome of nonverbal learning disabilities: Age differences in personality/behavioral functioning.* Manuscript in preparation.

Rourke, B. P., Dietrich, D. M., & Young, G. C. (1973). Significance of WISC Verbal-Performance discrepancies for younger children with learning disabilities. *Perceptual and Motor Skills, 36,* 275–282.

Rourke, B. P., & Finlayson, M. A. J. (1978). Neuropsychological significance of variations in patterns of academic performance: Verbal and visual-spatial abilities. *Journal of Abnormal Child Psychology, 6,* 121–133.

Rourke, B. P., & Gates, R. D. (1980). *Underlining Test: Preliminary norms.* Windsor, Ontario: Authors, University of Windsor, Department of Psychology.

Rourke, B. P., & Strang, J. D. (1978). Neuropsychological significance of variations in patterns of academic performance: Motor, psychomotor, and tactile–perceptual abilities. *Journal of Pediatric Psychology, 3,* 62–66.

Rourke, B. P., & Telegdy, G. A. (1971). Lateralizing significance of WISC Verbal–Performance discrepancies for older children with learning disabilities. *Perceptual and Motor Skills, 33,* 875–883.

Rourke, B. P., Young, G. C., & Flewelling, R. W. (1971). The relationships between WISC Verbal–Performance discrepancies and selected verbal, auditory–perceptual, visual-perceptual, and problem-solving abilities in children with learning disabilities. *Journal of Clinical Psychology, 27,* 475–479.

Rourke, B. P., Young, G. C., Strang, J. D., & Russell, D. L. (1986). Adult outcomes of central processing deficiencies in childhood. In I. Grant & K. M. Adams (Eds.), *Neuropsychological assessment in neuropsychiatric disorders: Clinical methods and empirical findings* (pp. 244–267). New York: Oxford.

Skinner, H. A. (1981). Toward the integration of classification theory and methods. *Journal of Abnormal Psychology, 90,* 68–87.

Strang, J. D., & Rourke, B. P. (1983). Concept-formation/nonverbal reasoning abilities of children who exhibit specific academic problems with arithmetic. *Journal of Clinical Child Psychology, 12,* 33–39.

Strang, J. D., & Rourke, B. P. (1985). Adaptive behavior of children who exhibit specific arithmetic disabilities and associated neuropsychological abilities and deficits. In B. P. Rourke (Ed.), *Neuropsychology of learning disabilities: Essentials of subtype analysis* (pp. 302–328). New York: Guilford Press.

Tranel, D., Hall, L. E., Olson, S., & Tranel, N. N. (1987). Evidence for a right-hemisphere developmental learning disability. *Developmental Neuropsychology, 3,* 113–127.

Voeller, K. K. S. (1986). Right-hemisphere deficit syndrome in children. *American Journal of Psychiatry, 143,* 1004–1009.

Wechsler, D. (1949). *Wechsler Intelligence Scale for Children.* New York: Psychological Corporation.

Weintraub, S., & Mesulam, M. M. (1983). Developmental learning disabilities of the right hemisphere: Emotional, interpersonal, and cognitive components. *Archives of Neurology, 40,* 463–468.

Werry, J. S., & Sprague, R. L. (1970). Hyperactivity. In C. G. Costello (Ed.), *Symptoms of psychopathology: A handbook* (pp. 397–417). New York: John Wiley & Sons.

Wirt, R. D., Lachar, D., Klinedinst, J. K., & Seat, P. D. (1977). *Multidimensional description of child personality: A manual for the Personality Inventory for Children.* Los Angeles: Western Psychological Services.

CHAPTER 14

Developmental Analysis of Children/Adolescents with Nonverbal Learning Disabilities: Long-Term Impact on Personality Adjustment and Patterns of Adaptive Functioning

Jerel E. Del Dotto, John L. Fisk, Gerald T. McFadden, and Byron P. Rourke

Professionals responsible for the evaluation and treatment of developmentally and neurologically handicapped children are all too familiar with the problem of responding unequivocally to questions posed by parents concerning etiologic, treatment, and prognostic issues. Next to the "hows" and "whys" of a disorder are those questions designed to gain some understanding of the child's potential for future academic growth, vocational adjustment, and socioemotional adaptation. These sorts of questions are especially difficult to answer for the learning-disabled child since, although there is some knowledge regarding the cause of these disorders, there is relatively little known regarding appropriate and meaningful intervention strategies. There is more known about prognoses than about treatment, and empirical evidence regarding the long-term outcome of learning disabilities is lacking. A review of the relevant literature suggests that the primary interest among researchers has been to evaluate suspected (including possible brain-related) causes for such disorders. More recently, a number of studies have begun to focus on the longitudinal tracking of children afflicted with a learning disability.

In reviewing relevant longitudinal studies, one is immediately struck by the fact that these investigations have focused almost exclusively on the long-term outcome of early *reading* disturbance. Although it must be granted that reading deficits undoubtedly constitute the major problem of learning-disabled children, many of the follow-up studies seem to have ignored the notion that there exist subtypes of academically impaired children. For example, one child may fail to display age-appropriate word recognition skills and written spelling skills yet demonstrate competent written arithmetic abilities, whereas a second child might exhibit adequate word recognition skills within the context of rather poorly developed written spelling and arithmetic abilities. So too, one child may fail to read single words because of language-related difficulties; another because of the visual–spatial features of the words.

To date, the most comprehensive review of follow-up studies of learning disability has been published by Schonaut and Satz (1983). In this review, clinical and psychometric data on 18 follow-up studies spanning a duration of 2 to 25 years are summarized. Since methodological shortcomings are obvious in many of the studies, some attempt is made by Schonaut and Satz to evaluate each study for methodological adequacy by utilizing and author-derived rating scale composed of the following five major criteria: length of follow-up; sample size; adequacy of sampling procedure; adequacy of controls; and criteria for defining learning disability. Although the authors readily admit that the scale provides at best only a crude index of methodological merit, nevertheless, this procedure did help to identify the better-designed studies from which one might derive some reasonable generalizations. Of the 18 investigations evaluated, five appeared to be methodologically superior. These five investigations (Howden, 1967; Lawson, 1968; Rutter, Tizard, Yule, Graham, & Whitmore, 1976; Satz, Taylor, Friel, & Fletcher, 1978; Spreen, 1978) are discussed at some length and are not reviewed extensively in the context of this chapter. However, several general conclusions regarding the long-term outcome of learning-disabled children can be drawn from the results of these five follow-up studies as follows:

1. In general, the academic prognosis for children with early learning problems appears to be rather poor. For the most part, only those children who are from families of higher socioeconomic status or who have been favored with intensive remedial programs display any sort of meaningful gain with respect to academic functioning.
2. Children with early learning disabilities appear to be slightly more "at risk" for terminating their academic studies prematurely, although the relative "drop-out" rates for learning-disabled and normal children are not actually known.
3. Although data on job satisfaction, salaries, and unemployment rates are sparse, it appears that few learning-disabled children are in occupations that demand extended education.

4. It is not at all clear whether and to what extent early identification and treatment of learning disabilities result in a better prognosis than does late identification.

5. Generally, the available reports are equivocal with respect to whether and to what extent the learning-disabled youngster is at greater risk for delinquency or for socioemotional maladjustment.

In keeping with the conclusions of Schonaut and Satz (1983), Hartzell and Compton (1984) have also reported that a 10-year retrospective study of 114 learning-disabled students revealed significantly lower levels of school attainment, academic success, and social success in these individuals compared to 144 siblings without learning disability. Poor outcome in each of these areas was strongly associated with severity of learning disability, presence of hyperactivity, and, of interest within the context of this chapter, with a concomitant disability in mathematics.

In addition to follow-up data on academic and vocational adjustment, several investigators have focused on "cognitive" outcomes of learning disability. For example, McCue and his associates (McCue, Goldstein, Shelly, & Katz, 1986; McCue, Shelly, & Goldstein, 1986) collected intellectual, academic, and neuropsychological test performances on 100 learning-disabled adults in an attempt to determine if patterns of learning disability "subtypes" that have been identified in children also persist into adulthood. Although from an academic perspective, most learning-disabled individuals do not appear to have specific disabilities (i.e., reading and spelling disabilities are usually accompanied by problems with arithmetic, whereas specific arithmetic disabilities seem to be rare), cognitive testing revealed that learning-disabled adults who perform poorly at reading but relatively better, although not normally, at arithmetic tend to exhibit deficiencies on linguistic-related tasks. On the other hand, learning-disabled adults who perform reasonably well at reading but poorly at arithmetic are seen to display deficits in visual–spatial, nonverbal problem-solving, and complex psychomotor domains. These "cognitive profiles" closely resemble cognitive subtypes found in learning-disabled children. (See McCue & Goldstein, Chapter 15, this volume, for more details regarding this and related studies.)

In another series of studies (Sarazin & Spreen, 1986; Spreen & Haaf, 1986), retesting of learning-disabled subjects 15 years after their initial evaluation revealed the long-term persistence of neuropsychological deficits as the child matures from middle childhood to early adulthood. Cluster-analytically derived neuropsychological subtypes found in both childhood and adult samples partially resembled subtypes reported in the literature. That is to say, both visuoperceptual and graphomotor subtypes could be identified in the adult sample, although a linguistic impairment subtype was no longer recognizable. Spreen (1988) has explained and expanded on this series of studies in considerable detail. For instance, when the learning-disabled sample was broken down into three groups according to degree of neurological impairment (definite impairment, Group 1; suggested impairment, Group 2; learning disability without clinically demonstrated neurological impairment, Group 3), the definitely brain-damaged group (Group 1) was found to exhibit the poorest outcome of all three groups on measures of educational, social, personal, and occupational adjustment. Children with evidence of minimal or questionable brain dysfunction (Group 2) showed poorer outcome than did those without neurological impairment (Group 3), whereas Group 3 children fared worse than a matched control group.

For the past several years, Rourke and his associates have been examining the neuropsychological significance of variations in patterns of reading, spelling, and arithmetic abilities and disabilities. Three groups of children have been studied in considerable detail. Group 1 is composed of children who are uniformly deficient in reading (word recognition), spelling, and arithmetic. Group 2 is composed of children who are relatively adept (although still impaired relative to age expectation) at arithmetic compared to reading and spelling. Group 3 is composed of children who display intact, and in some cases extraordinarily well-developed, reading and spelling skills within the context of poor arithmetic abilities. Group 3 children, in particular, are defined by a constellation of neurocognitive deficits, including compromised visual–spatial abilities, bilaterally impaired haptic perceptual skills, bilateral psychomotor deficits, organizational problems, writing difficulties, and impaired nonverbal problem-solving capacities (see Rourke, 1987, 1988, 1989; Rourke & Finlayson, 1978; Rourke & Strang, 1978; Strang & Rourke, 1983).

In the literature, these individuals have been described as having a nonverbal learning disability (NLD). Possibly because of some fairly well-developed auditory–verbal and language-related skills, this group is not typically viewed as being "at risk" for educational or socioemotional difficulties during early to middle childhood. However, as these children progress through the academic arena, it becomes apparent that their reading comprehension is vastly inferior to their well-developed word recognition skills. Moreover, more generalized problems with comprehension become salient, especially in situations that require an appreciable degree of inferential or higher-order conceptual reasoning. It is not uncommon to observe that older NLD children are clumsy and inept in social situations and inclined to befriend much younger children, remain friendless, and/or associate almost exclusively with adults. In general, they exhibit considerable difficulty with novel, complex, or unstructured situations, be these social or academic in nature.

Further investigation of children chosen so as to be similar to NLD children in terms of some of their neuropsychological attributes (Ozols & Rourke, 1985) found them to have some difficulty in interpreting visual–perceptual input (e.g., nonverbal social cues such as facial expressions, hand movements, body postures, and other physical gestures). Furthermore, parental estimates of personality functioning as measured by the Personality Inventory for Children (PIC; Wirt, Lachar, Klinedinst, & Seat, 1977) reveals that this particular group exhibits the most maladaptive patterns of socioemotional disturbance of any learning disability subtype investigated (Strang & Rourke, 1985a). It is also noteworthy that single-case follow-up studies of NLD individuals have suggested that this subtype of learning-disabled person may be at particular risk for depression and suicide (Rourke, Young, & Leenaars, 1989).

Much of our knowledge regarding long-term outcome in the NLD child is derived from individual case studies. However, with respect to developmental progression and long-term outcome, a cross-sectional study by Rourke, Young, Strang, and Russell (1986) is one investigation that sheds some light on this important issue. In this study, the performances of NLD children were compared with a group of clinic-referred adults on a wide range of neuropsychological variables. The adults presented with Weschsler Adult Intelligence Scale (WAIS; Wechsler, 1955) VIQ–PIQ discrepancies and Wide Range Achievement Test (WRAT; Jastak & Jastak, 1978) patterns that were virtually identical to the patterns in the NLD children. It was demonstrated that the patterns of age-related performance of the adults and the children on the neuropsychological variables were nearly identical. Furthermore, there was clear evidence of internalized forms of psychopathology in the adults—again reminiscent of the socioemotional difficulties displayed by NLD children.

In an attempt to expand the previously reported (Rourke et al., 1986) initial observations of apparent age-related changes in the presentation of the NLD syndrome in adults, Casey and Rourke (1989) conducted a study to determine the pattern of developmental change in a group of NLD children within the school age range of 7 to 15 years. Subjects were selected for study in accordance with the neuropsychological, academic, and socioemotional criteria of the NLD syndrome. These subjects were divided into two groups on the basis of age: a "young" group (7 to 8 years of age) and an "old" group (9 to 15 years of age). Based on the NLD model and previous research, it was expected that the older NLD subjects would exhibit (1) relative stability (i.e., age-appropriate advances) in rote verbal skills, word recognition, spelling, and simple motor skills;

(2) relative declines in visual–spatial–organizational skills, mechanical arithmetic, and complex psychomotor skills; and (3) increased severity of psychopathology, especially of the internalized variety, and a decrease in hyperactivity.

With the exception of finding no lessening of hyperactivity with advancing years, the results of these studies provided strong support for the predictions based on the hypothesized dynamics of the NLD syndrome.

In this chapter, we present the findings of a longitudinal investigation of children with outstandingly deficient arithmetic skills who possess many of the neuropsychological features of the NLD group. The study was conducted with two specific purposes in mind. First, an attempt was made to determine whether and to what extent the academic and neuropsychological ability repertoire of NLD individuals remains stable or changes over time. In this sense, a developmental analysis of such individuals provides a measure of predictive validity. A second aim was to gather further information on socioemotional and personality functioning in this particular type of learning-disabled individual.

Method

Subjects

Twenty-eight subjects were initially identified from a population pool of over 4,000 individuals who had been referred to a large urban children's clinic for comprehensive neuropsychological evaluation. These subjects were at least 16 years of age and right-handed with respect to name-writing preference. Each subject displayed centile scores greater than or equal to 50 on both the Reading and Spelling subtests of the WRAT and a centile score of less than or equal to 25 on the Arithmetic subtest at the time of initial testing. In addition, subjects had to display deficits in at least three of the five following areas: Wechsler Intelligence Scale for Children—Revised (WISC-R; Wechsler, 1974) PIQ less than VIQ by 10 points; bilateral deficits in psychomotor functioning; bilateral deficiencies in haptic perceptual skills; Tactual Performance Test (TPT) left-hand poorer than TPT right-hand score; poor nonverbal problem-solving skills (i.e., performance at least 1 standard deviation below the age-appropriate mean on the Category Test). Of the 28 subjects screened, we were able to locate five (two females and three males ranging in age from 16 to 23 years) who agreed to participate.

Procedure

Each subject was administered a neuropsychological test battery composed of the Wechsler Adult Intelligence Scale—Revised (WAIS-R; Wechsler, 1981), Auditory Closure Test, Speech-Sounds Perception Test, Finger Agnosia and Dysgraphesthesia examinations, Tactile Performance Test, Grooved Pegboard Test, and Trail Making Test—Parts A and B (Reitan & Davidson, 1974). The Booklet Version of the Adult Category Test was also administered (DeFilippis & McCampbell, 1979). Academic achievement status was measured by readministration of the WRAT. Personality adjustment was evaluated using the Minnesota Multiphasic Personality Inventory (MMPI; Hathaway & McKinley, 1967) and the Profile of Mood States (POMS; McNair, Loor, & Droppleman, 1971). Finally, adaptive functioning was assessed using the Vineland Adaptive Behavior Scales (VABS; Sparrow, Balla, & Cicchetti, 1984).

Results

Neuropsychological Data

Table 14.1 presents the means for age, WISC-R, WAIS-R, and WRAT scores for both the initial and follow-up evaluations. As is readily evident from this table, the mean VIQs and PIQs are comparable across testing sessions, with mean PIQ scores being consistently lower. Both testing sessions yielded eceptionally higher WRAT reading (word recognition) scores and above average spelling scores; performances on the Arithmetic subtest of the WRAT were at the 10th centile level at the time of initial evaluation and at the 16th centile level at the time of follow-up testing. These scores indicate that there is relative stability in this particular pattern of academic retardation over time.

Figure 14.1 depicts *T*-score means for the neuropsychological measures at both initial and follow-up testings. Visual inspection of this figure reveals a marked similarity between the initial and follow-up test findings, both from a level of performance as well as from configurational perspective. Pearson product–moment correlation analysis of these data yielded a coefficient in excess of .90. Thus, visual similarity of the profiles as well as the correlational value between the profiles attest to a near-perfect match between performance patterns generated at initial testing and those obtained at the time of follow-up evaluation.

TABLE 14.1. Mean Age, WISC-R/WAIS-R, and WRAT Scores
for Arithmetic-Disabled Sample

	Testing time	
Measure	1	2
Age (years)		
Mean	12.9	18.5
Range	9.5–15.5	16.3–23.4
VIQ		
Mean	105.6	98.00
Range	101–109	93–104
PIQ		
Mean	91.60	96.20
Range	75–103	80–104
WRAT Reading centile		
Mean	83.40	92.60
Range	88–99	94–97
WRAT Spelling centile		
Mean	75.80	69.40
Range	55–86	58–82
WRAT Arithmetic centile		
Mean	10.00	16.60
Range	4–16	5–37

Objective Personality Data

The MMPI profiles of the two female and three male subjects are depicted
in Figures 14.2 and 14.3 respectively. Examination of these figures reveals
that four out of the five profiles have scale elevations in the clinically
interpretive range. With respect to the female subjects, one is characterized by a 476(2) profile, whereas the other subject is characterized by a
high-point Scale 9. The first of these profiles is consistent with a charac-
terological disorder with associated poor impulse control and mild depression, whereas the second protocol is reflective of some type of mood
disorder, most likely hypomanic in nature.

Of the male subjects, one MMPI profile is defined by a high point
Scale 1, and a second is characterized by some mild elevation of Scale 0.
The third profile appears to be essentially within normal limits. Individuals who exhibit elevations on Scale 1 are usually seen to exhibit more
than average worry about bodily functioning, which may be suggestive of
a possible somatoform disturbance. Elevation on Scale 0 is commonly

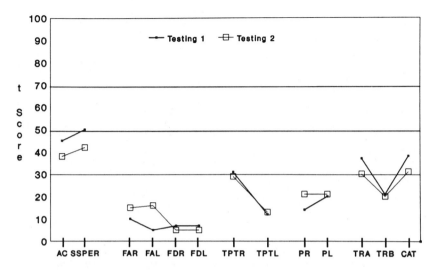

FIGURE 14.1. Plot of *T*-score means for neuropsychological measures.

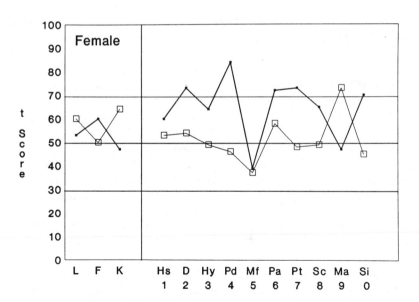

FIGURE 14.2. MMPI profiles for the two female subjects.

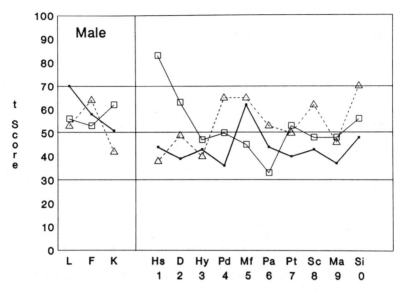

FIGURE 14.3. MMPI profiles for the three male subjects.

associated with social discomfort, with such individuals either being chronically schizoid or presenting a neurotic style of adjustment.

Secondary analysis of the MMPI profiles revealed that the Goldberg Index (Goldberg, 1965) was pathologically high on four subjects and indeterminate for one. This index (derived from a linear regression equation) is thought to be a good discriminator between psychotic and neurotic MMPI profiles. This index is also thought to be related to level of adjustment, with greater values indicating greater maladjustment.

Figure 14.4 depicts the POMS profiles for each subject. The POMS is an adjective-rating form that assesses present mood state. It is intended to provide a measure of an individual's emotional state in response to environmental changes and is not necessarily an index of more stable personality traits. A review of Figure 14.4 suggests some similarities across profiles in four of the five subjects. Although these four profiles appear to be essentially within normal limits, there was a trend for *T*-score values to be particularly low on the Tension–Anxiety, Depression–Dejection, Anger–Hostility, and Confusion–Bewilderment scales. Low scores on these particular scales are thought to be associated with individuals who view themselves as being relaxed and anxiety-free, euphoric in mood, easy-going in temperament, and intellectually and cognitively adaptable. One subject did exhibit clinically significant elevations on the Depression–Dejection and Anger–Hostility scales, reflecting the presence of a dysphoric mood that is characterized by feelings of personal worthlessness and emotional isolation as well as feelings of intense overt anger.

Adaptive Behavior Data

As indicated earlier, the VABS provides a measure of a person's adaptive functioning. In broad terms, it assesses personal and social sufficiency in four domains: Communication (language-related tasks), Daily Living Skills (personal, domestic, and community-related tasks), Socialization (interpersonal relationships, play and leisure, and coping skills), and Motor (gross and fine motor coordination). A global measure of adaptive functioning is also provided by the Adaptive Behavior Composite. A trained interviewer administers the instrument to the parent or primary caretaker of a suspected handicapped individual.

Figure 14.5 presents the mean standard score equivalents for the VABS Communication, Daily Living, and Socialization domains and the Adaptive Behavior Composite. These standard scores ranged from a low of 57.25 on the Socialization domain to a high of 76.25 on the Daily Living Skills domain. Whereas the perfomrance on the Daily Living

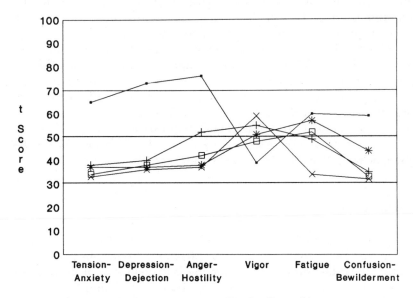

FIGURE 14.4. POMS profiles for five subjects.

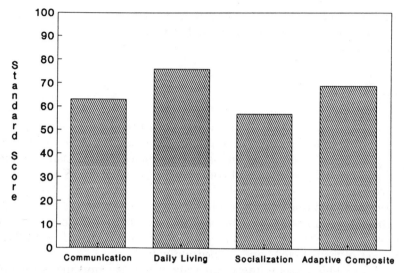

FIGURE 14.5. Mean scores: Vineland Adaptive Behavior Scales.

Skills domain represents a moderately low level of adaptive functioning, the remaining domain scores are classified as low. This pattern suggests that the capacity of these individuals to engage in self-care and domestic duties, albeit impoverished, is somewhat better developed than are their communication skills, which, in turn, are slightly more adequate than are their capacities for interpersonal and social sufficiency.

A score was also generated for each subject on the Maladaptive Behavior domain. This scale is designed to measure behaviors that may interfere with the individual's adaptive functioning; it is scored on the basis of frequency count. For two subjects, the maladaptive scale placed these individuals in the lowest 16% of individuals of the same age. An intermediate classification was obtained on this scale for two other subjects, suggesting that these subjects were reported to exhibit more maladaptive behaviors than at least 50% of same-age cohorts.

Discussion

Obviously, one must exercise caution in generalizing from such a limited sample size. The small sample size precluded the application of any sophisticated statistical analyses, forcing interpretations of the results to be carried out on the basis of inferential analysis of simple descriptive data. Lack of adequate comparisons, varying length of follow-up, and differences in age at time of initial testing could also be viewed as methodological shortcomings. Evaluated within the context of the limitations imposed by sampling considerations, however, the results of this study suggest the following.

The academic and neurocognitive ability repertoire in this sample of NLD individuals has remained remarkably stable over time. This is apparent both from a level of performance as well as from a configurational (pattern analysis) perspective. The subjects in this study continue to exhibit above-average word recognition and spelling abilities in the context of markedly deficient mechanical arithmetic skills. Their neuropsychological protocol continues to be characterized by bilaterally impaired haptic perceptual abilities, left-sided tactually guided problem-solving deficits, bilaterally deficient fine finger dexterity skills, poor nonverbal concept-formation capacities, and somewhat underdeveloped visual–spatial abilities. These findings are quite consistent with those reported by Rourke et al. (1986) in their retrospective study of eight NLD adults. As noted by this group of investigators, the academic problems of NLD adults seem to be associated with difficulties in perceptual–motor, visual–spatial, and problem-solving functioning. Many of the sorts of arithmetic errors (i.e., spatial disorganization, misreading of mathematical signs, and failure to shift "mental set") noted to occur with NLD children (Strang & Rourke, 1985b) were also evident in the protocols of this sample of NLD adults.

In the present study, although no consistent pattern of socioemotional disturbance is discernible on objective personality measures, it is interesting to note that four of the five subjects had MMPI profiles with scale elevations in the clinically interpretable range. Even more intriguing is the finding of a pathologically high Goldberg Index on four subjects and the endorsements by primary caretakers of a significant number of maladaptive behaviors (subsuming characteristics of anxiety, impulsivity, and social withdrawal) on the VABS. Similar to the findings of Rourke et al. (1986, 1989), the NLD subjects in this study manifest a meaningful degree of emotional and/or behavioral maladjustment. In contrast, however, they do not necessarily exhibit a cluster of internalized psychological difficulties (i.e., depression).

As suggested by Rourke and his associates, perhaps the most parsimonious explanation for this behavioral and socioemotional maladjustment lies within the NLD individual's deficient nonverbal logical reasoning capacities and his/her inability to deal effectively with cause-and effect relationships. Moreover, their ineptness in fully appreciating the subleties of various forms of nonverbal communication (e.g., facial and emotional recognition, personal social distance) may render them all but social outcasts in most social milieux.

Just as new social situations may pose serious problems for NLD individuals because of the large number of complex verbal and nonverbal social cues that must be interpreted properly in order to understand fully social interactions, an "ideational" handicap may be one explanation for what appears to be a rather "Polyannaish" presentation on the POMS. In other words, the ability to engage in abstract levels of thought clearly influences a particular individual's self-insight and self-understanding. Deficiencies in this area, therefore, might well eventuate in situations wherein the individual possesses little, if any, awareness of his/her problems.

The results of the parentally derived VABS data are thought-provoking. They highlight what seems to be markedly underdeveloped communication and socialization skills in this group of individuals. Although the immediate significance of these findings is unclear, they nevertheless draw attention to the inefficiencies exhibited by NLD individuals in the performance of daily activities. In addition to appearing to be somewhat inadequate in terms of their ability to function and maintain themselves independently, this particular group of individuals seems to lack the ability to meet culturally imposed demands of personal and social responsibility, at least as described by parents. And, as adaptation to real-world demands is likely to become more problematic for NLD individuals with the passage of time (i.e., as a function of increased occupational, vocational, and social challenges), the risk for psychopathology in those individuals so afflicted may be expected to increase. Such a state of affairs may be the most parsimonious explanation for the differences in socioemotional adjustment noted between our "younger" NLD cases and those "older" NLD individuals described by Rourke et al. (1986, 1989).

Finally, our current understanding of the complex relationship between patterns of cognitive strengths and weaknesses on the one hand and socioemotional functioning on the other is primitive at best. In the case of some subtypes of learning-disabled children (e.g., NLD individuals), it may be that their neurocognitive deficits lead directly to personality maladjustment as an adult outcome. In contrast, other patterns of neurocognitive strengths and weaknesses, such as are seen in reading-disabled children with psycholinguistic deficits, may not be sufficient to produce emotional maladjustment in isolation (i.e., in the absence of other psychosocial stressors). Future longitudinal studies of learning-disabled children must take into account the relationship between variations in cognitive function as they potentially relate to personality functioning. Failure to do so will only lead to broad generalizations (e.g., learning-disabled children are at significant risk for emotional disturbance) that are scientifically unjustified and of limited use in clinical application.

References

Casey, J. E., & Rourke, B. P. (1989, August). *Developmental manifestations of the nonverbal learning disability syndrome in children.* Paper presented at the annual meeting of the American Psychological Association, New Orleans.

DeFilippis, N. A., & McCampbell, E. (1979). *Manual for the Booklet Category Test.* Odessa: Psychological Assessment Resources.

Goldbrg, L. R. (1965). Diagnosticians vs. Diagnostic signs: The diagnosis of psychosis vs. neurosis from the MMPI. *Psychological Monographs, 79* (Whole No. 602).

Hartzell, H. E., & Compton, C. (1984). Learning disability: 10-year follow-up. *Pediatrics, 74,* 1058–1064.

Hathaway, S. R., & McKinley, J. C. (1967). *The Minnesota Multiphasic Personality Inventory manual.* New York: Psychological Corporation.

Howden, M. E. (1967). *A nineteen year follow-up study of good, average and poor readers in the fifth and sixth grades.* Unpublished doctoral dissertation, University of Oregon.

Jastak, J. F., & Jastak, W. (1978). *WRAT manual.* Wilmington, DE: Jastak Associates.

Lawson, M. (1968). *Developmental language disability: Adult accomplishments of dyslexic boys.* Baltimore: Johns Hopkins University Pess.

McCue, M., Goldstein, G., Shelly, C., & Katz, L. (1986). Cognitive profiles of some subtypes of learning disabled adults. *Archives of Clinical Neuropsychology, 1,* 13–23.

McCue, P. M., Shelly, M. A., & Goldstein, G. (1986). Intellectual, academic, and neuropsychological performance levels in learning disabled adults. *Journal of Learning Disabilities, 19,* 233–236.

McNair, D. M., Loor, M., & Droppleman, L. F. (1971). *Profile of Mood States.* San Diego: EDITS/Educational and Industrial Testing Service.

Ozols, E. J., & Rourke, B. P. (1985). Dimensions of social sensitivity in two types of learning-disabled children. In B. P. Rourke (Ed.), *Neuropsychology of learning disabilities: Essentials of subtype analysis* (pp. 281–301). New York: Guilford Press.

Reitan, R. M., & Davison, L. A. (Eds.). (1974). *Clinical neuropsychology: Current status and applications.* Washington, DC: Winston.

Rourke, B. P. (1987). Syndrome of nonverbal learning disabilities: The final common pathway of white matter disease/dysfunction? *The Clinical Neuropsychologist, 1,* 209–234.

Rourke, B. P. (1988). Syndrome of nonverbal learning disabilities: Developmental manifestations in neurological disease, disorder, and dysfunction. *The Clinical Neuropsychologist, 2,* 293–330.

Rourke, B. P. (1989). *Nonverbal learning disabilities: The syndrome and the model.* New York: Guilford Press.

Rourke, B. P., & Finlayson, M. A. J. (1978). Neuropsychological significance of variations in patterns of academic performance: Verbal and visual–spatial abilities. *Journal of Abnormal Child Psychology, 6,* 121–133.

Rourke, B. P., & Strang, J. D. (1978). Neuropsychological significance of variation in patterns of academic performance: Motor, psychomotor, and tactile–perceptual abilities. *Journal of Pediatric Psychology, 3,* 62–66.

Rourke, B. P., Young, G. C., & Leenaars, A. A. (1989). A childhood learning disability that predisposes those afflicted to adolescent and adult depression and suicide risk. *Journal of Learning Disabilities, 22,* 169–187.

Rourke, B. P., Young, G. C., Strang, J. D., & Russell, D. L. (1986). Adult outcomes of central processing deficiencies in childhood. In I. Grant & K. M. Adams (Eds.), *Neuropsychological assessment of neuropsychiatric disorders* (pp. 244–267). New York: Oxford University Press.

Rutter, M., Tizard, J., Yule, W., Graham, P., & Whitmore, K. (1976). Research report: Isle of Wight studies, 1964–1974. *Psychological Medicine, 6,* 313–332.

Sarazin, F., & Spreen, O. (1986). Fifteen-year stability of some neuropsychological tests in learning disabled subjects with and without neurological impairment. *Journal of Clinical and Experimental Neuropsychology, 8,* 190–200.

Satz, P., Taylor, H. G., Friel, J., & Fletcher, J. M. (1978). Some developmental and predictive precursors of reading disabilities: A six year follow-up. In A. Benton, & D. Pearl (Eds.), *Dyslexia: An appraisal of current knowledge* (pp. 313–347). New York: Oxford University Press.

Schonaut, S., & Satz, P. (1983). Prognosis for children with learning disabilities: A review of follow-up studies. In M. Rutter (Ed.), *Developmental neuropsychiatry* (pp. 542–563). New York: Guilford Press.

Sparrow, S., Balla, D. A., & Cicchetti, D. V. (1984). *Vineland Adaptive Behavior Scales.* Circle Pines, MN: American Guidance Service.

Spreen, O. (1978). *Learning-disabled children growing up* (Final report to Health and Welfare, Canada, Health Programs Branch). Ottawa: Health and Welfare, Canada.

Spreen, O. (1988). *Learning disabled children growing up: A followup into adulthood.* London: Oxford University Press.

Spreen, O., & Haaf, R. G. (1986). Empirically derived learning disability subtypes: A replication attempt and longitudinal patterns over 15 years. *Journal of Learning Disabilities, 19,* 170–180.

Strang, D. D., & Rourke, B. P. (1983). Concept formation/nonverbal reasoning abilities of children who exhibit specific academic problems with arithmetic. *Journal of Clinical Child Psychology, 12,* 33–39.

Strang, J. D., & Rourke, B. P. (1985a). Adaptive behavior of children with specific arithmetic disabilities and associated neuropsychological abilities and deficits. In B. P. Rourke (Ed.), *Neuropsychology of learning disabilities: Essentials of subtype analysis* (pp. 302–320). New York: Guilford Press.

Strang, J. D., & Rourke, B. P. (1985b). Arithmetic disability subtypes: The neuropsychological significance of specific arithmetic impairment in childhood. In B. P. Rourke (Ed.), *Neuropsychology of learning disabilities: Essentials of subtype analysis* (pp. 167–183). New York: Guilford Press.

Wechsler, D (1955). *WAIS manual.* New York: Psychological Corporation.

Wechsler, D. (1974). *WISC-R manual.* New York: Psychological Corporation.

Wechsler, D. (1981). *WAIS-R manual.* New York: Psychological Corporation.

Wirt, R. D., Lachar, D., Klinedinst, J. K., & Seat, P. D. (1977). *Multidimensional description of child personality. A manual for the Personality Inventory for Children.* Los Angeles: Western Psychological Services.

Adult Studies

Neuropsychological Aspects of Learning Disability in Adults

Michael McCue and Gerald Goldstein

Statement of the Problem

It now seems reasonably well established that the common wisdom that children outgrow their learning disabilities is not actually the case. Learning disabilities often persist into adulthood and may provide individuals having such conditions with substantial adaptive difficulties. These difficulties are not typically identified by limited academic progress, because the school years are over for most of these people. Rather, they are seen mainly in the area of attainment and maintenance of employment.

Commonly occurring scenarios involve such matters as inability to fill out an application for employment properly because of poor reading or spelling skills, difficulties in maintaining employment when a job that did not previously require more than rudimentary academic skills is changed such that these skills become required, and the reemployment of the industrial worker whose job was lost because the factory was closed and who now must compete for new employment that may require substantial academic skill levels. Also common is the occurrence of job-related difficulties caused by other characteristics commonly associated with learning disability, such as language comprehension and expression difficulties, social skills deficits, and inattention. Correspondingly, the major referral source of individuals with adult learning disability is not the school system but vocational rehabilitation agencies that provide counseling, rehabilitative, and placement services for individuals experiencing problems in gaining or maintaining employment. Self-referral to agencies known to provide services to learning-disabled adults, such as the Association for Children and Adults with Learning Disabilities (ACLD), is also not uncommon.

Recently, an entire volume has appeared related to learning disabilities in adults (Johnson & Blalock, 1987), and there have been follow-up studies into adulthood of children identified as having learning disabilities in childhood (Kline & Kline, 1975; Horn, O'Donnell, & Vitulan, 1983; Spreen, 1987). One of Spreen's conclusions based on follow-up of subjects into their mid-20s was as follows: "Learning problems reflected in academic achievement tests were clearly not overcome, but put LD youngsters at a disadvantage in finding advanced education and vocational opportunities" (p. 134). Johnson (1980) and Bowen and Hynd (1988) reported on the persistence of auditory dysfunction in learning-disabled adults, whereas Kronick (1978) studied psychosocial aspects in individuals with learning disabilities that persisted into adolescence. Learning disability has been identified in college students, and special programs have been designed to meet their needs (Birely & Manley, 1980; Cordoni, 1979; Kahn, 1980).

For the purposes of this chapter, the term learning disability is used to describe a heterogeneous group of developmentally based disorders that include, but are not limited to, academic skills disorders. The National Joint Committee for Learning Disabilities presents the following definition of learning disabilities:

> Learning disabilities is a generic term that refers to a heterogeneous group of disorders manifested by significant difficulties in the acquisition and use of listening, speaking, reading, writing, reasoning, or mathematical abilities, or of social skills. These disorders are intrinsic to the individual and presumed to be due to central nervous system dysfunction. Even though a learning disability may occur concomitantly with other handicapping conditions (e.g., sensory impairment, mental retardation, social and emotional disturbance), with socioenvironmental influences (e.g., cultural differences, insufficient or inappropriate instruction, psychogenic factors), and especially with attention deficit disorder, all of which may cause learning problems, a learning disability is not the direct result of those conditions or influences. (Kavanagh & Truss, 1988, pp. 550–551)

Of particular importance is that learning disabilities include disturbances of language comprehension and expression, including nonverbal language and social skills. The DSM-III-R (American Psychiatric Association, 1987) categorized Specific Developmental Disorders into several categories including Academic Skills Disorders (Reading Disorder, Arithmetic Disorder, Expressive Writing Disorder); Language Skills Disorders (Expressive Language Disorder, Receptive Language Disorder, Articulation Disorder); Motor Skills Disorders; and Developmental Disorders, Not Otherwise Specified. The adults described in this chapter may be categorized using any of these diagnostic possibilities and are not limited to specific disorders of reading, spelling, and arithmetic.

Theoretical Issues

Neuropsychologically related issues in adult learning disability obviously have a great deal of overlap with those matters extensively studied with learning-disabled children. In essence, the neuropsychology of learning disability in children provides the foundation for understanding adult learning disability. However, certain questions may be raised that are specific to adults. First, can the observation that learning disability sometimes persists into adulthood be objectivly verified? Specifically, are there adults of roughly average intelligence, who have had the opportunity to receive an adequate education, who nevertheless are significantly deficient in one or more academic, language, or other developmentally based skills relative to their intellectual level? A series of questions concerns the matter of resemblances between learning disability in adults and children. First, it is well established that learning disability in childhood is not a unitary condition but is divided into numerous subtypes (Rourke, 1985). One may then ask whether the subtypes found in children are the same as those found in adults. Spreen (1987) points out that not all subtypes appear with similar frequencies at all ages, and in his longitudinal study, he found that not all of his cluster-analysis-based subtypes that appeared in children also appeared in adults. Nevertheless, he reports that some similarity is evident.

A related question concerns whether the neuropsychological profiles that accompany subtypes identified in childhood persist into adulthood. There are several logical possibilities here. First, the subtype and the neuropsychological profile may both persist into adulthood. Alternatively, the learning disability characteristics could persist but the neuropsychological profile could normalize, or the academic deficiences could be resolved without a significant change in the neuropsychological profile. In the first case, nothing has changed since childhood. In the second, neurological or neuropsychological deficits may have been associated with the period of acquisition of the learning disability and produced permanent damage to mechanisms for acquiring academic skills even though they eventually resolved. The third instance would obtain for the individual who has improved academically despite the persistence of neuropsychological deficits. Such individuals may have benefited significantly from remedial education or compensated in some way for the detrimental effects their neuropsychological deficits were having on their learning of academic skills. Rourke (1987) has pointed out that certain brain structures appear to be important for both the development and maintenance of a function, whereas other structures are only required during the development of the function.

Evidence for the Persistence of Learning Disability into Adulthood

The major sources for documentation of persistence of learning disability in adulthood are a series of controlled longitudinal studies of children identified as learning-disabled and followed into adulthood (Bruck, 1985; Spreen, 1987; Vetter, 1983; White, Schumaker, Warner, Alley, & Deshler, 1980). Rather than attempt to duplicate here the extensive work reported in these studies, we simply indicate that it seems clear that children with a learning disability often grow into adulthood with that disability and that it remains problematic for them in regard to advancing their education or seeking and maintaining employment. Clearly the most comprehensive and well-designed study was that of Spreen (1987). Phase II of Spreen's longitudinal study conducted with subjects in their mid-20s found that his learning-disabled subjects continued to do less well than controls with regard to type of employment, income level, and personal adjustment. Neurological impairment, when it was initially present, tended to persist.

Another method of documenting the persistence of learning disability into adulthood is to examine characteristics of individuals who meet diagnostic criteria for learning disability (DSM-III or DSM-III-R criteria of Specific Development Disorders). In our own work (McCue, Shelly, & Goldstein, 1986), we were able to identify a sample of 100 young adults who, as a group, met psychometric and diagnostic criteria for learning disability. Their mean Wechsler Adult Intelligence Scale (WAIS; Wechsler, 1955) Verbal IQ was 87.1 ($SD = 10.2$), their mean WAIS Performance IQ was 92.4 ($SD = 11.0$), and their mean Full Scale IQ was 88.64 ($SD = 9.2$). Their scores on the Wide Range Achievement Test (WRAT; Jastak & Jastak, 1965) in Reading, Arithmetic, and Spelling ranged with the fourth to fifth grade level, and the mean score on the Gates–MacGinitie Reading Comprehension Test (MacGinitie, 1978) was also at the fifth grade level. Thus, we identified a group of young adults (mean age = 24.4 years; $SD = 7.9$ years) of slightly below-average range general intelligence but average-range performance intelligence with a lower Verbal IQ than Performance IQ and an apparent discrepancy between intellectual capacity and academic achievement levels. This suggests that there are adults who meet the psychometric criteria for learning disability established for children. These subjects were mainly unemployed and were referred for testing by the state vocational rehabilitation agency as part of an effort being made to seek employment or training for them. Another descriptive study (Minskoff, Hawks, Steidle, & Hoffman, 1989) utilizing the revised Wechsler Adult Intelligence Scale (WAIS-R; Wechsler, 1981) and a battery of neuropsychological tests administered to 145 learning-disabled adults arrived at findings that were very similar to those reported in the McCue, Shelly, and Goldstein study.

Since learning-disabled individuals in the United States are sometimes eligible for publicly funded rehabilitation services, some information is available with regard to the prevalence of the disorder among referred clients in various states. In California, 2.5% of referred clients were characterized as learning disabled (Gerber, 1981). In a nationwide study of successful vocational rehabilitation case closures during 1985, Mars (1986) found that 2.6% of those cases had a primary disability classification of learning disability. Currently, national caseload data indicate that 3% to 5% of the disabled population served by state vocational rehabilitation agencies are eligible on the basis of a learning disability. Some states report the prevalence of adult learning disability as high as 10% of the population (McCue, 1988).

In summary, there is abundant evidence that learning disability persists into adulthood. Furthermore, it appears to be generally definable by the same psychometric criteria developed for children. Finally, just as learning-disabled children experience significant academic and psychosocial difficulties in school, so do learning-disabled adults experience difficulties in advanced educational and employment contexts.

Prototype Neuropsychological Profiles of Learning-Disabled Adults

The matter dealt with here concerns the generic neuropsychological test profile of learning-disabled adults derived from administration of standard neuropsychological test batteries. The profiles of subtypes are addressed in a later section. Several studies have employed achievement tests in combination with intelligence tests and the Halstead–Reitan Neuropsychological Test Battery (Reitan & Wolfson, 1985). Some years ago, Selz and Reitan (1979a, 1979b) showed that the Halstead–Reitan battery could discriminate effectively among older brain-damaged, learning-disabled, and normal children. O'Donnell, Kurtz, and Ramanaiah (1983) provided a similar comparison for young adults. With regard to general level of performance, they found that 36% of the learning-disabled subjects had an impairment index that was greater than or equal to 0.4, a value generally accepted as signifying possible impairment of brain function.

The mean scores of the learning-disabled subjects on the component tests used always fell between those obtained by the brain-damaged subjects and those obtained by the controls.

Similar results were obtained by McCue, Shelly, et al. (1986) in their descriptive study of 100 learning-disabled adults. The mean Average Impairment Rating was 1.72 which falls into the mildly impaired range according to Russell, Neuringer, and Goldstein (1970) norms. Table 15.1 presents impairment ratings for the sample. If modal Russell, Neuringer, and Goldstein ratings are used as the measure of central tendency, these subjects did relatively poorly on the Location component of the Tactual Performance Test, Finger Tapping, the Speech-Sounds Perception Test, and the Seashore Rhythm Test. They did relatively well on the performance time and memory components of the Tactual Performance Test, both Parts A and B of the Trail Making Test, and the Reitan Aphasia Screening Test. As indicated above, those subjects had a mean Verbal IQ that was lower than their mean Performance IQ (87 versus 92). Their worst WAIS subtest scaled score was on Arithmetic (6.57), and their best subtest scaled score was on Object Assembly (9.33).

There have been several studies in which the Luria–Nebraska Neuropsychological Battery (LNNB; Golden, Hammeke, & Purisch, 1980) was used to assess learning-disabled adolescents and adults (Harvey & Wells, 1989; Lewis & Lorion, 1988; McCue, Shelly, Goldstein, & Katz-Garris, 1984). Data obtained from these studies are summarized in Figures 15.1 and 15.2. Figure 15.1 contains the mean LNNB profiles, while Figure 15.2 contains Wide Range Achievement Test—Revised (WRAT-R) and WAIS-R summary scores, With regard to the LNNB, the profiles obtained by Harvey and Wells and by Lewis and Lorion were almost identical, with that of McCue et al. deviating somewhat, particularly in the Rhythm scale. In all three cases, mean scores on the Writing, Reading, Arithmetic, and Intellectual Processes scales were elevated relative to the remaining scales. On the WRAT-R, the subjects in the Harvey and Wells study did somewhat better than did the other groups, but the IQ values were quite comparable. Lewis and Lorion did not report Verbal and Performance IQs, but the Verbal IQ was lower than the Performance IQ in both of the other studies. There was approximately a 2-point discrepancy in both cases.

Both the Harvey and Wells (1989) and the McCue et al. (1984) studies were descriptive and did not include comparison or control groups. However, Lewis and Lorion (1988) had an age-, education-, and intelligence-matched control group. They found that the learning-disabled subjects did significantly less well than the controls on 10 of the 12 LNNB scales compared. Only the Tactile and Receptive Speech scales were not associated with significant differences. A discriminant function

TABLE 15.1. Percentage Distribution for Russell, Neuringer, and Goldstein Ratings of Selected Halstead-Reitan Tests

Test	Excellent 0	Average 1	Mildly impaired 2	Moderately impaired 3	Severely impaired 4	Very severely impaired 5	n	M	Mode	SD
Tactual Performance Test—total time	7	35	29	21	3	5	100	1.93	1	1.19
Tactual Performance Test—Memory component	22	47	25	3	2	1	100	1.19	1	.95
Tactual Performance Test—Location component	13	25	16	33	12	1	100	2.09	3	1.3
Finger Tapping (number of taps)	19	27	34	20	0	0	100	1.56	2	1.02
Trail Making A (sec)	3	48	31	12	5	0	100	1.68	1	.91
Trail Making B (sec)	13	39	26	16	4	2	100	1.65	1	1.14
Speech Perception (number of errors)	4.4	17.8	47.8	24.4	2.2	3.3	94	2.12	2	.99
Rhythm (number correct)	17.2	19.2	41.4	14.1	6.1	2.1	97	1.79	2	1.19
Aphasia Screening Test (summary score)	4.9	32.8	31.1	23	8.2	0	65	1.97	1	1.05
Average Impairment Rating	0–.9 8	1–1.9 57	2–2.9 33	3–3.9 2	4–4.9 0	5 0	100	1.72	1.3	.12

Note. From McCue, Shelly, and Goldstein (1986). Reprinted by permission.

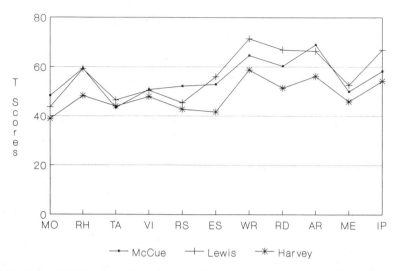

FIGURE 15.1. Mean LNNB profiles for three independent studies of adult learning disability. MO, Motor Scale; RH, Rhythm Scale; TA, Tactile Scale; VI, Vision Scale; RS, Receptive Speech Scale; ES, Expressive Speech Scale; WR, Writing Scale; RD, Reading Scale; AR, Arithmetic Scale; ME, Memory Scale; IP, Intellectual Processes Scale.

analysis correctly classified 90% of the sample. McCue et al. did not have a control group, but they compared the data they obtained on the LNNB factor scales (McKay & Golden, 1981) with published data obtained for adult patients with localized lesions in the left and right temporal and parietooccipital areas. They found that the learning-disabled subjects had the same levels of impairment on the factor scales related to academic skills, such as Reading Polysyllabic Words, as did the left temporal lesion cases, but they did better than those cases on the factor scales assessing more basic language functions, such as Word Comprehension and Motor Writing Skills. A similar picture emerged in the comparison with the left parietooccipital lesion cases. With regard to the comparison between the learning-disabled subjects and patients with right hemisphere lesions, the learning-disabled subjects actually performed worse than the subjects with structural lesions on several of the factor scales including Relational Concepts, Verbal–Spatial Relations, Word Comprehension, Logical Grammatical Relations, and essentially all of the factor scales involving reading or calculation.

In summary, as a group, learning-disabled adults demonstrate neuropsychological deficits. Evidence for this assertion comes from both Halstead–Reitan and LNNB data. Consistent with the findings of Selz and Reitan (1979a, 1979b), levels of performance tend to fall between those of normal individuals and individuals with structural brain damage. Intelligence test data indicate that there is often a slightly lower verbal than performance IQ that in group data does not reach the point of statistical significance. Three studies reviewed (Harvey & Wells, 1989; Lewis & Lorion, 1988; O'Donnell et al., 1983) reported finding average-range Full Scale IQs in their samples, whereas McCue et al. (1984) reported finding a slightly below average Full Scale IQ. There was clear evidence in all studies of marked discrepancies between educational levels and performance on academic achievement tests. Across studies, WRAT-R standard scores ranged from the high 70s to the low 80s, although most of the subjects had received at least some education at the high school level. Differences between learning-disabled subjects and controls were seen not only on tests of academic achievement but also on tests of motor function, abstract reasoning, attention, and auditory discrimination. Tests of nonverbal memory and problem solving that derive from the Halstead–Reitan battery and the LNNB did not tend to discriminate between learning-disabled subjects and controls.

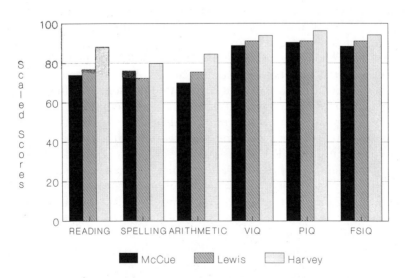

FIGURE 15.2. Mean WAIS-R and WRAT performance for three independent studies of adult learning disability. VIQ, Verbal IQ; PIQ, Performance IQ; FSIQ, Full Scale IQ.

Neuropsychological Subtypes
of Learning-Disabled Adults

The extensive study of subtypes of learning-disabled children reviewed by Rourke (1985) has barely begun in the case of adults. Spreen and Haaf (1986) concluded on the basis of their longitudinal studies that there is a rough correspondence between the typologies found among children and adults. That is, they found adults who grouped into generally impaired, reading-impaired, and arithmetic-impaired subtypes. However, they could not find the clear "linguistic" type described by Mattis, French, and Rapin (1975), who divided dyslexic children and adults into "visual-perceptual," "articulo-graphomotor," and "linguistic" types. Spreen and Haaf found that learning-disabled children of the linguistic type evolved into a group with more generalized impairment. These findings suggest that individuals with severe linguistic deficits as children have particularly poor prognoses, since they apparently go on to develop more global impairment that may worsen in adolescence and adulthood. Spreen's (1988) review of several studies of subtypes in adults indicates that visual-perceptual and graphomotor subtypes can be identified in adulthood. A linguistic subtype could not be identified. Learning-disabled subjects with visual–spatial deficits during childhood maintained those deficits in adulthood and continued to have difficulties with reading and arithmetic. The subgroup with linguistic impairment during childhood seemed to evolve into a group with more generalized low performance.

McCue, Goldstein, et al. (1986) conducted an investigation of whether a group of subtypes described by Rourke (1985) could be identified in adults. The subtypes were based on WRAT or WRAT-R performance and involved discrepancies between Reading and Arithmetic subtest scores. One group was identified as having relatively well-developed reading but very poor mechanical arithmetic skills (Group A), and another as having very poor reading skills with better, but still deficient, mechanical arithmetic skills (Group B). The remaining subjects, who did not have a major discrepancy in their WRAT-R scores, were called Group R members. The basis for classification was a 1.5-year grade-level discrepancy between Reading and Arithmetic subtests. Subjects without such a discrepancy were placed into Group R. Rourke, Young, Strang, and Russell (1986) summarized a series of studies of learning-disabled children that demonstrated many significant cognitive, perceptual, and motor differences among these subgroups. For example, Group A subjects had a cognitive profile characterized by good basic language and perceptual–motor skills but relatively poor visual–spatial, fine rapid psychomotor, and higher-level conceptual skills. Group B members had poor linguistic but relatively good visual-spatial, psychomotor, and conceptual skills.

McCue, Goldstein, et al. (1986) found 32 Group A subjects, 17 Group B subjects, and 51 Group R subjects. Cognitive profiles of these subjects wee described on the basis of their performances on the WAIS-R and components of the Halstead–Reitan battery. With regard to the WAIS-R findings, Groups B and R had higher Performance than Verbal IQs. There was a 9-point discrepancy in the case of Group B and a 6-point discrepancy for Group R. Group A had a mean Verbal IQ that was 2 points higher than the Performance IQ. WAIS-R subtests were compared among the groups by directly comparing the actual standard scores and by comparing deviation scores based on differences between subtest standard scores and the individual's general level of performance. When the direct method was used, Group A was found to do significantly better on the Information and Vocabulary subtests than did the other groups. When the deviation scores were used, it was found that Group A did significantly better than its own generel level of performance on Information and Vocabulary, while Groups B and R did worse. Furthermore, Groups B and R did significantly better than their own general levels of performance on Block Design, while Group A did significantly worse.

With regard to the Halstead–Reitan data, it was first noted that the three subgroups did not differ from each other with regard to general level of impairment, using the Average Impairment Rating as the impairment index. Group A did significantly worse than Groups B and R on the total performance time measure of the Tactual Performance Test, while Group A did significantly better than the other groups on the Aphasia Screening Test. In summary, the McCue, Goldstein, et al. (1986) study led to the identification of the subtypes described by Rourke and his colleagues in adults and demonstrated that the neuropsychological profiles found to characterize those subtypes during childhood also obtain in adulthood. Thus, one might hypothesize that neither the academic deficits nor the associated cognitive dysfunctions were "outgrown" in the individuals studied.

Comparable studies have been carried out with the LNNB. Harvey and Wells (1989) divided their learning-disabled subtypes into groups based on WAIS-R Verbal–Performance IQ discrepancies, and they examined academic achievement and LNNB scores within each of those groups. We do not summarize all of the findings for each subtype here but provide some examples. One group was defined in terms of having a Verbal IQ that was 10 or more points higher than the Performance IQ. This group had its major academic deficit in arithmetic and had an LNNB profile that was characterized by impaired scores on the Arithmetic and Intellectual Processes scales. The mean scores on the LNNB Tactile Sensation, Visual–Spatial Organization, and Arithmetic Calculations factor scales also fell into impaired ranges in the case of this group.

Another group was defined in terms of having a Performance IQ 4–9 points higher than the Verbal IQ. Academically, this group was characterized as having moderate deficits in reading, severe deficits in spelling, and mild deficits in arithmetic. On the LNNB, this group showed significant impairment on the Rhythm, Writing, Reading, and Arithmetic scales. On the LNNB factor scales, significantly impaired mean scores were noted for the Rhythm and Pitch Perception, Verbal–Spatial Relationships, Reading Polysyllabic Words, Spelling, Motor Writing, and Arithmetic Calculation scales. In general, the Harvey and Wells study found meaningful correspondence among data obtained from the WAIS, measures of academic achievement, and the LNNB.

McCue, Goldstein, Shelly, and Katz-Garris (1985) reanalyzed their LNNB descriptive data (McCue et al., 1984) in an attempt to identify preliminary subtypes of adult learning disability through a cluster analysis of the LNNB. The major clinical scales of the LNNB classified the sample into three relatively distinct groups. Figure 15.3 contains the mean LNNB profile for the three groups. Cluster 1 reflected a combination of deficit areas involving both the Rhythm scale and the three academic scales. Cluster 2 had a somewhat poorer mean score than did Cluster 1 on the Rhythm scale but was better on the academic scales. Cluster 3 was approximately equivalent to Cluster 2 with regard to the academic scales but did not show impairment on the Rhythm scale. If we interpret the Rhythm scale as a measure of nonverbal auditory attention, it appears that Cluster 1 had a combination of substantial nonverbal attentional deficits and academic difficulties; Cluster 2 exhibited even greater nonverbal attentional deficits but less profound academic disability; and Cluster 3 had only academic disabilities, without a significant nonverbal attention deficit. However, all three groups had some degree of verbal attention deficit.

All comparisons made for WAIS-R IQ and WRAT achievement scores yielded statistically significant results indicating that cluster membership is associated with general level of intelligence and academic achievement. Table 15.2 presents ANOVA results for WAIS-R and WRAT comparisons. Considering the clusters individually, the first group demonstrated substantial impairment of verbal intelligence relative to performance intelligence. These subjects exhibited very low levels of academic achievement, which did not exceed the fourth grade level despite the fact that their Full Scale IQ level was not in the mentally retarded range. The second group had substantially impaired performance intelligence relative to that of the other two groups and to its own level of verbal intelligence. However, they exhibited a mean Full Scale IQ comparable to that of the first group. Academically, the WRAT grade levels of this second group were depressed, but not to the extent found for the first

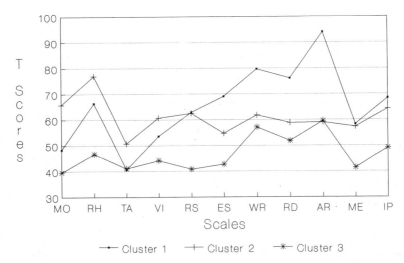

FIGURE 15.3. Mean LNNB profiles for three clusters (from McCue, Goldstein, Shelly, & Katz-Garris, 1985). MO, Motor Scale; RH, Rhythm Scale; TA, Tactile Scale; VI, Vision Scale; RS, Receptive Speech Scale; ES, Expressive Speech Scale; WR, Writing Scale; RD, Reading Scale; AR, Arithmetic Scale; ME, Memory Scale; IP, Intellectual Processes Scale.

group. The relative elevation on the Motor scale in this group suggests that a component of their learning disability may have involved some degree of deficiency in perceptual–motor coordination. The third group showed no substantial difference between levels of verbal and performance intelligence, both of which were somewhat superior to those found for the other two groups. They also exhibited lesser degrees of academic disability than was the case for the other groups.

An examination of pertinent LNNB factor scales essentially confirmed that the first group had substantially greater academic disability than did the other two groups. It was noted that, although the three clusters did not differ with regard to age, $F(2,22) = .84$, $p > .05$, they did differ with regard to education level, $F(2,22) = 6.7$, $p > .01$, with Cluster 1 having the lowest level. It is unlikely, however, that limited education was primarily responsible for the poor academic achievement of the Cluster 1 members, since their mean level of education was 10 years ($SD = 2.1$). It seems more likely that their learning disabilities, which were probably longstanding in nature, played a major role in engendering the limited educational levels of Cluster 1 members relative to the other subgroups.

TABLE 15.2. Means, Standard Deviations, and Analysis of Variance Results for Comparisons of the Three Clusters on WAIS-R and WRAT Variables

| | Cluster | | | | | | | |
| | 1 | | 2 | | 3 | | | |
Variable	M	SD	M	SD	M	SD	F	p
WAIS-R Verbal IQ	77.0	3.9	89.7	10.6	95.7	8.9	11.0	<.001
WAIS-R Performance IQ	88.6	11.4	73.5	9.1	97.8	15.4	6.8	<.01
WAIS-R Full Scale IQ	81.3	4.3	80.8	7.1	96.0	10.5	9.7	<.001
Information (SS)	5.1	1.8	8.5	1.5	8.4	2.2	7.4	<.01
Digit Span (SS)	6.0	2.5	5.8	1.0	7.3	1.6	1.7	>.05
Vocabulary (SS)	5.3	1.0	7.7	3.0	9.1	2.0	7.3	<.01
Arithmetic (SS)	5.3	.8	7.7	2.0	7.9	1.3	8.7	<.01
Comprehension (SS)	6.7	2.0	7.8	2.7	11.3	3.0	7.6	<.01
Similarities (SS)	6.3	1.5	8.7	3.6	10.3	3.1	4.1	<.05
Picture Completion (SS)	8.0	2.4	6.2	1.7	10.3	3.1	5.2	<.05
Picture Arrangement (SS)	8.4	2.3	6.5	3.7	9.9	1.8	3.8	<.05
Block Design (SS)	8.4	1.8	5.8	1.5	10.1	2.2	9.8	<.001
Object Assembly (SS)	9.7	1.9	5.8	2.0	9.7	2.1	8.2	<.01
Digit Symbol (SS)	5.7	2.2	5.2	2.3	9.0	2.5	6.9	<.01
WRAT Reading (GE)	4.0	1.1	6.9	1.0	8.4	1.6	23.6	<.001
WRAT Arithmetic (GE)	3.6	.6	5.7	1.5	6.7	1.5	12.9	<.001

Note. SS, scaled score; GE, grade equivalent. From McCue, Goldstein, Shelly, and Katz-Garris (1985).

Speculating on the nature of the basis for the cluster differences, one could suggest that the first group had difficulty primarily in the language development area itself. The second group may have had developmental difficulties with those nonverbal visual–spatial and perceptual skills that support language learning. It may not be necessary to postulate any form of specific developmental difficulty in the case of the third group. The relatively mild degree of disability of this group might not be associated with any kind of neuropsychological deficit or asymmetry of verbal versus performance intellectual function. Speculating further, it could be suggested that the first group had its difficulties in the area of left (language-dominant) cerebral hemisphere function, whereas the second group had its major problems with abilities thought to be mediated largely by the right hemisphere.

In summary, the differing patterns evident between the identified groups may be based to some extent on asymmetries in information-processing skill levels mediated by the two cerebral hemispheres. The results of this study, therefore, provide some support for the view that it is possible to classify learning-disabled individuals on the basis of the LNNB with satisfactory external validity. However, the internal validity of the clustering procedure remains to be established through the utilization of larger samples. Furthermore, the small sample used here only provides suggestive evidence of the existence of the three subgroups described.

In a more general study of the capacity of the LNNB to classify cases into diagnostically specific categories, Goldstein, Shelly, McCue, and Kane (1987) included in their sample 40 adult learning-disabled individuals in addition to subgroups of patients with diffuse and lateralized acquired brain damage. Cluster analysis was used to produce the classifications. Ideally, if the LNNB-based classification mapped directly onto established diagnostic classification, there would be clusters predominantly containing members of the various diagnostic groups (i.e., a left hemisphere brain-damage cluster, an adult learning disability cluster, etc.). That did not occur. Although a four-cluster solution seemed well justified, cluster membership bore little resemblance to diagnostic category. In this chapter, we only consider the classifications of the learning-disabled subjects. The LNNB profile for Cluster 1 was entirely normal, with an elevation on the Writing scale approaching, but not exceeding, the age- and education-adjusted cut-off score for impairment. Sixteen of the 40 learning-disabled subjects fell into that cluster. The LNNB profile for Cluster 2 was characterized by impaired level performance on the Expressive Speech, Writing, Reading, Arithmetic, and Intellectual Processes scales. Nineteen of the learning-disabled subjects were classified into that cluster. Cluster 3, containing the remaining five learning-disabled subjects, had a mean LNNB profile characterized by mild but impaired level elevations on numerous scales, including the Motor, Rhythm, Writing, Arithmetic, Memory, and Intellectual Processes scales.

Thus, the LNNB clinical scales classified the 40 learning-disabled subjects into two large subgroups and one small subgroup. One of the large subgroups had a normal LNNB profile, with an elevation on the Writing scale, which subsequent ipsative analysis revealed to be statistically significant. The authors concluded that this subgroup was likely to have a specific academic disability in spelling. The other large subgroup was placed into a cluster with an LNNB profile that clearly suggested generalized language dysfunction but substantially more impairment of academic skills than of basic linguistic functions. The remaining five learning-disabled subjects fell into a cluster with an LNNB profile that would be more consistent with the presence of mild generalized acquired brain dysfunction than with learning disability. In any event, it appeared to be a rather unusual neuropsychological profile for learning-disabled individuals. It is interesting to note that 10 of the 26 subjects with documented diffuse structural brain damage were also classified into Cluster 3. Goldstein et al. (1987) did not suggest that the LNNB-based classification of learning disabled cases was coextensive with any established subtyping system but only that the heterogeneity of learning disability could have provided some basis for the diversity in cluster assignments.

In conclusion, Spreen (1987) has indicated that there is a rough correspondence between child and adult subtypes except for the absence of a linguistic subtype in adults. Our own work is in agreement with his first conclusion, but it is uncertain whether or not we have identified a linguistic subtype. Although we clearly did not identify an adult group with specific syntactic, sound-blending, auditory processing, and naming deficits, groups with language-based deficits were obtained. Most of the evidence suggests that neuropsychological deficits accompany the academic disabilities into adulthood, with the possible exception of individuals who have mild academic deficits and at least average-level general intelligence. It is noted that more detailed studies involving such matters as specific aspects of particular disabilities, and specific dispositional conditions, such as left-handedness, have not been investigated as yet.

Summary and Implications for Rehabilitation

Evidence from follow-up studies into adulthood of children diagnosed as learning disabled and cross-sectional studies of adults who meet criteria for learning disability support the notion that significant patterns of deficits (and strengths) are identifiable through the use of standardized neuropsychological tests. From a diagnostic standpoint, neuropsychological tests have demonstrated adequate discriminative validity in distinguishing individuals with learning disabilities from other disability groups and from normals (Lewis & Lorion, 1988; O'Donnell et al., 1983; Selz & Reitan, 1979a, 1979b) and have yielded prototypic patterns of performance on the basis of which learning disability in an individual might be identified. In this fashion, the application of neuropsychological assessment to individuals suspected of learning disability may assist in the identification and diagnostic process. This is particularly relevant for adults because of the lack of adequate normative data on psychoeducational instruments beyond high school age.

Studies that have described subtypes of adults with learning disability indicate clearly that learning disabilities do not constitute a homogeneous group from the standpoint of cognitive function. These findings are certainly preliminary at this point and should not be overinterpreted to suggest that all adults with learning disabilities fall into one of the subgroups described. However, from a clinical standpoint, the capacity of neuropsychological approaches to identify differential patterns of strengths and weaknesses serves as a source of information on which to develop a rehabilitation program. With respect to remediation and rehabilitation, the assessment process may yield information about what the individual can or cannot do as a result of the learning disability. Neuropsychological test results may facilitate planning with respect to identification of a realistic vocational goal, delineation of remedial or compensatory strategies that are required, identification of areas in need of skill development (e.g., social skills), and identification of vocational training and placement needs. From a prescriptive standpoint, neuropsychological assessment may be used to identify best and worst learning and communication modality, define the optimal environmental considerations that fit the individual, and provide some information regarding the prognosis of involvement in rehabilitation services.

References

American Psychiatric Association. (1987). *Diagnostic and statistical manual of mental disorders* (3rd ed., revised). Washington, DC: Author.

Birely, M., & Manley, E. (1980). The learning disabled student in a college environment: A report of State University's program. *Journal of Learning Disabilities, 13,* 12–15.

Bowen, S. M., & Hynd, G. W. (1988). Do children with learning disabilities outgrow deficits in selective auditory attention? Evidence from dichotic listening in adults with learning disabilities. *Journal of Learning Disabilities, 21,* 623–631.

Bruck, M. (1985). The adult functioning of children with specific learning disabilities: A follow-up study. In I. E. Sigel (Ed.), *Advances in applied developmental psychology* (pp. 91–127). Norwood, NJ: Ablex.

Cordoni, B. (1979). Assisting dyslexic college students: An experimental program designed at a university. *Bulletin of the Orton Society, 29,* 263–268.

Gerber, P. J. (1981). Learning disabilities and eligibility for vocational rehabilitation services: A chronology of events. *Learning Disability Quarterly, 4,* 422–425.

Golden, C. J., Hammeke, T. A., & Purisch, A. D. (1980). *The Luria–Nebraska neuropsychological battery: A manual for clinical and experimental uses.* Lincoln, NE: University of Nebraska Press.

Goldstein, G., Shelly, C., McCue, M., & Kane, R. L. (1987). Classification with the Luria–Nebraska Neuropsychological Battery: An application of cluster and ipsative profile analysis. *Archives of Clinical Neuropsychology, 2,* 215–235.

Harvey, J. R., & Wells, M. (1989, February). *Diagnosis of adult learning disabilities and vocational rehabilitation: A descriptive analysis.* Paper presented at the ACLD International Conference, Miami, FL.

Horn, W. F., O'Donnell, J. P., & Vitulano, L. A. (1983). Long-term follow-up studies of learning disabled persons. *Journal of Learning Disabilities, 16,* 542–555.

Jastak, J. F., & Jastak, S. P. (1965). *The Wide Range Achievement Test manual of instructions.* Wilmington, DE: Guidance Associates.

Johnson, D. (1980). Persistent auditory disorders in young dyslexic adults. *Bulletin of the Orton Society, 30,* 269–276.

Johnson, D. J., & Blalock, J. W. (1987). *Adults with learning disabilities: Clinical studies.* Orlando, FL: Grune & Stratton.

Kahn, M. (1980). Learning problems of the secondary and junior college learning disabled student: Suggested remedies. *Journal of Learning Disabilities, 13,* 445–449.

Kavanagh, J. F., & Truss, T. J. (1988). *Learning disabilities: Proceedings of the national conference.* Parkton, MD: York Press.

Kline, C., & Kline, C. (1975). Follow-up study of 216 children. *Bulletin of the Orton Society, 25,* 127–144.

Kronick, D. (1978). An examination of psychosocial aspects of learning disabled adolescents. *Learning Disability Quarterly, 1,* 86–93.

Lewis, R. D., & Lorion, R. P. (1988). Discriminative effectiveness of the Luria–Nebraska Neuropsychological Battery for LD adolescents. *Learning Disabilities Quarterly, 11,* 62–69.

MacGinitie, W. H. (1978). *Manual for the Gates–MacGinitie Reading Tests* (2nd ed.). Boston: Houghton Mifflin.

Mars, L. I. (1986). Profile of learning disabled persons in the rehabilitation program. *American Rehabilitation, 12,* 10–13.

Mattis, S., French, J., & Rapin, I. (1975). Dyslexia in children and young adults: Three independent neuropsychological syndromes. *Developmental Medicine and Child Neurology, 17,* 150–163.

McCue, M. (1988). Survey of state VR agencies. [Unpublished raw data]

McCue, M., Goldstein, G., Shelly, C., & Katz, L. (1986). Cognitive profiles of some subtypes of learning disabled adults. *Archives of Clinical Neuropsychology, 1,* 13–23.

McCue, M., Goldstein, G., Shelly, C., & Katz-Garris, L. (1985, August). *Cluster analysis of the Luria–Nebraska with learning disabled adults.* Paper presented at the American Psychological Association Convention, Los Angeles, CA.

McCue, M., Shelly, C., Goldstein, G., & Katz-Garris, L. (1984). Neuropsychological aspects of learning disability in young adults. *The International Journal of Clinical Neuropsychology, 6,* 229–233.

McCue, M., Shelly, C., & Goldstein, G. (1986). Intellectual, academic and neuropsychological performance levels in learning disabled adults. *Journal of Learning Disabilities, 19,* 233–236.

McKay, S. E., & Golden, C. J. (1981). The assessment of specific neuropsychological skills using scales derived from factor analysis of the Luria–Nebraska Neuropsychological Battery. *International Journal of Neuroscience, 14,* 189–204.

Minskoff, E. H., Hawks, R., Steidle, E. F., & Hoffman, F. J. (1989). A homogeneous group of persons with learning disabilities: Adults with severe learning disabilities in vocational rehabilitation. *Journal of Learning Disabilities, 22,* 521–528.

O'Donnell, J. P., Kurtz, J., & Ramanaiah, N. V. (1983). Neuropsychological test findings for normal, learning-disabled, and brain-damaged young adults. *Journal of Consulting and Clinical Psychology, 51,* 726–729.

Reitan, R. M., & Wolfson, D. (1985). *The Halstead–Reitan Neuropsychological Test Battery.* Tucson, AZ: Neuropsychology Press.

Rourke, B. P. (Ed.). (1985). *Neuropsychology of learning disabilities: Essentials of subtype analysis.* New York: Guilford Press.

Rourke, B. P. (1987). The syndrome of nonverbal learning disabilities: The final common pathway of white-matter disease/dysfunction? *The Clinical Neuropsychologist, 1,* 209–234.

Rourke, B. P., Young, G. C., Strang, J. D., & Russell, D. L. (1986). Adult outcomes of central processing deficiencies in childhood. In I. Grant & K. M. Adams (Eds.), *Neuropsychological assessment of neuropsychiatric disorders* (pp. 244–267). New York: Oxford University Press.

Russell, E. W., Neuringer, C., & Goldstein, G. (1970). *Assessment of brain damage: A neuropsychological key approach.* New York: Wiley-Interscience.

Selz, M., & Reitan, R. M. (1979a). Rules for neuropsychological diagnosis: Classification of brain function in older children. *Journal of Consulting and Clinical Psychology, 47,* 258–264.

Selz, M., & Reitan, R. M. (1979b). Neuropsychological test performance of normal, learning-disabled, and brain damaged older children. *Journal of Nervous Mental Disorders, 167,* 298–302.

Spreen, O. (1987). *Learning disabled children growing up: A follow-up into adulthood.* Lisse, Netherlands: Swets & Zeitlinger.

Spreen, O., & Haaf, R. (1986). Empirically derived learning disability subtypes: A replication attempt and longitudinal patterns over 15 years. *Journal of Learning Disabilities, 19,* 170–180.

Vetter, A. A. (1983). *Comparison of the characteristics of learning disabled and non-learning disabled young adults.* Doctoral dissertation, University of Kansas.

Wechsler, D. (1955). *Manual for the Wechsler Adult Intelligence Scale.* New York: Psychological Corporation.

Wechsler, D. (1981). *Manual for the Wechsler Adult Intelligence Scale—Revised.* New York: Psychological Corporation.

White, W. J., Schumaker, J. B., Warner, M. M., Alley, G. R., & Deshler, D. D. (1980, January). *The current status of young adults identified as learning disabled during their school career* (Research Report No. 21). Lawrence, KS: University of Kansas Institute for Research in Learning Disabilities.

CHAPTER 16

Subtypes of Arithmetic-Disabled Adults: Validating Childhood Findings

Robin D. Morris and L. Warren Walter

Because of the greater value Western society places on verbal skills, there have been fewer societal pressures placed on mathematics compared to reading (Cohn, 1968; Houck, Todd, Barnes, & Engelhard, 1980; Rourke & Strang, 1983) in academic training. Further, many professionals in education and psychology have traditionally viewed mathematics skills as a specific type of language activity (Levy, 1981); this has promoted the view that remediative language training would increase deficient mathematics skills (Rourke & Strang, 1983). More recently, it has been shown that mathematical abilities are based on a unique set of skills (Bohlen & Mabee, 1981; Lerner, 1976; Logue, 1977; Ross, 1976) and that some arithmetic disabilities are largely the result of nonverbal deficits (Rourke, 1978, 1988b; Rourke & Strang, 1983).

There is a relatively long history of the study of arithmetic disorders. As early as 1920, Henschen used the term "dyscalculia" to describe a syndrome in which the skills of calculation and copying from dictation were specifically deficient and suggested that the angular gyrus was involved. Gerstmann (1940; see also Benton, 1987) described a syndrome of dyscalculia in which finger agnosia and right–left confusion co-occurred with mathematical deficits. Kinsbourne and Warrington (1963) used the term "developmental Gerstmann syndrome" to describe children with difficulties in learning mathematics. Cohn (1968) has even described a very specific disorder in which the ability to multiply was deficient. Most recently, the concept of specific mathematics disabilities (SMD; Walter, 1987) has been used to describe a specific type of developmental learning disability in the areas of arithmetic and mathematics.

Research on arithmetic/mathematics abilities has focused on many types of skills thought to be important for competence performance. In particular, spatial, visual–spatial, visual–perceptual, and visual–perceptual–motor abilities have been considered by many to be the foundations necessary for the successful development of arithmetic/mathematics skills (Bohlen & Mabee, 1981; Fabian & Jacobs, 1981; Greenstein & Strain, 1977; Kaliski, 1962; Kosc, 1974, 1981; McLeod & Crump, 1978; Rourke, 1975; Rourke & Finlayson, 1976, 1978; Rourke & Strang, 1983; Saxe & Shaheen, 1981). Mathematical calculations, at minimum, require the ability to orient properly (Hartje, 1987; Kaliski, 1962) and to align (Hartje, 1987; Wagner, 1981) numbers and symbols and the ability to form and copy numerals. Because many written math operations include up–down, right–left, and/or diagonal components (Kaliski, 1962), directionality has also been considered a foundational skill necessary for competency in mathematics/arithmetic (Dean, Schwartz, & Smith, 1981; Greenstein & Strain, 1977; Kosc, 1974; McLeod & Crump, 1978; Saxe & Shaheen, 1981; Wagner, 1981). Memory and attentional abilities have also been deemed necessary for learning and performing mathematical skills (Brainerd, 1987; Cohn, 1961; Lerner, 1976; Ross, 1976).

Houck et al. (1980) suggested that mathematics-related memory could be separated into three different abilities: (1) recall of previously learned information in order to make viable estimations of space, weight, time, etc.; (2) the ability to remember the steps in a specific task based on a general model that must be retrieved from memory; and (3) the ability to recall the meaning of graphic symbols and numerical concepts (see also Brainerd, 1987). Higher-order mathematical–quantitative reasoning and mathematical–conceptual skills have also been a focus of study in researchers' attempts to understand the development and performance of mathematics-related skills (Greenstein & Strain, 1977; Houck et al., 1980; Kosc, 1974, 1981; McLeod & Crump, 1978; Rourke & Strang, 1983; Strang & Rourke, 1983).

Deficits in Mathematics-Related Abilities

It has been suggested that difficulties with any of the basic abilities mentioned above can be exhibited by persons with SMD. For example, Rourke and Finlayson (1978) found that subjects who scored markedly better on the Wide Range Achievement Test (WRAT; Jastak & Jastak, 1965, 1978) Spelling and Reading subtests as compared to their Arithmetic subtest performance exhibited specific deficits on tasks assessing their visual–spatial and visual–perceptual abilities. Wagner (1981) has suggested that these visual–spatial deficits can easily be observed if one performs an error analysis of such students' computations. A directionality problem exists when a student goes in the wrong direction during a step of the process (e.g., going from left to right when multiplying two three-digit numbers). Mirror writing occurs when a student writes down the answer in the opposite order (e.g., the answer is "12," and the student writes "21"). Visual misperception of signs results when the student, especially during multiplication or addition, misperceives the operational symbol, usually because of a perceptual rotation. Some of these errors may also be due to attentional problems, which may influence the perceptual process. Measurements of such deficiencies have often been used as classification variables in studies of SMD children.

Rourke and Strang (1983) have discussed three different orientations to the study of children with SMD. These include the following: (1) the study of children with brain damage who exhibit mathematics deficits; (2) syndrome analysis (the search for a constellation of symptoms common to children with mathematics deficits); and (3) the study of the errors that children make in order to discover their underlying processing problems. Each of these approaches has been used to assist in the differentiation of children with SMD from those with other types of learning disabilities and to form subclassifications (i.e., subtypes) of children with SMD.

A well-known problem in the study of learning-disabled children has been the use of heterogeneous or ill-defined groups of subjects (Morris, 1988; Morris & Fletcher, 1988; Satz & Morris, 1981). In a study of well-defined, homogeneous groups, Kosc (1974) utilized syndrome analysis to describe six subtypes of developmental dyscalculia. These included the following: (1) verbal dyscalculia; (2) practognostic dyscalculia; (3) lexical dyscalculia; (4) graphic dyscalculia; (5) ideognostical dyscalculia; and (6) operational dyscalculia. Rourke and Strang (1983) assessed neuropsychological abilities thought to be subserved primarily by each of the two cerebral hemispheres in order to establish subtypes of SMD that were represented by differential ability patterns.

Subjects in the series of studies on SMD by Rourke and colleagues (Rourke, 1975; Rourke & Finlayson, 1976, 1978; Rourke & Strang, 1978, 1983; Strang & Rourke, 1983, 1985a, 1985b) were first classified into three learning-disabled subtypes on the basis of their performance patterns on the Reading, Spelling, and Arithmetic subtests of the WRAT. One subtype (Group 1) was uniformly deficient in all three academic areas. Another subtype (Group 2) was also deficient in all three areas, but their Arithmetic subtest performance was significantly superior to their performance on the Reading and Spelling subtests. The third was deficient in Arithmetic only (Group 3).

Aspects of the battery of neuropsychological tests on which these three subtypes were compared included measures of verbal, auditory-perceptual, visual–perceptual, visual–spatial, and psychomotor abilities.

Rourke and Finlayson (1978) pointed out that, although two of the subtypes did not differ in their level of performance on the Arithmetic subtest, they differed greatly in their neuropsychological ability patterns, which are believed to underlie their arithmetic performances. They concluded that "it is essential to continue to specify more precisely the patterns of abilities and deficits exhibited by differing types of learning-disabled children" (p. 421). Whether such patterns of abilities and deficits are exhibited by adults has rarely been addressed.

SMD in Adults

Recently, Cordoni, O'Donnell, Ramaniah, Kurtz, and Rosenshein (1981) provided empirical evidence to address the question of whether learning disabilities continue into adulthood. The results of their research provided support for the existence of specific learning disabilities in college-aged adults. They performed analyses to determine the efficacy of the ACID pattern (outstandingly low Arithmetic, Coding, Information, and Digit Span on the Wechsler Adult Intelligence Scale [WAIS]) in identifying learning-disabled adults. Discriminant function analyses of the ACID pattern correctly identified 88% of the controls and 82% of the learning-disabled adults in their sample. These results were interpreted as supporting the hypothesis that learning disabilities continue into the college years and that the same patterns of cognitive abilities/disabilities observed in younger LD children are seen in learning-disabled college adults.

Unfortunately, there are few studies that deal specifically with SMD in college-aged adults. That there are individuals with such mathematics/arithmetic disabilities is certainly plausible in light of the work by Cordoni et al. (1981). Whether they would exhibit the same types of abilities or disabilities as, say, the children in the Rourke studies was the focus of interest in our present investigation.

Based on Rourke's previous findings in children, it was hypothesized that (1) college-aged adults could be identified who showed a specific deficit in Arithmetic on the WRAT (similar to Rourke's Group 3 children), which would suggest an SMD, and (2) that college-aged adults who exhibited such a deficit pattern on the WRAT (Rourke, Yanni, McDonald, & Young, 1973) would show specific deficits in visual–spatial skills (Rourke & Strang, 1983). To address this latter hypothesis, it was specifically predicted that the WAIS-R VIQ of the SMD subtype subjects would be significantly greater than their PIQ and that the SMD subtype subjects would perform below average on other visual–spatial, visual–perceptual–motor, and fine motor tasks.

Study of SMD in College Students

Subjects in a study designed to address these hypotheses (Walter, 1987) were volunteers from a population of college students. They were enrolled in a program created for students who, on admission to a large urban university, were determined to need remediation in certain subject areas before they could matriculate into regular college courses. All subjects met the following criteria to participate in the study: (1) WAIS-R FSIQ between 85 and 115; (2) no need of psychiatric care; and (3) no history of brain injury or disease. Criteria 2 and 3 were determined during an initial screening interview.

One hundred four ($n = 104$) subjects with a variety of documented academic difficulties were administered the WRAT as the academic screening instrument following the model for children established by Rourke and associates. The following criteria, adapted from Rourke's studies with children aged 9 to 14, were used as *a priori* classification criteria for all subjects: Type 1 (Global Deficit Group; GDG), WRAT Reading, Spelling, and Arithmetic Standard Scores (SS) of 85 or below; Type 2 (Reading Deficit Group; RDG), WRAT Reading and Spelling SSs at least 15 points below WRAT Arithmetic SS; and Type 3 (Arithmetic Deficit Group; ADG), WRAT Reading and Spelling SSs exceed WRAT Arithmetic SS by at least 15 points. Type 1 or Type 2 subjects were not found in the college sample.

Subjects placed in the Type 3 group were administered a screening battery of neuropsychological tests that encompassed three ability areas: (1) auditory–verbal, (2) visual–perceptual and spatial, and (3) psychomotor. These measures were considered to be viable adult versions or alternatives of the same tests used by Rourke and Finlayson (1978) and by Rourke et al. (1973). These measures included WAIS-R (Wechsler, 1981); Peabody Picture Vocabulary Test—Revised (Dunn & Dunn, 1981); Halstead–Wepman Aphasia Screening Test (Reitan & Davison, 1974); Sentence Repetition Test (Spreen & Benton, 1968); Trail Making Test, Parts A and B (Army Individual Test Battery, 1944); Rey–Osterrieth Complex Figure Test, copy, immediate, and delayed recall trials (Osterrieth, 1944; Rey, 1941); Visual Form Discrimination Test (Benton, Hamsher, Varner, & Spreen, 1983); and the Finger-Tapping Test (Reitan & Davison, 1974). All tests were administered and scored using standardized procedures.

Although the original purpose of this study was to replicate Rourke and associates' SMD subtyping system in an adult college sample, there were also questions regarding whether the WRAT could independently yield meaningful learning disability subtypes in this population. Because cluster analysis is designed to produce subtypes with homogeneous characteristics (Morris, Blashfield, & Satz, 1981), it was also utilized as a method to form subtypes in a *post hoc* manner. The three subtests of the WRAT were used as the variables for clustering all 104 subjects. The choice of which clustering methods to use was based on guidelines described by Morris et al. (1981). The average-linkage, minimum-variance (Ward's), furthest-neighbor (complete linkage), and centroid methods of clustering (SAS Institute, 1985) were used for multimethod replication with squared euclidean distance the choice of similarity/dissimilarity metric. In theory, if the clustering procedures were effective, and the Rourke *a priori* definitions were useful, then the *a priori*-defined ADG subjects should cluster together, non-ADG (nADG) subjects should cluster together, and there should be very little overlap between different types of subjects.

Study Results

As previously described, the current study used Rourke's original criteria to place subjects in the Arithmetic Deficit Group (ADG). However, neither the Reading Deficit Group (RDG) nor the Global Deficit Group (GDG) was found in the present sample of college students with a variety of academic difficulties. Out of 104 WRATs administered, no subject met the requirements to be placed in either the RDG or the GDG. Thirty-six subjects (35%) met the original criteria to be placed in the ADG. Because of this limited coverage of the college sample, the original score requirements were slightly relaxed (discrepancy between Arithmetic and lower of Reading and Spelling decreased to 11 SS points from 15) in order to provide a broader sample. As a result, 15 additional subjects (total = 51, 49%) met ADG eligibility requirements. Of these 51, 30 students chose to participate further in the study by taking the neuropsychological screening test battery. There were few significant demographic or achievement differences between those participating in the additional testing and those who did not. Descriptive statistics and demographic characteristics for the total sample ($n = 104$), for the participating ADG ($n = 30$), and for the nonclassifiable ($n = 53$) groups are presented in Tables 16.1 and 16.2.

Because most currently accepted definitions of specific learning disabilities require both academic *and* related cognitive deficits, the identification of a group of college students with a relatively low WRAT Arithmetic score only partially identified potential SMD subjects. In order to be clinically diagnosed as having SMD, all ADG subjects' test data were reviewed, and those meeting the following criteria were considered to be SMD: (1) history of problems with arithmetic/math since elementary school; (2) math problems not primarily resulting from anxiety (measured by self-report and analysis of the several relevant tasks); (3) a relative weakness on the Block Design subtest of the WAIS-R; (4) a below-average performance

TABLE 16.1. Demographic Characteristics and WRAT Subtest Standard Scores for Subjects in Total Sample ($n = 104$), ADG ($n = 30$), and Nonclassified (nClass; $n = 53$)

	Total sample		ADG		nClass	
	M	*SD*	*M*	*SD*	*M*	*SD*
Age (years)	23.6	8.2	23.7	8.2	24.1	9.0
WRAT Reading	110.81	9.6	115.17	8.5	107.70	10.6
WRAT Spelling	108.76	8.8	113.50	6.7	105.57	10.4
WART Arithmetic	97.99	10.5	93.63	8.9	102.87	10.6
Percentage males	38.5		26.7		49.1	

on the copy and delayed-recall portions of the Rey–Osterrieth Complex Figure Test; and (5) a below-average performance on fine motor tasks. Those ADG students who did not meet these criteria showed an onset of problems with arithmetic/math after elementary school, did not show evidence of an area of specific cognitive deficit, and reported that anxiety appeared to play an important role in hampering their math performance.

With this approach, 21 of the 30 subjects were clinically diagnosed as having SMD; 6 of the 21 had Arithmetic subtest discrepancy scores of between 11 and 15 points. These data do question the study's original *a priori* definition of a student with an SMD. Had the original ADG membership criterion (Arithmetic subtest at least 15 points lower than lower of Reading and Spelling) been strictly followed, a number of subjects clinically diagnosed as SMD would not have been included in the ADG sample. The increase in numbers of subjects becoming eligible for ADG membership because of this slight criteria alteration suggests that Rourke and his associates' original WRAT criteria for identifying children with ADG may be overly strict for identifying college students with actual SMDs using such screening achievement measures.

The question of whether such *a priori* criteria are actually identifying a naturally occurring subgroup of students with specific mathematics disabilities or just arbitrarily dichotomizing a group of students into groups can begin to be addressed by comparing these results with those obtained using clustering methods. The initial clustering procedure was performed using the average-linkage clustering method. Three types of results were then examined to determine the number of homogeneous clusters in the sample: the hierarchical tree, clustering coefficients, and cluster-profile means.

A visual analysis of the hierarchical tree for the average-linkage method indicated possible solutions of between two and six clusters.

Clustering coefficients indicate the amount of variance accounted for as the clustering procedure forms clusters. Arguments for between two and four clusters could be made on the basis of the review of clustering coefficients. Examination of the cluster profile means indicated that solutions for between two and five clusters were of interest. Canonical correlation-graphing methods used to visualize the two-, three-, five-, and six-cluster solutions suggested that the best cluster differentiation was a two-cluster solution.

Multimethod comparisons (Morris et al., 1981) were used in the reanalysis of the 104 participants' WRAT scores using the minimum variance, furthest neighbor, and centroid clustering methods. For each of

TABLE 16.2. Descriptive Statistics for Neuropsychological Measures for ADG ($n = 30$) Subjects

Variable	M	SD
WAIS-R FSIQ	99.53	11.62
WAIS-R VIQ	100.80	11.82
WAIS-R PIQ	98.00	12.36
WAIS-R subtests		
Information SS	8.98	2.37
Digit Span SS	10.30	3.10
Vocabulary SS	10.50	2.53
Arithmetic SS	8.37	1.92
Comprehension SS	9.83	2.94
Similarities SS	9.47	2.47
Picture Completion SS	9.73	3.10
Picture Arrangement SS	9.20	2.57
Block Design SS	8.63	2.43
Object Assembly SS	8.70	2.87
Digit Symbol SS	11.20	2.12
PPVT-R SS	105.77	12.73
Sentence Repetition Test (number correct)	15.66	1.82
Trail Making, Part A (time)	26.16	8.22
Trail Making, Part B (time)	51.70	16.05
Benton Visual Form Discrimination (number correct)	29.80	2.00
Finger Tapping, right hand	44.10	7.78
Finger Tapping, left hand	40.37	6.79
Rey–Osterrieth Complex Figure		
Copy—raw score	29.25	4.67
Immediate recall—raw score	20.12	6.23
Delayed recall—raw score	19.21	6.97

Note. SS, standard score.

the clustering methods, hierarchical tree analysis, clustering coefficients, plots, and profile means data provided support for the two-cluster solution.

One method for evaluating cluster homogeneity is the use of iterative partitioning methods that assess the relative stability of subject placement into a specific cluster. Multimethod comparison of results based on the original cluster solutions indicated that for five- and six-cluster solutions, over 50% of the participants were reassigned to different clusters using iterative partitioning methods. The three-cluster solution fared better, but 21% of the participants were still reassigned to different clusters. The two-cluster solution proved to be the best solution; all participants were assigned to the same clusters across all four clustering methods.

Of the subjects meeting the original ADG criteria, 14 (28%) were placed in cluster 1, and a majority (37, 72%) were placed in cluster 2. The SMD and nSMD subjects were spread evenly between the two clusters. Nine of the 21 clinically diagnosed SMD participants (43%) were placed in cluster 1, and 12 of the 21 (57%) were placed in cluster 2. Therefore, these clustering results only partially confirmed the *a priori* ADG grouping based on the WRAT scores, but they were not very sensitive to the clinically defined SMD groups. This latter result is not surprising, given that these clustering methods did not use all the data available to the clinicians to classify these subjects. Which results are more valid and useful was not addressed by the current study.

Besides the basic classification and definitional issues, additional hypotheses were also empirically tested. One prediction stated that college-aged adults who exhibited the ADG deficit pattern on the WRAT should show deficits in visual–spatial and related (e.g., psychomotor) functions. This hypothesis was partially supported, as ADG subjects performed in the below-average range on the direct-copy and delayed-recall conditions of the Rey–Osterrieth Complex Figure Test, which measures visual–perceptual–motor and visual–spatial abilities. On the other hand, they did not show a pattern of relative deficits in PIQ, or Performance subtests, when compared to VIQ, or Verbal subtest scores. The ADG did perform significantly below average on the Finger-Tapping Test, a measure of fine motor ability.

Case Illustrations

To describe further the differences between the clinically classified SMD and nSMD groups with the college-aged ADG, two brief cases are presented as exemplars of each group's characteristics:

Case 1

Like the majority of those in her subgroup, A.R. had a history of math problems dating back to elementary school. Her test performances suggested a relative weakness in nonverbal concept-formation, constructional, and spatial skills (Block Design), deficits in visual–perceptual-motor skills (Rey–Osterrieth), as well as a weakness in psychomotor speed (Finger-Tapping Test). Her math errors on the Arithmetic subtest of the WRAT were mainly indicative of not understanding basic arithmetic algorithms. This was evidenced by answers that were clearly improbable. For example, A.R. made a subtraction error on the second problem of the subtest, which is $94 - 64$ presented in columnar form. Her answer was 60. The fifth problem is $2\frac{1}{2} + 1\frac{1}{2}$, in horizontal form. A.R.'s answer was 1. The complexity of an algorithm, as measured by the number of steps required to accomplish it, did not seem to be a factor. For example, A.R. successfully subtracted $7\frac{2}{3}$ from $10\frac{1}{4}$, an operation requiring six separate steps.

Case 2

B.D. had problems with mathematics starting late in junior high school. She reported that anxiety was always a problem in taking mathematics tests. Her performance suggested that anxiety was the main factor in her obtained standard score of 83 on the WRAT Arithmetic subtest. Her errors on the Arithmetic subtest of the WRAT could be labeled "mental errors"; that is, she knew how to do the problems, but, because of the interference of anxiety or time pressure, she rushed through and made careless errors. For example, she misadded on two 3×2 multiplication problems but correctly added a four-entry addition problem of more visual and arithmetic complexity. Her errors on the multiplication problems were single carrying errors, which are often observed in the work of anxious students who rush through their work.

Discussion

In summary, some of the general ideas, concepts, and work on which this project was based were able to be partially supported. Rourke and colleagues (e.g., Rourke & Strang, 1983) have carried out numerous studies demonstrating the relationship between visual–perceptual–motor and visual–spatial skills and right hemisphere functioning, and the necessity of these skills for successful achievement in arithmetic and mathematics.

Although the range of cognitive deficits appeared to be narrower in SMD college students compared to the population of children from which Rourke drew, some support for Rourke's findings was found. For example, both SMD and nSMD subjects reported varying amounts of anxiety surrounding mathematics performance. Similarly, recent studies by Rourke and associates (Rourke, 1987, 1988a, 1988b, 1989; Rourke, Young, & Leenaars, 1989; Strang & Rourke, 1985a, 1985b) showed that anxiety is one of several personality variables that differentiates SMD children from the Global Deficit, and Reading and Spelling Deficit groups.

Although children in Rourke's studies have not been reported to have complained of "math anxiety" (i.e., anxiety caused specifically by having to perform mathematics) as did the adults in the current study, it is quite plausible that such anxiety could develop during the latency and adolescent years. Regarding SMD children, Rourke (1988b) pointed out that "excessive anxiety . . . [as well as other] forms of socioemotional disturbance tend to increase with advancing years" (p. 303). Another similarity between this project and Rourke's work has to do with educational history. Because most of the students diagnosed as SMD had a long history of moderate to severe math problems, it is highly probable that these SMD adults had been SMD children.

Differences between results of Rourke's earlier work and this study were also found. Even though 104 subjects were administered the WRAT, no subject performed in the manner required to be placed in the general-deficit or reading- and spelling-deficit groups (in Rourke's studies, Group 1 and Group 2, respectively). Also, the cognitive skill patterns of the members of the ADG group were somewhat different from children aged 9 to 14 who scored similarly on the WRAT. Performance subtests were generally low in ADG children, but all Performance subtests fell within the average range for the ADG adults in this study.

In retrospect, it is not surprising that GDG subjects (all WRAT subtest scores of 85 or less) were not found in a college sample. Students with such low achievement scores would likely have had an unrewarding academic experience in elementary and secondary schools (Rourke & Strang, 1983) and would have opted not to attend college. Furthermore, their academic achievement levels and cognitive abilities would mitigate against successful entry into, or continued success at, the college level. The fact that no RDG subjects (WRAT Arithmetic standard score 15 points higher than the greater of Spelling and Reading) were found was a little more surprising. This group was consistently represented in Rourke's child studies. One possible reason for its absence is that college is, first and foremost, based on reading-related verbal abilities, and students with reading problems may have been steered toward vocations and fields based on skills of a nonverbal nature. Alternatively, it is probable that RDG college students exist but were not in the current sample, which was drawn from a liberal arts institution. Such students would be drawn toward schools emphasizing fields such as engineering, art and design, and technical fields.

The subgroup of students who were not classified by the WRAT raises interesting questions; the 53 subjects in this subgroup are an enigma. Over 90% of the subjects in the nonclassified subgroup were taking remediative math classes, and it would be expected that many of them would have been classified into the ADG. These students possibly fall into two groups. One group would be those students whose anxiety militates against successful math course work or who had poor math backgrounds and will catch up with special assistance. The other group would be those students whose specific math problems are not picked up by the limited WRAT math assessment.

It had been hypothesized that ADG subjects would perform below the normative means on (1) the WAIS-R Performance scale subtests, (2) other measures of visual–perceptual–motor and visual–spatial abilities, and (3) tasks of fine motor skills. Only parts of this hypothesis were unequivocally supported; the ADG performed significantly below the population mean on the Finger-Tapping Test. Rourke and Strang (1983) reported that their ADG children displayed depressed scores for both hands on the Grooved Pegboard Test, which is a fine motor test correlated with the Finger-Tapping Test. ADG subjects also performed at below-average levels on the Rey–Osterrieth Complex Figure Test, which assesses visual–perceptual–motor, planning, and nonverbal memory abilities, although they did not show deficient performances on other visual–spatial tasks.

From the preceding discussion, a profile of the college student with math problems (not necessarily an SMD) can be developed. He/she probably has WRAT standard scores within the average range. His/her performance on the Finger-Tapping Test would probably be more than 1 standard deviation below the normative mean for each hand. His/her anxiety related to mathematics could range from nonexistent to practically debilitating. Finally, he/she would probably have had a history of mathematics problems beginning some time between the early elementary school years and junior high. The test measures factors that seem best to differentiate SMD from nSMD students are a relative weakness on the Block Design subtest and below-average performance on the three subtests of the Rey–Osterrieth Complex Figure.

There were other interesting findings. Rourke's ADG was comprised of 50% boys and 50% girls. The ADG identified in this project was comprised of 73% females. Anxiety specifically related to mathematics performance seemed to be an important factor in the mathematical performances of ADG adults, but anxiety is not specifically mentioned as a critical factor in performing mathematics in Rourke's child studies. In addition, although there were self-report data that ADG and SMD adults were ADG and SMD children or adolescents, the evidence is anecdotal.

Rourke and Strang (1983) made the important point that most earlier studies of math disorders of children suffered from heterogeneous samples. Because no efforts had been made to differentiate among subjects, clear patterns of math disabilities had not been found. To combat this problem, Rourke administered the WRAT as a screening instrument. On the basis of such an evaluation, Rourke and Finlayson (1978) and Rourke and Strang (1983) reported that ADG children exhibited a "specific arithmetic disorder" (p. 328). In contrast, the ADG adults in this project, all of whom have WRAT subtest patterns similar to Rourke's ADG children, did not form such a homogeneous group. There appeared to be at least two groups, which can best be described as SMD and nSMD.

As a group, Rourke's ADG children performed well on auditory-perceptual and verbal tasks and poorly on visual–perceptual, visual-spatial, and psychomotor tasks. This is exemplified by their performance on the WISC, which showed a statistically significant difference between VIQ and PIQ favoring the VIQ, and by their deficient performance on the Target Test, a test of visual memory. The ADG adults of this project exhibited neither a statistically significant VIQ–PIQ difference nor deficiencies in visual–spatial or visual–perceptual tasks (except on the Rey-Osterrieth Complex Figure). On the Finger-Tapping Test, they did perform well below the mean.

The clinically identified SMD adults ($n = 21$), however, did exhibit more of the expected visual–spatial problems. As mentioned above, this group of SMD adults performed poorly on the three subtests of the Rey-Osterrieth Complex Figure and on WAIS-R Block Design. Because the SMD subjects performed at average levels on other WAIS-R tasks involving visual–spatial skills (e.g., Picture Arrangement, Digit Symbol), the deficit(s) observed in their poor performance on the Block Design subtest and the Rey–Osterrieth Complex Figure Test appear to be more than just visual–spatial in nature. These tasks are more complex and require more spatial planning and motor integration than do the other spatial tasks presented.

Why are there differences between ADG children and adults? One possible answer to this question is that some of the adults' visual–spatial skills have been strengthened. This could have occurred through enrollment in remediative courses and/or self-contained special education classes. Another possible process may be related to concepts from the field of cognitive development. It may have taken longer for the visual–spatial skills tapped by the various tests to develop, and, during the early phases of learning arithmetic, these individuals were not mature enough to insure accurate, successful mathematics performances. Once behind, the child never caught up in basic mathematics skills. Piaget (1972) also suggests that there is the possibility that a person might reach a stage of formal operations in only one specific cognitive area.

Rourke and Strang (1983) report that ADG children make qualitatively different errors on the WRAT Arithmetic subtest in comparison to GDG and RDG children. The main class of error is an apparent deficiency in arithmetical concepts. An example of such an error is giving an answer that is larger than the minuend (number from which the subtrahend is subtracted) in a subtraction problem (Rourke & Strang, 1983). Barring misreading or overlooking the sign, this would signify what could be termed an "algorithmic–conceptual" error. Such an error would result from not understanding an algorithm because of an inability to grasp fully the concept underlying it. SMD adults exhibited these errors more consistently than did the nSMD adults.

One conjecture about this difference is that children who have ADGs might develop a specific "math anxiety" over time (Rourke, 1988b), as they would be punished by the aversive event of doing arithmetic and continually failing. By the time they are college-aged adults, anxiety would have become a strong response to having to perform arithmetic and would therefore have become a decided factor in their mathematics performance. At this point, it is unclear how anxiety plays a role in the mathematics performance of ADG adults. In general, quantifiable anxiety measures should be used in any assessment or study of college-aged adults with reported mathematics problems in order to begin to describe the part anxiety may play in their mathematics performances.

References

Army Individual Test. (1944). Washington, DC: War Department, Adjutant General's Office.

Benton, A. L. (1987). Mathematical disability and the Gerstmann syndrome. In G. Deloche & X. Seron (Eds.), *Mathematical disabilities* (pp. 111-120). Hillsdale, NJ: Lawrence Erlbaum.

Benton, A. L., Hamsher, K., Varner, N. R., & Spreen, O. (1983). *Contributions to neuropsychological assessment.* London: Oxford University Press.

Bohlen, K., & Mabee, W. S. (1981). Math disabilities: A limited review of causation and remediation. *Journal for Special Educators, 17,* 270-280.

Brainerd, C. J. (1987). Sources of working-memory error in children's mental arithmetic. In G. Deloche & X. Seron (Eds.), *Mathematical disabilities* (pp. 87-110). Hillsdale, NJ: Lawrence Erlbaum.

Cohn, R. (1961). Dyscalculia. *Archives of Neurology, 4,* 301-307.

Cohn, R. (1968). Developmental dyscalculia. *The Pediatrics Clinics of North America,* 651-668.

Cordoni, B. K., O'Donnell, J. P., Ramaniah, N. V., Kurtz, J., & Rosenshein, K. (1981). WAIS score patterns for learning disabled young adults. *Journal of Learning Disabilities, 14*, 404–407.

Dean, R. L., Schwartz, N. H., & Smith, L. S. (1981). Lateral preference patterns as a discriminator of learning difficulties. *Journal of Consulting and Clinical Psychology, 49*, 227–235.

Dunn, L., & Dunn, B. (1981). *Peabody Picture Vocabulary Test—Revised.* Circle Pines, MI: American Guidance Service.

Fabian, J. J., & Jacobs, U. W. (1981). Discrimination of neurological impairment in the learning disabled adolescent. *Journal of Learning Disabilities, 14*, 594–596.

Gerstmann, J. (1940). Syndrome of finger agnosia, disorientation for right and left, agraphia and acalculia. *Archives of Neurology and Psychiatry, 44*, 398–408.

Greenstein, J., & Strain, P. S. (1977). The utility of the Key Math Diagnostic Arithmetic Test for adolescent learning disabled students. *Psychology in the Schools, 14*, 275–281.

Hartje, W. (1987). The effects of spatial disorders on arithmetical skills. In G. Deloche & X. Seron (Eds.), *Mathematical disabilities* (pp. 121–136). Hillsdale, NJ: Lawrence Erlbaum.

Henschen, S. E. (1920). *Klinische und pathologische beitrage zur pathologie des gehirns.* Stockholm: Nordiske Bokhandeln.

Houck, C., Todd, R. M., Barnes, D., & Engelhard, A. (1980). LD and math, is it the math or the child? *Academic Therapy, 15*, 557–570.

Jastak, J., & Jastak, S. (1965). *The Wide Range Achievement Test.* Wilmington, DE: Guidance Associates.

Jastak, J., & Jastak, S. (1978). *The Wide Range Achievement Test* (rev. ed.). Wilmington, DE: Jastak Associates.

Kalisiki, D. (1962). Arithmetic and the brain-injured child. *Arithmetic Teacher, 9*, 245–250.

Kinsbourne, M., & Warrington, E. K. (1963). The developmental Gerstmann syndrome. *Archives of Neurology, 8*, 490–501.

Kosc, L. (1974). Developmental dyscalculia. *Journal of Learning Disabilities, 7*, 165–177.

Kosc, L. (1981). Neuropsychological implications of diagnosis and treatment of mathematical learning disabilities. *Topics in Learning and Learning Disabilities, 1*, 19–30.

Lerner, J. W. (1976). *Children with learning disabilities* (pp. 292–302). Boston: Houghton-Mifflin.

Levy, W. K. (1981). How useful is the WISC-R Arithmetic subtest? *Topics in Learning and Learning Disabilities, 1*, 81–87.

Logue, G. (1977). Learning disabilities and math inadequacy. *Academic Therapy, 12*, 309–319.

McLeod, T. M., & Crump, W. D. (1978). The relationship of visuo-spatial skills and verbal ability to learning disabilities in mathematics. *Journal of Learning Disabilities, 11*, 237–241.

Morris, R. (1988). Classification of learning disabilities: Old problems and new approaches. *Journal of Clinical and Consulting Psychology, 56*, 789–794.

Morris, R., Blashfield, R. K., & Satz, P. (1981). Neuropsychology and cluster analysis: Potentials and problems. *Journal of Clinical Neuropsychology, 3*, 79–99.

Morris, R., & Fletcher, J. M. (1988). Classification in neuropsychology: A theoretical framework and research paradigm. *Journal of Clinical and Experimental Neuropsychology, 10*, 640–658.

Osterrieth, P. A. (1944). Le test de copie d'une figure complexe. *Archives de Psychologie, 30*, 206–256.

Piaget, J. (1972). Intellectual evolution from adolescence to adulthood. *Human Development, 15*, 1–12.

Reitan, R. M., & Davison, L. A. (Eds.). (1974). *Clinical neuropsychology: Current status and applications.* Washington, DC: Winston.

Rey, A. (1941). L'examen psychologique dans les cas d'encephalo-pathie traumatique. *Archives de Psychologie, 28(112),* 286-340.

Ross, A. O. (1976). *Psychological aspects of learning disabilities and reading disorders.* New York: McGraw-Hill.

Rourke, B. P. (1975). Brain-behavior relationships in children with learning disabilities: A research program. *American Psychologist, 30,* 911-920.

Rourke, B. P. (1978). Reading, spelling, arithmetic disabilities: A neuropsychologic perspective. In H. R. Myklebust (Ed.), *Progress in learning disabilities* (Vol. 4, pp. 97-120). New York: Grune & Stratton.

Rourke, B. P. (1987). Syndrome of nonverbal learning disabilities: The final common pathway of white-matter disease/dysfunction? *The Clinical Neuropsychologist, 1,* 209-234.

Rourke, B. P. (1988a). Socioemotional disturbances of learning disabled children. *Journal of Consulting and Clinical Psychology, 56,* 801-810.

Rourke, B. P. (1988b). The syndrome of nonverbal learning disabilities: Developmental manifestations in neurological disease, disorder, and dysfunction. *The Clinical Neuropsychologist, 2,* 293-330.

Rourke, B. P. (1989). Nonverbal learning disabilities, socioemotional disturbance, and suicide: A reply to Fletcher, Kowalchuk and King, and Bigler. *Journal of Learning Disabilities, 22,* 186-187.

Rourke, B. P., & Finlayson, M. A. J. (1976). Neuropsychological significance of variations in patterns of performance on the Trail Making Test for older children with learning disabilities. *Journal of Abnormal Psychology, 84,* 412-421.

Rourke, B. P., & Finlayson, M. A. J. (1978). Neuropsychological significance of variations in patterns of academic performance: Verbal and visual-spatial abilities. *Journal of Abnormal Psychology, 6,* 121-133.

Rourke, B. P., & Strang, J. D. (1978). Neuropsychological significance of variations in patterns of academic performance: Motor, psychomotor, and tactile-perceptual abilities. *Journal of Pediatric Psychology, 3,* 62-66.

Rourke, B. P., & Strang, J. D. (1983). Subtypes of reading and arithmetical disabilities: A neuropsychological approach. In M. Rutter (Ed.), *Developmental neuropsychology* (pp. 473-488). New York: Guilford Press.

Rourke, B. P., Yanni, D., McDonald, G., & Young, G. (1973). Neuropsychological significance of lateralized deficits on the Grooved Pegboard Test for older children with learning disabilities. *Journal of Consulting and Clinical Psychology, 41,* 128-134.

Rourke, B. P., Young, G. C., & Leenaars, A. A. (1989). A childhood learning disability that predisposes those afflicted to adolescent and adult depression and suicide risk. *Journal of Learning Disabilities, 22,* 169-185.

SAS Institute Inc. (1985). *SAS user's guide: Statistics, version 5 edition.* Cary, NC: Author.

Satz, P., & Morris, R. (1981). Learning disability subtypes: A review. In F. J. Pirozzolo & McC. Wittrock (Eds.), *Neuropsychological and cognitive processes in reading* (pp. 109-141). New York: Academic Press.

Saxe, G. B., & Shaheen, S. (1981). Piagetian theory and the atypical case: An analysis of the developmental Gerstmann syndrome. *Journal of Learning Disabilities, 14,* 131-135.

Spreen, O., & Benton, A. L. (1968). Sentence repetition test. *Neurosensory Center Comprehensive Examination for Aphasia.* Victoria, BC: Neuropsychology Laboratory, Department of Psychology, University of Victoria.

Strang, J. D., & Rourke, B. P. (1983). Concept formation and non-verbal reasoning abilities of children who exhibit specific academic problems with arithmetic. *Journal of Clinical Child Psychology, 12*, 33–40.

Strang, J. D., & Rourke, B. P. (1985a). Adaptive behavior of children with specific arithmetic disabilities and associated neuropsychological abilities and deficits. In B. P. Rourke (Ed.), *Neuropsychology of learning disabilities: Essentials of subtype analysis* (pp. 302–328). New York: Guilford Press.

Strang, J. D., & Rourke, B. P. (1985b). Arithmetic disability subtypes: The neuropsychological significance of specific arithmetical impairment in childhood. In B. P. Rourke (Ed.), *Neuropsychology of learning disabilities: Essentials of subtype analysis* (pp. 167–183). New York: Guilford Press.

Wagner, R. F. (1981). Remediating common math errors. *Academic Therapy, 16*, 449–453.

Walter, L. W. (1987). *Mathematics learning disabilities in college-aged adults.* Unpublished master's thesis, Georgia State University, Atlanta, GA.

Wechsler, D. (1981). *Wechsler Intelligence Scale—Revised.* New York: Psychological Corporation.

Dimensions of
Clinical Validity

In this section there are seven case studies presented: three dealing with adults, two with adolescents, and two with children. The adult cases are the work of Linas Bieliauskas (Chapter 19); the adolescent cases, John De Luca (Chapter 18); and the child cases, Sara Sparrow (Chapter 17). Names of all individuals and details specific to their identities have been changed to insure confidentiality.

The cases are presented with the sole aim of providing evidence regarding the "clinical" or "ecological" validity of the syndrome of nonverbal learning disabilities (NLD). This syndrome, which is one subtype of learning disabilities, has been described extensively by Rourke (1987, 1988, 1989). Its principal manifestations have been presented by Casey and Rourke (Chapter 13, this volume). Those readers who are unfamiliar with the original formulations of Rourke may wish to consult Chapter 13 for the specifics of the syndrome and the model that was developed in conjunction with it.

References

Rourke, B. P. (1987). Syndrome of nonverbal learning disabilities: The final common pathway of white-matter disease/dysfunction? *The Clinical Neuropsychologist, 1*, 209-234.

Rourke, B. P. (1988). The syndrome of nonverbal learning disabilities: Developmental manifestations in neurological disease, disorder, and dysfunction. *The Clinical Neuropsychologist, 2*, 293-330.

Rourke, B. P. (1989). *Nonverbal learning disabilities: The syndrome and the model.* New York: Guilford Press.

CHAPTER 17

Case Studies of Children with Nonverbal Learning Disabilities

Sara S. Sparrow

Consistent with Rourke's theory of the syndrome of nonverbal learning disabilities (NLD), the following cases are prototypic examples. In children with nonverbal learning disabilities, which are hypothesized to result from impairment of the right hemisphere capacities and/or generalized disturbance of white-matter functioning, we see deficiencies in visual–spatial and perceptual abilities, graphomotor abilities, nonverbal problem solving, visual memory, and motor abilities. In addition, problems in arithmetic are frequently found, whereas relatively more adequate and near-adequate verbal expressive capacities and auditory-processing skills are often evident.

Case Study 1

The first case is a 6½-year-old girl, M, who was born prematurely (1,500 g) and spent 3 weeks in intensive care. She had had an intraventricular hemorrhage and hydrocephalus. Several months before the evaluation, she developed leukemia, for which she was receiving chemotherapy and for which a bone marrow transplant was currently planned. M was referred for testing in order to obtain baseline data before further medical treatments were carried out. M had received extensive medical treatment and hospitalizations for her various medical conditions, but she had never had any formal developmental or psychological testing. Even at age 6, she was not enrolled in a formal school program.

M was very friendly with people in the waiting room, even indiscriminately so. M came to the testing easily and in an overly friendly manner was exceedingly eager to please. During testing, M had great difficulty maintaining interest and responded impulsively with poor attention and concentration. She needed frequent reminders to work slowly and carefully. M alternated between using right and left hand and had a clumsy gait. Table 17.1 shows the test results obtained.

Visual–Spatial Organization Abilities. The Kaufman Assessment Battery for Children (K-ABC) is particularly sensitive to difficulties in these areas, as can be seen by M's scaled scores. The significant weakness of Simultaneous compared with Sequential Processing is indicative of a relative weakness in visual–spatial processing and poor organizational skills. Her performance on Spatial Memory was under the 3-year age level, and on Gestalt Closure, she achieved an age score of 3 years, 3 months.

Nonverbal Problem Solving. M's level of performance in the Nonverbal Problem Solving area ranged from 3 years, 9 months on Triangles to 4 years, 6 months on Matrix Analogies, so that on all Nonverbal Problem Solving tasks she was at least 2 years below age-appropriate levels. She was unable to complete any items on Photo Series.

Motor and Graphomotor Skills. M exhibited serious difficulties in both fine and gross motor skills on the McCarthy motor tasks. She showed inconsistencies in use of right and left hand. M was much more awkward with her left hand than with her right hand. Her performance on the Developmental Test of Visual–Motor Integration was also at a very low level (age equivalent = 3 years, 2 months). She was able to pass only the first two designs. M had difficulty holding the pencil and controlling it.

Academic Achievement. Although M is severely delayed in all academic areas, she is most deficient in arithmetic. M did not recognize a circle or a triangle and only had one-to-one correspondence to five.

Memory. M's significant strength in Sequential Processing indicates her superiority on tasks that require rote performance, particularly on Number Recall, where she had an age equivalent of 6 years, 9 months. She performed less well on the two sequential tasks that required visual cues.

Speech and Language. M exhibited some sound substitutions but performed adequately, with significant strength on the Riddles subtest of the K-ABC. Her Peabody score reflecting listening vocabulary was above her overall level of psychometric intelligence. M's standard score of 84 on the Verbal Reasoning Factor of the Stanford–Binet Intelligence Scale (4th ed.) is further evidence of her relative strength in verbal over nonverbal areas.

TABLE 17.1. Test Results for M, a 6½-Year-Old Girl

Kaufman Assessment Battery for Children	Standard score	%	Scaled score
Mental Processing Composite	70	2	
Sequential Processing	81	10	
Hand Movements			6
Number Recall			9 S[a]
Word Order			6
Simultaneous Processing	67	1	
Gestalt Closure			4
Triangles			5
Matrix Analogies			6
Spatial Memory			4
Photo Series (raw score = 0)			5
Achievement	64	1	
Faces and Places			70
Arithmetic			55 W[b]
Riddles			91 S[c]
Reading Decoding			65

Developmental Test of Visual–Motor Integration	Standard score	Age equivalent	%
	55	3–2	1

McCarthy Scales of Children's Abilities	Standard score
Motor Scale Index	23
	($M = 50$; $SD = 10$)

Stanford–Binet Intelligence Scale (4th ed.)	Standard score
	($M = 50$; $SD = 8$)
Verbal Reasoning	
Vocabulary	42
Comprehension	44
Absurdities	43
Verbal Reasoning Composite	84
	($M = 100$; $SD = 16$)

Peabody Picture Vocabulary Test —Revised	Standard score
	76

Vineland Adaptive Behavior Scales	Standard score	Adaptive level	%
Communication	75	Moderate	5
Daily Living	67	Low	1
Socialization	58	Low	0.3
Adaptive Behavior Composite	61	Low	0.5
Maladaptive level			Significant

[a]Denotes significant strength relative to all other mental processing subtests.

[b]Denotes significant weakness relative to overall subtest performance.

[c]Denotes significant strength relative to overall subtest performance.

Social Skills and Social-Emotional Functioning. M's Vineland scores indicate significant weakness in Socialization, which is at the "low" level. Her Communication score also indicates some practical difficulties in the more social aspects of communication. On the Maladaptive Behavior domain, M was reported as having difficulty in controlling her temper, having poor eye contact, and being negativistic and stubborn. M's parents reported on the Vineland that she is overly friendly with strangers. This is similar to the behavior that was seen in the waiting room when she arrived.

The results of this assessment fit many of the clinical features of the NLD syndrome. M's significant relative strength in verbal ability coupled with her deficits in visual-spatial abilities, her poor graphomotor skills, her poor number and arithmetic ability, and her lack of development of social skills present a picture of a child with nonverbal learning disabilities.

Case Study 2

P is a 9½-year-old boy who was referred to an outpatient clinic for what his mother termed "bouts of depression." P's mother was also concerned, as was the school, with P's academic achievement, particularly in the area of mathematics. His mother reported that he was a good reader but had always had difficulty with numbers. P's mother felt that he was very intelligent and that this interfered with his getting along with peers. She also reported that he exhibited behavioral difficulties at home.

During the evaluation, P, who presented as a somewhat overweight boy, occasionally exhibited unusual behavior such as banging his head with the palm of his hand, squinting, grunting, and grabbing his face with one hand. He began hitting his head with his hand in the waiting room before each testing session. He seemed tense throughout the testing, yet he put forth excellent effort and seemed invested in doing well. His motor behavior, both fine and gross, was quite awkward. He held a pencil awkwardly and walked with an unusual gait.

During the assessment, P obtained the scores shown in Table 17.2.

Visual-Spatial Organization Abilities. On the Wechsler Intelligence Scale for Children—Revised (WISC-R), P's Performance IQ was generally at the average level but was significantly below his Verbal IQ. If P's Arithmetic subtest had not been so low, the difference between Verbal and Performance IQs would have been considerably greater.

Nonverbal Problem Solving. Again, those subtests on the WISC-R that measure Nonverbal Problem Solving were average.

Motor and Development. P is a right-handed boy who performed at average or slightly below-average levels on the motor task (Developmental Test of Visual–Motor Integration). His pencil holding was awkward. His significantly low score on Coding reveals a serious weakness in graphomotor skills. His gait was clumsy. P still has great difficulty with cursive script, and his printing is immature.

Academic Achievement. P's Reading Decoding and Comprehension were well above average. His Spelling was below average, but since he used a phonetic approach the words were easily read. His level of performance on the math test of the Kaufman Test of Educational Achievement was at the low end of average. Furthermore, P obtained an Arithmetic scaled score on the WISC-R of 5.

Memory. P had scaled scores ranging from 13 to 18 on the Information, Vocabulary, and Digit Span subtests of the WISC-R. His Memory for Sentences was above average.

Speech and Language. The WISC-R VIQ (other than the significant weakness on the Arithmetic subtest) indicates excellent speech and language for P. Boston Naming and Verbal Fluency confirm sound verbal skills.

Social Skills and Social–Emotional Functioning. The profile of P obtained from his mother completing the PIC indicates serious emotional difficulties. The Adjustment index indicates that a comprehensive psychological evaluation should be undertaken. On the Personality Inventory for Children (PIC), the Depression index indicates inordinate sadness, while the Family Relations score reflects serious difficulties in this area. The Withdrawal, Anxiety, and Psychosis indices were all exceedingly high, and the effects of these are probably reflected in the Social Skills index, which indicates severe impairment.

P's scores on the Vineland Adaptive Behavior Scales support those obtained on the PIC. Although P's Communication domain was age-appropriate (partly as a result of his high reading level), he exhibited severe deficits in the Daily Living and the Socialization domains. His greatest deficit on the Vineland was in the Interpersonal Relationship subdomain, where he obtained an age score of 4 years, 1 month. In addition, the Maladaptive Behavior domain score of 24 is highly significant. P's mother reports that he is withdrawn, overly dependent, and extremely anxious, that he has poor eye contact and is excessively unhappy, and that he is also negativistic, defiant, and stubborn.

TABLE 17.2. Test Results for P, a 9½-Year-Old Boy

Wechsler Intelligence Scale for Children—Revised	
Full Scale IQ	108
Verbal IQ	115
Performance IQ	98

	Scaled score
Verbal Tests	
Information	14
Similarities	18
Arithmetic	5
Vocabulary	13
Comprehensive	13
Performance Tests	
Picture Completion	10
Picture Arrangement	11
Block Design	11
Object Assembly	11
Coding	6

Kaufman Test of Educational Achievement	Standard score
Math Applications	100
Math Computation	94
Math Composite	96
Reading Decoding	123
Reading Comprehension	124
Reading Composite	124
Spelling	89
Battery Composite	115

Vineland Adaptive Behavior Scales	Standard score	Adaptive level	%
Communication	98	Adequate	45
Daily Living	58	Low	0.3
Socialization	67	Low	1
Adaptive Behavior Composite	69	Low	2
Maladaptive level		Significant	

Personality Inventory for Children	*T*-score
Lie	42
F	87
Defensiveness	37
Adjustment	99
Achievement	53
Intellectual Screening	37
Development	51
Somatic Concern	58
Depression	110

(*continued*)

TABLE 17.2. (Continued)

Personality Inventory for Children	*T*-score
Family Relations	75
Delinquency	80
Withdrawal	100
Psychosis	112
Hyperactivity	43
Social Skills	90

Developmental Test of Visual–Motor Integration	Standard score	%
	92	30

Stanford–Binet Intelligence Scale (4th ed.)	Standard score
Memory for Sentences	58
	($M = 50$; $SD = 8$)

	Level
Boston Naming	Above average
Verbal Fluency	Above average

In summary, P's performance on the tests completed in this evaluation, as well as the reports of his parents, indicate that P has a relative weakness in his nonverbal problem-solving and perceptual organizational skills as compared to his highly developed verbal skills. He is also experiencing serious social–emotional and adaptive difficulties. This profile, combined with a relative weakness in mathematics, supports a classification of nonverbal learning disability (NLD syndrome).

CHAPTER 18

Case Studies of Adolescents with Nonverbal Learning Disabilities

John W. DeLuca

Introduction

Two adolescents exhibiting the nonverbal learning disabilities (NLD) syndrome are presented in this chapter. While both case presentations illustrate rather severe manifestations of the NLD syndrome, Case 1 occurs within the context of a relatively intact family. Case 2 exemplifies the occurrence of the NLD syndrome within the context of a dysfunctional family system. As a result, the second adolescent must cope with the resulting personality disorder and psychopathology arising from his developmental–environmental situation as well as with the limitations of the NLD syndrome. While both of the latter are considered to be independent entities, they do interact and exacerbate one another. That is, his neuropsychological limitations prevent him from gaining insight into his emotional problems.

Case Study 1

Referral

George was a 12-year, 10-month-old boy referred for assessment because it was felt that previous testing did not adequately describe his capabilities. He was said to evidence problems with number concepts, numerical reasoning, and visual–motor output. His self-esteem was poor, and there were indications of underlying anxiety. George was also characterized as being highly distractible and had difficulty concentrating. He often failed to complete his schoolwork, and he engaged in frequent fighting with his peers.

History

When George was quite young, he liked to be held tightly. With the exception of some allergies for grass, trees, and mold, his medical history was unremarkable. George's behavior problems (e.g., low tolerance for frustration and poor social skills) were first evident when he was enrolled in a day-care program. He had some type of mental health intervention since the first grade. Ritalin® was prescribed at age 5, and Mellaril® at age 11.

George was placed in a split regular/learning-disabled class at the third grade level. His behavior problems were thought to interfere with his academic progress, and he was later placed in a fourth grade self-contained class. At age 11, he was said to evidence dyscalculia. George also had problems with telling time, language concepts, and "survival" skills. He was often disruptive in school, and he tried to play the class clown. He became fearful that he could not finish his schoolwork, and, as a result, some degree of avoidance and withdrawal were noted. George began to be belligerent around home, and he often refused to complete his chores. He had few friends around home, and he tended to befriend children younger than himself. His mother contended that his problems were solely the result of his poor concentration skills and distractibility.

George was first evaluated at our facility (a large metropolitan child psychiatric hospital) at 12 years of age. In a psychiatric interview with his parents, George was described as being affectionate, happy, quiet, generous, and concerned about his family. Poor impulse-control skills and a low tolerance for frustration were also noted. His family situation appeared to be stable. In an interview with George, he admitted having few friends and having trouble maintaining long-term relationships. Psychological testing revealed a Wechsler Intelligence Scale for Children— Revised (WISC-R) Verbal IQ of 90, Performance IQ of 75, and Full Scale IQ of 81. His Bender–Gestalt drawings were at the 7- to 8-year level. He was diagnosed (ICD-9-CM) as exhibiting a mixed developmental disorder and an overanxious disorder. He was admitted to the outpatient Day School program at our facility 8 months after the initial outpatient evaluation.

At the time of admission to the Day School, George underwent further projective testing. Reality testing and perceptual accuracy were said to be intact. His Thematic Apperception Test (TAT) stories were considered to be logical and coherent. However, there were indications of idiosyncratic thought processes that appeared to be "neurological" (i.e., organic). He was thought to have poor impulse-control skills, and his drives and instincts were said to outnumber his delay mechanisms and resources. George was found to be egocentric and in need of immediate gratification. He appeared to be highly aroused by affective stimuli, and he had difficulty in modulating his emotions. He tended to force affect into some situations.

George was said to perceive his environment as aggressive and malevolent. There were indications of unpredictability, possible tragic episodes or experiences in his past, and a perceived loss of precious things or loved ones. Although George was found to have adequate object relations, he did exhibit problems in interacting directly with his environment. He had high expectations about his performances and behavior, and he was said to feel inadequate when failure ensued. As a result, George harbored some hostility and resentment associated with social relationships. High levels of psychic tension and distress were noted.

On the Achenbach Child Behavior Checklist, Personality Inventory for Children—Revised, and Conners Parent Questionnaire, George was said to evidence poor social skills, immaturity, anxiety, and some degree of hyperactivity. Most important, a high level of psychopathology was evident. On the basis of these additional test data, he was diagnosed as exhibiting a mixed emotional disturbance with attention deficit disorder/hyperactivity.

Course of Day School Treatment

On admission, George had difficulty focusing on tasks and completing his work. He was disruptive in class, and he required constant individual supervision and/or monitoring. He isolated himself from his peers, and he often set himself up to play the role of scapegoat.

As treatment progressed, George's academic performance improved somewhat; however, he continued to require constant monitoring in the classroom. He also became quite defensive and evidenced "idiosyncratic verbalizations." The latter were said to be quite bizarre, and it was considered that he may have been developing a thought disorder. Following minimal gains during the first 2 months of treatment, his behavior deteriorated. He was seen as being less focused and more depressed. Norpramin® was prescribed; it provided only minimal improvement. In individual psychotherapy, George expressed feelings of hopelessness and worthlessness. He had difficulty in understanding those aspects of his behavior that alienated his peers. His therapist was unsure of how much George was actually able to use "support and mild interpretation" (i.e., insight). As a result of his poor progress in the outpatient program, inpatient hospitalization was recommended.

Course of Inpatient Hospitalization

George initially evidenced obsessive behaviors, and he overreacted to comments by his peers. George began to talk to and answer himself on a regular basis. He often became defensive and agitated when he was told to stop. His behavior was characterized as being very loose and disorganized. He appeared "scattered," and his concentration skills were poor. Other problem behaviors included agitating or threatening peers, provoking others, mimicking speech and gestures, profanity, and sexually inappropriate gestures.

After 2 months of hospitalization, he was characterized as exhibiting an "atypical psychosis," and Haldol® (initially 0.5 mg p.o. and later 1.5 mg p.o.) was prescribed. George's behavior remained loose and disorganized. Argumentativeness increased, and he continued to talk to himself.

Test Behavior

George was assessed just prior to inpatient hospitalization; at that time, he was receiving 75 mg/day of Norpramine®. Although George was generally cooperative, rapport was somewhat difficult to establish with him. He tended to respond quite slowly. He was distractible in the sense that questions often had to be restated, or he tried, albeit unsuccessfully, to anticipate what to do before it was fully explained to him. His coordination skills were somewhat poor. Overall, however, his level of motivation appeared adequate.

Summary of Impressions and Recommendations

George evidenced several neuropsychological deficiencies within the context of other age-appropriate skills. In short, his overall pattern of test performances was quite similar to those children evidencing a nonverbal learning disability. The following report adds some specification to these generalizations. Table 18.1 presents a summary of George's scores on intellectual and academic measures.

George was exclusively right-handed, right-footed, and right-eyed. He evidenced considerable difficulty with both hands on various tests of tactile–perceptual functions (i.e., tactile suppression, finger agnosia, finger dysgraphesthesia, and tactile form recognition for coins). Although he performed somewhat poorly on simple motor tasks (finger tapping and kinetic motor steadiness with the right hand), most evident was his

TABLE 18.1. Neuropsychological Test Results for
George, a 12-Year, 10-Month-Old Boy

Wechsler Intelligence for Children—Revised	
Verbal IQ	88
Performance IQ	73
Full Scale IQ	80
Information	9
Comprehension	6
Arithmetic	5
Similarities	11
Vocabulary	10
Digit Span	5
Picture Completion	7
Picture Arrangement	6
Block Design	6
Object Assembly	8
Coding	3
Peabody Picture Vocabulary Test—Revised	
Standard score	92
Centile rank	30
Age equivalent	11 yr, 7 mo
Wide Range Achievement Test—Revised	
Reading (grade equiv.)	7E
Spelling (grade equiv.)	5B
Arithmetic (grade equiv.)	<3
Peabody Individual Achievement Test	
Reading comprehension (grade equiv.)	5.5

severely impaired performance on a test of complex psychomotor skills (i.e., speeded eye–hand coordination) with both hands.

He also performed in a clearly impaired manner on a test of "hands-on" learning (i.e., the Tactual Performance Test; TPT) that involves strategy generation, psychomotor coordination, and the ability to benefit from tactile input and kinesthetic feedback. His performance on the second trial (when using his left hand) on the TPT was especially poor. His incidental memory for information gleaned from this test was severely impaired.

Overall, George evidenced considerable difficulty on tasks involving tactile perception and fine psychomotor skills. It is believed that such restricted sensory–motor experiences during earlier developmental periods often diminish a child's capacity to "get in touch with his/her world." Thus, such children often rely overly much on verbal (as opposed to nonverbal) modes of interacting and responding to the world.

George's rote verbal and basic auditory–verbal component skills (i.e., appreciation of the phonological aspects of language, sound–symbol matching, attention to and discrimination of auditory rhythms, verbal fluency, and short- and long-term memory for paragraphs of information) were generally age-appropriate. He performed in a normal manner on tests requiring attention to and discrimination of auditory–verbal input. Although George did perform rather poorly on some of the WISC-R subtests associated with attentional deployment, it is likely that his poor Arithmetic subtest performance was primarily caused by his lack of understanding of basic mathematical processes. His poor Digit Span performance was primarily the result of his difficulty on the Digits Backwards portion of this test. George also performed poorly on the Comprehension subtest. The latter may be a reflection of his difficulty in abstraction. Overall, he obtained a WISC-R Verbal IQ of 88.

On the Reitan–Indiana Aphasia Screening Test, George had difficulty in spelling the word "triangle," in pronouncing a multisyllabic word, in completing a mental and a written arithmetic problem, and in understanding verbal directions. He evidenced no errors in naming common items, in reading, or in writing. In fact, his receptive language vocabulary (i.e., PPVT-R) was roughly age-appropriate. In contrast, George performed quite pooly on a test requiring him to remember or code words into, and to retrieve these same words from, long-term memory. However, his poor performance on the latter task was likely the result, at least in part, of his trouble in understanding the requirements of the test even after repeated instruction over several trials.

This boy's reading (single-word recognition) skills were age-appropriate. However, he performed poorly on tasks of spelling to dictation, mechanical arithmetic, and reading comprehension. He obtained the following standard (centile) scores on the Wide Range Achievement Test—Revised (WRAT-R) subtests and Peabody Individual Achievement Test (PIAT) Reading Comprehension subtest: Reading, 100 (50); Spelling, 87 (19); Arithmetic, 50 (0.07); Reading Comprehension, 89 (23). Although George was able to decode single words, his actual understanding of the material he read was well below age-expectation. Inspection of his spelling performances revealed that his errors were generally of a phonetically accurate variety. However, they were also characterized by letter additions, insertions, substitutions, and letter-sequencing problems. On the arithmetic subtest, he was able to complete simple one- and two-digit addition and subtraction problems. However, he did not complete any multiplication or division problems, and he had difficulty with multidigit addition and subtraction problems. He did not take the time to attempt problems that he perceived to be beyond his capability.

Although George's graphomotor productions and his renderings of simple geometric figures were relatively age-appropriate, his drawings of more complex figures were quite poor.

On the WISC-R, he obtained a Performance IQ of 73. In a relative sense, he performed better on tasks requiring the perception of visual detail and puzzle completion than he did on other subtests involving the appreciation of cause-and-effect relationships presented pictorially, visual–spatial organization and synthesis, and the transcription of nonverbal symbols. His performance was considerably impaired when he was required to remember and reproduce simple visual–spatial sequences. Moreover, his ability to remember and reproduce simple line drawings in both immediate and half-hour-delay conditions was mildly to moderately impaired.

George had considerable difficulty on a task involving conceptual flexibility under symbolic shifting conditions (i.e., Trail Making Test, Part B). The latter suggests that he has trouble planning his behavior effectively, keeping more than one idea in his mind at the same time, and controlling his impulses.

He also performed poorly on another test of conceptual flexibility under nonverbal and more ambiguous conditions (i.e., Wisconsin Card-Sorting Test). He was unable to discern all of the concepts, and the number of perseverative errors he evidenced was in the severely impaired range. Moreover, he performed in a considerably impaired manner on one complex nonverbal test involving concept formation, the ability to benefit from immediate positive and negative informational feedback, hypothesis testing, and deductive reasoning skills (i.e., Category Test). The latter performance suggests that George will likely experience trouble in gaining insight into his own or others' behaviors, in dealing with abstract, complex, or novel information, and in understanding the nature of things in a more general sense.

This pattern of performances is similar, in almost all respects, to that evidenced by children who exhibit the NLD syndrome (see Casey & Rourke, Chapter 13, this volume). Furthermore, his mother's ratings of his behavior on the Personality Inventory for Children—Revised were clearly indicative of greater internalized (as opposed to externalized) psychopathology consistent with the NLD syndrome. Elevations on the Depression, Anxiety, Psychosis, and Social Skills scales were especially prominent. His rating on the Hyperactivity scale was unremarkable. Children exhibiting the NLD syndrome often use language as a principal means for social relating, information gathering, and relief from anxiety. It may very well be the case that George's constant talking and answering himself was a reflection of this coping mechanism. It was clear that medication had little effect in decreasing or eliminating this behavior. In short, George's learning disability appears to be chronic and longstanding; the prognosis remains poor.

The following recommendations, in addition to those proposed by Rourke (1989), were suggested:

1. It is quite clear that George will require a placement in a setting that provides him with a very structured environment with clear, concrete, and consistent rules, limits, and expectations. He will likely perform better in situations when he is provided with increased feedback. At the same time, hold George responsible and/or accountable for his actions and provide him with immediate consequences for negative behaviors. Given George's difficulty in gaining insight into his own or others' behaviors, a behavior modification approach to treatment is recommended. If an insight-oriented approach to treatment is utilized, keep information at a concrete level.

2. Some of George's verbal skills are quite well developed and may serve to make him appear to be better off than is actually the case. Although his speech may appear fluent, he will likely evidence poor psycholinguistic pragmatic and abstraction skills. When George becomes too verbal, extinguish extraneous verbalizations and bring him back to the task at hand.

3. In addition, George may need extra time to warm up to complex, novel, or social situations. More specifically, social and problem-solving strategies that would be helpful in daily living situations should be taught in a direct manner. Various metacognitive strategies would be helpful in teaching him to "talk himself through" particular tasks. The aim would be to improve self-control, self-monitoring, attention, and concentration skills. However, the degree to which he can generalize these skills and strategies to situations outside of the training milieu may be quite poor.

Case Study 2

Referral

Dan was a 17-year, 9-month-old youth who was referred for a neuropsychological assessment in order to facilitate placement following his anticipated release from a state-funded facility for juvenile offenders. His past adjudicated offenses included arson, carrying a concealed weapon, car theft, and failure to obey a police officer. According to the referral information, Dan had been experiencing command hallucinations concerning homicidal and suicidal themes. He was on suicide precaution at the time of this assessment, and he had been prescribed Prolixin® and

Cogentin®. The latter were thought to have a positive therapeutic effect on this boy's behavior.

History

Dan was abused by his biological parents at a very early age. In one instance, his father threw him against a wall. He was subsequently removed from the home by protective services and placed in foster care. Dan was adopted 9 months later, at 1 year of age. In this placement, he exhibited problem behaviors, including aggressive acting out and fire setting. Neither parent set effective limits for Dan; he was overindulged, emotionally neglected, and subject to inconsistent disciplinary action. At age 9, he returned home to find his adoptive mother dead as the result of a myocardial infarction. His adoptive father continued to care for Dan in spite of his significant behavior problems. However, he told Dan that his mother's death was Dan's fault. At age 10, Dan found his father dead of an overdose of prescription medication. Dan was placed with a relative, but his behavior was uncontrollable; he was omnipotent, defiant, aggressive, and frequently truant. Dan was made a ward of the state, and he was placed in several different facilities.

Dan has a history of self-mutilative behavior (which was thought to be manipulative, in part), aggressive acting out, and fire setting. He had been placed in numerous mental health facilities. Several medications have been utilized, including carbamazepine, Elavil®, lithium, Stelazine®, and Thorazine®. According to reports, there was only minimal success with carbamazepine; none was reported for the other medications. A psychiatric evaluation undertaken in our clinic eventuated in a diagnosis to the effect that Dan was seen as exhibiting an undersocialized aggressive conduct disorder with antisocial, narcissistic, borderline, and hysterical traits (DSM-III-R). Medication trials of Tegretol®, Haldol®, and Prolixin Decanoate® were attempted as part of treatment within our clinic.

Several psychological examinations of Dan were undertaken between the ages of 10 and 16 years. Full Scale IQs in these ranged from a low of 61 to a high of 87. Verbal IQs ranged from 77 to 103; Performance IQs from 49 to 73. A neuropsychological evaluation undertaken at one facility suggested that Dan suffered from bilateral parietal lobe damage.

A psychiatric follow-up in our clinic approximately 1 year after the initial evaluation indicated that Dan continued to report homicidal and suicidal ideation. He also experienced command hallucinations, which were telling him to kill himself and staff members. According to the psychiatric evaluation, Dan's thinking remained well organized, and his memory and orientation were within normal limits. However, the psychiatrist noted evidence of a "perceptual disturbance" and the fact that Dan perceived himself as the anti-Christ.

Course of Treatment

Dan was seen at least weekly for individual psychotherapy by a staff psychiatrist for approximately 12 months. He continued to experience violent fantasies as well as homicidal and suicidal thoughts. There were numerous occasions of self-mutilation requiring medical attention. These ranged from inserting staples in his urethra to inserting staples, paper clips, and other metal objects into his abdomen and arms. In one instance, major surgery was required because a metal object had lodged near his abdominal aorta. Dan required constant and vigilant one-to-one staff supervision on a 24-hour basis. He was restrained during the day and monitored visually during sleep. He continued to experience command hallucinations with homicidal and suicidal themes. Both Tegretol® and Haldol® were prescribed at various times with no positive effect. Some positive results were obtained with doses of Prolixin® (up to 25 mg weekly). However, he continued to experience hallucinations and to exhibit self-mutilative behaviors.

During the later stages of treatment, Dan continued to be depressed and anxious. Although his thinking was said to be well organized, his judgment and insight were limited. For example, Dan wrote a threatening letter to the judge at a waiver hearing. Dan claimed that the letter was illegally seized and that he never intended to send it. Dan's discharge diagnosis was undersocialized conduct disorder of the aggressive type, atypical psychosis to paranoid schizophrenia—subchronic with acute exacerbation. He was later waived to an adult forensic mental health facility.

Test Behavior

Dan presented with a somewhat disheveled and unkept appearance. He sported a "skinhead"-type haircut. He exhibited an odd, shuffling gait, and he walked in a hunched-over position. He was friendly at times; however, rapport with him was minimal. Although Dan engaged in some spontaneous conversation, he did not elaborate in responding to most verbal questions. Dan tended to respond slowly, and he was hypoactive.

General motor coordination skills appeared to be poor. Overall, however, he was attentive to the tasks at hand. He exhibited a low level of tolerance for frustration, and he was sometimes careless. His level of motivation was variable and related to task demands. For example, Dan was much better motivated during verbal, as opposed to nonverbal, tasks. With respect to his low tolerance for frustration, Dan would often refuse to attempt to answer or complete difficult test items even when he had sufficient time to do so. This was especially true for nonverbal items. Overall, it is clear that we can place more confidence in the reliability of this boy's adequate performances than we can in those that were deficient. However, it is felt that we obtained a good estimate of his neuropsychological functioning in this examination.

Summary of Impressions and Recommendations

Dan evidenced some areas of adequate functioning within the context of other skill areas that were quite deficient. Given the variability in Dan's levels of performance on this test battery, his Wechsler Adult Intelligence Scale—Revised (WAIS-R) Full Scale IQ of 79 provides little, if any, information regarding his current level of functioning. Table 18.2 presents a summary of Dan's scores on intellectual and academic measures.

With respect to basic auditory–perceptual skills and language functioning, language component skills were at least age-appropriate. He had no difficulty in attending to or in discriminating auditory rhythms, in matching sounds and symbols, in verbal fluency, or in remembering auditory–verbal input in short- or long-term memory. He made no aphasic errors on the Aphasia Screening Test. Although his receptive language vocabulary and rote-verbal skills were somewhat deficient, these performances were likely the result of some form of language and/or environmental deprivation (e.g., poor investment in the educational process, inconsistent educational opportunities, and/or poor language models during earlier developmental periods). On the other hand, his difficulty on the WAIS-R Comprehension subtest may be attributed to his poor abstraction skills.

In addition to adequate performances on tests of attention and memory for auditory–verbal input, Dan's performances on tests of reading (i.e., single-word recognition) and spelling to dictation were above average and average, respectively. However, it was also clear that his reading comprehension and mechanical arithmetic skills were quite deficient. His poor performance in mechanical arithmetic probably reflected a combination of his difficulty in understanding or comprehending mathematical processes and a lack of adequate instruction in this area.

Dan evidenced considerable difficulty on a task involving tactile perception (i.e., fingertip number writing). Also, he was quite deficient

TABLE 18.2. Neuropsychological Test Results for
Dan, a 17-Year, 9-Month-Old Youth

Wechsler Adult Intelligence Scale—Revised	
Verbal IQ	95
Performance IQ	67
Full Scale IQ	79
Information	6
Comprehension	7
Arithmetic	9
Similarities	8
Vocabulary	7
Digit Span	9
Picture Completion	5
Picture Arrangement	5
Block Design	4
Object Assembly	3
Digit Symbol	6
Peabody Picture Vocabulary Test—Revised	
Standard score	82
Centile rank	12
Age equivalent	13 yr, 8 mo
Wide Range Achievement Test—Revised	
Reading (grade equiv.)	>12
Spelling (grade equiv.)	12B
Arithmetic (grade equiv.)	7B
Peabody Individual Achievement Test	
Reading comprehension (grade equiv.)	7.2

on a task requiring "hands on" learning, psychomotor coordination, and strategy generation (i.e., Tactual Performance Test). The usual positive practice effect expected on repeated trials of this test was not evident. His incidental memory for information gleaned from the latter test was also quite poor.

Dan performed in a moderately impaired manner on tests of simple motor functioning (i.e., finger tapping, grip strength) with the right hand; his performances on these measures with the left hand were severely impaired. His performance on a test of speeded eye–hand coordination was severely impaired with both hands.

In addition to tactile–perceptual and motor deficiencies, Dan performed in a clearly impaired manner on tasks of a visual–spatial nature. The latter included the perception of visual detail, appreciation of cause-and-effect relationships presented pictorially, visual–spatial organization and synthesis, visual–motor output, and short- and long-term memory for simple line drawings.

Dan's performance on a test of conceptual flexibility under symbolic shifting conditions was quite poor; the latter was indicative of problems in visual scanning, in planning, in keeping more than one idea in his mind at the same time, and in impulse control. He also had trouble on a nonverbal test of conceptual flexibility under more ambiguous conditions (i.e., Wisconsin Card-Sorting Test). The number of perseverative errors he evidenced was in the mildly to moderately impaired range. Dan had difficulty in maintaining psychological set. The latter performance suggested that Dan has difficulty in shifting and in maintaining thoughts or ideas.

Dan also performed in a mildly to moderately impaired manner on one complex nonverbal test involving concept formation, ability to benefit from immediate positive and negative informational feedback, hypothesis testing, and deductive reasoning skills (i.e., Category Test). His performance on this test suggests that Dan would be expected to experience marked problems in gaining insight into his own or others' behaviors, in seeing things from alternate perspectives, or in understanding complex, abstract, or novel informational input.

Dan's projective drawings were marked by clear evidence of emotional immaturity, a pathological difficulty in being accessible to others, overdefensiveness, and a felt lack of psychological warmth and/or emotional stimulation in the home. Very strong indications of hostility and aggression were noted, and, when repressed, these feelings would be the cause of considerable inner tension. Feelings of ambivalence, indecision, impotence, and futility were evident, as was a tendency to withdraw from social relationships. Dan tended to fixate on the past and to fear future events. He evidenced a precarious personality balance that was unable to assist in satisfying strong, basic needs. Dan had a desire to secure frank, immediate emotional satisfaction through behaving in an impulsive manner. His feelings of inadequacy, coupled by castration-like fears, were a strong source of anxiety for him. His projective drawings also provided indications of urethral eroticism, auditory hallucinations, and schizoid tendencies.

Although certainly not diagnostic of any active neuropathological condition, Dan's particular pattern of test results is consistent with the presence of cerebral impairment. However, these findings do *not* support those of a previous neuropsychological examination, which suggested left parietal lobe involvement. Although Dan does have poorly developed rote verbal skills (e.g., general information, word definition skills, comprehension of common social problem situations, and receptive word vocabulary), he performed quite well on tests of reading, spelling, sound–symbol matching, and verbal fluency. His poor rote verbal skills were likely the result of some form of language deprivation rather than of brain dysfunction. More to the point, Dan evidenced a pattern of abilities and deficits indicative of a nonverbal learning disability. These deficiencies appear to be of a longstanding, static, and chronic nature.

Dan exhibited both emotional problems and neuropsychological deficiencies that serve to interact and exacerbate one another. For instance, his preverbal and later physical and emotional traumas may have been a primary cause of anger, hostility, and other unresolved transference issues, sexual identity confusion, impulsiveness, and a poor capacity for emotional attachments. These emotional problems, when coupled with neuropsychological deficiencies in the areas of abstract thinking, conceptual flexibility, nonverbal skills, sensorimotor functioning, and social skill development, put Dan in the worst of all possible scenarios. Clearly, prognosis for this youth is quite poor. Given his poor abstract reasoning skills and ability to gain insight into his own or others' behaviors, it is unlikely that insight-oriented individual psychotherapy would be beneficial. Rather, a behavior modification approach to management may be more successful. The latter would be especially helpful in decreasing negative and self-injurious behaviors. Other recommendations appropriate to treatment are provided by Rourke (1989).

Acknowledgments

The author would like to thank Mary L. Stewart and Byron P. Rourke for their thoughtful comments and editorial expertise.

Reference

Rourke, B. P. (1989). *Nonverbal learning disabilities: The syndrome and the model.* New York: Guilford Press.

CHAPTER 19

Case Studies of Adults with Nonverbal Learning Disabilities

Linas A. Bieliauskas

The syndrome of nonverbal learning disabilities (NLD) is seen as predisposing for the development of psychopathology in adolescents and adults, especially depression and suicidal tendencies (Rourke, Young, & Leenaars, 1989). This is felt to result from the handicap NLD deficits impose on dealing effectively with complex novel situations, determining appropriate behavior in rapidly shifting social contexts, and efficiently planning behaviors and constructing behavioral hierarchies in seeking academic and occupational achievement. Individuals with NLD are generally frustrated with their inability to succeed in life even though their scholastic preparation and general intellectual abilities suggest a far greater potential. It is thus possible that NLD may be a general contributor to significant subgroups of psychopathology that heretofore have been regarded as having only psychological/behavioral etiologies.

Case descriptions of adults with NLD are limited because of the relative recency of the recognition of this syndrome (Rourke, 1982, 1988, 1989) as well as the additional diagnostic complications that arise in neuropsychological assessment of adults as a result of their extended developmental, social, and academic histories. Because of such complications, it should not be expected that diagnostic findings will necessarily be as clean or singular as might be seen in children; frequently, the determination of NLD contributions to presentations of psychopathological syndromes will be a clinical judgment of relative impact rather than an identification of a singular etiology.

In the section below, we describe three adult individuals whom we have diagnosed as having NLD. All three have had lifelong social difficulties and many contacts with mental health professionals over the years. They present with significant learning and work difficulties and clinically significant distress and depression on psychological testing. For all these patients, the identification of NLD provided valuable diagnostic insight and, in two of these cases, resulted in effective treatment referrals or programs.

Case 1

This individual is a right-handed 45-year-old married male with 12 years of education (no graduation) who has worked as a refrigeration maintenance worker. As a child, he had a febrile episode, at which time he reports "the doctors said I was dead" and after which he was resuscitated with the comment that "I was brain damaged." The patient had a history of psychiatric problems since age 28, which he describes as "nerves." Since the plant for which he had worked closed a year earlier, the patient has been unemployed. The patient's siblings were highly successful, one a physician and another an attorney.

Of particular interest for this patient were complaints of memory difficulties for the past 1 to 2 years. The patient's father had died a year earlier of presumed progressive dementia, although an autopsy had not been performed. Concern was expressed that this patient was manifesting a familial expression of primary degenerative dementia.

As can be seen in Figure 19.1, the patient showed a pattern of cognitive difficulties that resembled NLD: Performance IQ < Verbal IQ; lowered Arithmetic achievement test scores; and decreased nonverbal memory. He also evidenced significant psychological distress, as can be seen on the Minnesota Multiphasic Personality Inventory (MMPI).

Analysis of additional neuropsychological test data did not suggest the presence of a primary progressive dementia. The patient's cognitive difficulties were felt to result from expected NLD characteristics, with acute exacerbation from depression and distress related to environmental factors.

In this case, recognition of the patient's risk for, and exhibition of, the NLD syndrome aided in a differential diagnosis from a progressive dementia. It also aided in the provision of recommendations to continue psychiatric treatment and referral for verbal psychotherapeutic intervention (as illustrated in Case 3, below), which can be particularly valuable for these patients.

Case 2

The second individual is a single 24-year-old male who has been variously diagnosed as having minimal brain dysfunction, dyscalculia, left hemisphere dysfunction, etc. throughout his life. He was born prema-

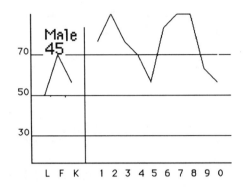

WAIS-R: VIQ = 93
PIQ = 82
FSIQ = 87

WMS: Logical Memory = 5
Memory for Designs = 6
Paired Associates = 18
MQ = 94

WRAT-R GRADE LEVELS: Reading = 7E
Spelling = 4B
Arithmetic = 5E

FIGURE 19.1. MMPI and cognitive scores for 45-year-old male. WAIS-R, Wechsler Adult Intelligence Scale—Revised; VIQ, Verbal IQ; PIQ, Performance IQ; FSIQ, Full Scale IQ; WMS, Wechsler Memory Scale; MQ, Memory Quotient; WRAT-R, Wide Range Achievement Test—Revised.

turely and evidenced multiple medical problems, including allergies, strabismus, and delayed milestones for walking and talking. Currently, he was neither employed nor studying. He was a junior in a special college program for dyslexics. He was not able to continue studies, primarily because of difficulty with math but also because of general academic difficulties.

This patient was the youngest of four siblings, with the others being quite successful, obtaining professional degrees. The patient, in addition to his academic difficulties, was described as extremely clumsy, having suffered job injuries in even simple tasks. Evaluation was requested to clarify the nature of the patient's learning difficulties.

This patient's test data, as seen in Figure 19.2, represent a classic NLD picture, with decreased Performance IQ, and nonverbal memory, visuospatial abilities, and arithmetic achievement being disproportionately deficient. Of particular interest for this patient, test data were available from the age of 6.5 (also in Figure 19.2), which showed mild tendencies in the direction of NLD, although extensive testing in this regard was not done at the time.

Based on this evaluation, we were able to recommend placement in a day hospital psychiatric program that emphasized development of social skills and verbal processing of contextual social and environmental information. The patient is currently entering such a treatment program. More specific identification of use and rationale for such strategies is provided in the description of the next patient.

Case 3

This patient was a married 29-year-old attorney who, although having completed law school, was essentially functioning as a legal clerk in a large firm. He had an extensive psychiatric history, having been in psychotherapy for the previous 10 years. He was socially awkward and could not understand why learning and achieving were labored for him.

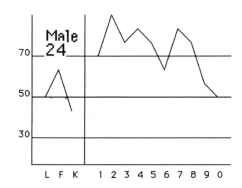

WAIS-R: VIQ = 112   WMS: Logical Memory = 12.5
        PIQ = 88   Memory for Deigns = 8.0
        FSIQ = 104   Paired Associates = 21.0
                                     MQ = 106

WRAT-R Grade Levels: Reading = 12
                        Spelling = 11
                        Arithmetic = 6

Scores at Age 6.5

WISC: VIQ = 86   WRAT GRADE LEVEL: Reading = 1.3
      PIQ = 87   Spelling = K-7
      FSIQ = 104   Arithmetic = K-4

FIGURE 19.2. MMPI and cognitive scores for 24-year-old male. Abbreviations as in Figure 19.1.

He complained that he was having a difficult time getting along with his boss because "he says I ask too many questions." He also complained of difficulty in understanding what he was reading. After assessment by another psychologist, the possibility of an unusual "learning disability" was raised, following which a time-limited treatment program was devised for the patient.

As can be seen in Figure 19.3, this patient also demonstrated an NLD-like syndrome with decreased PIQ, decreased nonverbal memory, and slightly decreased arithmetic abilities. Based on the NLD interpretation and the patient's reported difficulties, a time-limited, 10-week therapeutic program was devised to aid the patient in using his strengths to compensate for his weaknesses:

1. Hypnotic/relaxation procedures were instituted to teach the patient to relax in stressing situations. This was based on the logic that, if the patient had to employ unusual cognitive strategies in given circumstances, lowered arousal levels would aid judgment.

2. Syllogistic logic was taught to the patient. This approach was used because, in NLD right hemisphere functions are deficient, whereas left hemisphere functions remain intact. Thus, the individual with NLD has difficulty dealing with novel gestalt-like situations (including social interactions), although the systematic employment of overlearned strategies is unaffected. Based on the proposal by Semmes (1968) that the left hemisphere has focal representation integration of similar sensorimotor units that are necessary for behaviors such as speech, it was felt that the use of logic, which requires specific language-related rules, should also be preferentially regulated by the left hemisphere. Our approach was to teach the patient to make a syllogistic, logical analysis of a variety of social and work situations and to check his conclusions against his premises. Thus, it was hoped that left hemisphere functions could be used to compensate for deficient right hemisphere functions. After initial drills in the use of syllogistic logic, the patient was taught to employ it in the following manner: He was to delay immediate responding in as many situations as he could, relaxing, and making a logical analysis before engaging in behaviors; he was to do this particularly when he felt unsure about how to act or felt awkward; he was to order perceptual hierarchies clearly when making a logical analysis; he was to decide what was important as opposed to not important in a given situation and to let the important aspects of a situation guide him in deciding on his behavior.

3. The patient was instructed to use his wife as a "sounding-board" in social situations. He was to listen to her guidance and to look at her behavior when guiding his own.

4. He was instructed to read material in a paragraph-by-paragraph fashion and to construct a sentence summarizing each paragraph. Again,

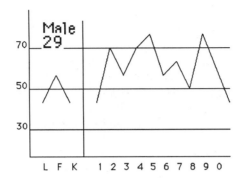

WAIS-R: VIQ = 112
PIQ = 84
FSIQ = 99

WMS: Logical Memory = 10
Memory for Designs = 6
Paired Associates = 11.5
MQ = 99

WRAT-R GRADE LEVELS: Reading = 11-2
Spelling = 10-7
Arithmetic = 10-4

FIGURE 19.3. MMPI and cognitive test data for 29-year-old male. Abbreviations as in Figure 19.1.

this strategy was designed to take advantage of purportedly unaffected language and processing of more discrete elements (left hemisphere functions).

5. The patient was instructed to obtain practice books for the Graduate Record Exam and the Law School Aptitude Test and to concentrate on reading comprehension and logical analysis sections, checking his own answers against the given ones. He was to practice with these books one-half hour per day.

6. Finally, the patient was instructed to read short stories and then to watch video representations of those stories (e.g., Hemingway's *The Old Man and the Sea*).

The patient was drilled in these procedures on a daily basis for a 10-week period. He made records of his syllogistic analyses and paragraph summaries, and these were reviewed and corrected as necessary. This procedure was done, of course, in the context of a supportive therapeutic setting.

The patient felt that his work and social contact were much easier as the result of his treatment, and he reported that his boss was not irritated with him any more. He also felt that he was understanding what he read much better and more quickly. He did not feel that the viewing of videos and reading stories were of great benefit, and he did not feel he had the time to continue effectively with reviews of practice books for exams.

Several months after the termination of treatment, the patient's primary therapist indicated that he felt that the patient's program had provided immense benefits and the patient had made significant progress during this brief period within the context of his years of therapy. The patient has contacted us occasionally since then, indicating that he continues to practice his skills and benefit from the procedures suggested.

Conclusions

The identification of NLD in adults has tremendous potential in identifying cognitive deficits that may subtly predispose individuals to a variety of forms of psychopathology and lifelong coping difficulties. Further understanding of how NLD interacts with other psychological variables may help explicate the development of behavioral disturbance in a wide variety of individuals. Certainly, identification of NLD is an aid in differential diagnoses, especially in older individuals. And, as we have suggested, it provides a logical basis for development of effective treatment strategies, even for persons who are older and have multiple contributing factors to their presenting difficulties.

References

Rourke, B. P. (1982). Central processing deficiencies in children: Toward a developmental neuropsychological model. *Journal of Clinical Neuropsychology, 4*, 1–18.

Rourke, B. P. (1988). The syndrome of nonverbal learning disabilities: Developmental manifestations in neurological disease, disorder, and dysfunction. *The Clinical Neuropsychologist, 2*, 293–330.

Rourke, B. P. (1989). *Nonverbal learning disabilities: The syndrome and the model.* New York: Guilford Press.

Rourke, B. P., Young, G. C., & Leenaars, A. A. (1989). A childhood learning disability that predisposes those afflicted to adolescent and adult depression and suicide risk. *Journal of Learning Disabilities, 22*, 169–187.

Semmes, J. S. (1968). Hemispheric specialization: A possible clue to mechanism. *Neuropsychologia, 6* 11–25.

Current Status and Future Directions

CHAPTER 20

Neuropsychological Validation Studies in Perspective

Byron P. Rourke

In Chapter 1, validity was defined as truth. Now that we have come to the conclusion of this work, it is reasonable to ask: What truth has been discovered? What do we know now, with some degree of certainty, that we did not know, or knew only vaguely, before? Although the contents of this volume cannot be summarized adequately in a few words, the following are some of the major dimensions of validity that emerge from these investigations. These conclusions regarding the validity of neuropsychological subtypes are especially necessary to frame, because the significant questions yet to be answered flow from them.

Conclusions

1. The manner in which measures of psychometric intelligence are employed in the definition of learning disabilities has an important effect upon the definition of learning disabilities. In consequence, the manner in which measures of psychometric intelligence are used, in conjunction with other criteria, to define learning disability in the individual case will have an important impact upon whether a child will be designated as eligible for special educational and other services. More generally, the identification of the learning-disabled population itself is dependent upon such definitions. Thus, this issue is of both clinical and scientific importance, and the analysis presented in Chapter 2 is a significant step forward in the resolution of this problem.

2. Profile analysis is a potentially powerful statistical tool for the determination of the reliability and validity of learning disability subtypes. Because it appears that *patterns* of performance are much more relevant than are *levels* of performance in such determinations, the ability

to evaluate such patterns (profiles) in a systematic and objective fashion is of considerable potential import.

3. Unless iterative relocation procedures used in the designation of learning disability subtypes are deployed with care, spurious conclusions may be drawn regarding the number and characteristics of subtypes that obtain in a given data set. This dimension of reliability has important implications for the validation of learning disability subtypes. For example, the failure to produce reliable subtypes may lie at the root of the failure to validate them against external criteria. It may also be the case that the investigator will attribute erroneously high levels of reliability to a particular subtype solution if iterative relocation and related procedures are deployed in a less than systematic and thoughtful fashion. In such cases, the investigator would do well to examine the reliability of the subtype classification that is being used rather than to continue the search for validity.

4. Phonetic accuracy of misspellings can serve as a very robust marker of neuropsychological integrity in the child with learning disabilities. The very large amount of variance accounted for by this easily measured variable is particularly impressive. Both the concurrent and the predictive validity of this dimension have been established.

5. The mnestic problems of some subtypes of learning-disabled youngsters vary in a rather predictable manner. In some cases, these differences are rather dramatic. One implication of these findings is that methods of academic intervention would, presumably, need to be quite different for these different subtypes of learning-disabled children. The theoretical implications of such findings, if replicated, are significant.

6. Relatively young (i.e., 7- and 8-year-old) children classified into subtypes on the basis of patterns of academic achievement in word recognition, spelling, and arithmetic exhibit patterns of performance that are somewhat similar to those of older (9- to 14-year-old) children who are subtyped on the same basis. However, it is abundantly clear that the differences evident between the two age groups far outweigh their similarities. This is another demonstration of the rather fragile (i.e., unreliable) nature of subtypes that are studied at tender ages.

7. There is considerable evidence to suggest that the L- and P-type dyslexia subtypes are reliable and valid. This evidence arises from a variety of sources, including studies employing electrophysiological recordings as dependent measures. There is emerging evidence to suggest that there are varying degrees of concurrent, predictive, and clinical validity for this classification method. There is also some evidence of construct validation for this typology.

8. The reliability and validity of learning disability subtypes appears to have a fairly sound cross-cultural basis.

9. There are reliable subtypes of psychosocial functioning exhibited by learning-disabled children. Furthermore, there is emerging evidence for the concurrent validity of these subtypes.

10. It is possible to discern reliable differences between subtypes of children who exhibit relatively normal levels of word recognition and impaired levels of mechanical arithmetic performance. Furthermore, there is evidence for the concurrent validity of these subtypes when their patterns of cognitive and personality functioning are examined.

11. Although fraught with numerous methodological and logistical difficulties, evidence supporting the concurrent and clinical validity of subtypes of children with reading disabilities is emerging. This evidence suggests strongly that the aptitude × treatment interaction has validity when the aptitude dimension is specified in terms of reliable subtyping procedures.

12. Adults with learning disabilities can be subtyped in a reliable fashion. These subtypes bear a strong resemblance to those isolated in children, and the initial concurrent validity studies of these adult subtypes are encouraging.

13. Large-scale studies of adults with various subtypes of learning disabilities suggest that the aptitude × treatment interaction is also valid.

14. Subtypes of arithmetic-disabled adults are quite similar to those identified in arithmetic-disabled children. Several dimensions of subtype validity in this domain are beginning to emerge.

15. The process of construct validation of the nonverbal learning disabilities (NLD) subtype is proceeding apace. Initial results suggest strong support for deductions based upon the NLD model.

16. The long-term impact of the NLD syndrome (subtype) on personality adjustment and patterns of adaptive functioning appears to be profound. This demonstration of the predictive validity of the NLD model is particularly important for treatment planning.

17. Initial studies of the clinical validity of the NLD syndrome have borne fruitful results in several different laboratories. These studies suggest that the proposed dynamics of the NLD syndrome and the model that was designed to encompass its complex manifestations have an important bearing on assessment and intervention with children, adolescents, and adults who exhibit the syndrome.

Future Directions

1. It is clear that important questions surrounding the definition of learning disabilities are not yet resolved. However, as has been suggested on a number of occasions (Rourke, 1983a, 1983b, 1985), the situation

regarding definition(s) is likely to be resolved satisfactorily only insofar as the issues regarding the reliability and validity of learning disability subtypes are resolved. We have generic definitions with which the vast majority of investigators can agree. What is required at this point are several definitions—one for each reliable and valid subtype. (For an attempt to do just that, the interested reader is referred to Rourke, 1989, Chap. 7.) It is clear that the systematic investigation of the validity of specific subtypes is a fruitful path to follow if we are to generate such definitions. A good start has been made in the case of the NLD subtype with respect to concurrent, predictive, construct, and clinical validity, and with the subtypes generated by Lyon and his colleagues with respect to concurrent, predictive, and clinical validity. The L and P typology of Bakker is another example of subtypes wherein rigorous investigation can lead to the specification of valid classifications (whose quintessential features are the dimensions of valid definitions). The promise shown to this point in this pursuit should encourage investigators to pursue this tack with even more vigor.

2. Although filled with considerable promise, we have yet to demonstrate the potential of profile-analytic techniques in the subtyping enterprise. It is clear that systematic application of such techniques will proceed at a vigorous pace during the next few years. Efforts to apply confirmatory factor analysis and structural equation methods to tests commonly used in the measurement of neuropsychologically relevant dimensions of human performance (e.g., Francis, Fletcher, & Rourke, 1988) should also be of considerable assistance in determining the validity of learning disability subtypes.

3. More generally, it will be the case that more in-depth analysis of statistical techniques, such as cluster analysis, will continue unabated. Unless we understand fully the potential pitfalls in the application of such techniques to learning disability subtyping, our efforts to use them in the initial stages of hypothesis generation will come to naught.

4. Dimensions relating to the phonetic accuracy of misspellings and various types of mnestic assets and deficits in learning disability subtypes should be the subject of intense investigation over the next few years. These appear to be prototypical dimensions of neuropsychological functioning that lie at the very heart of the central processing assets and deficits that characterize many learning disability subtypes. It is not possible to underestimate the importance of the specification of the extent to which assets and deficits in various phonological, visual–spatial, and executive processes are involved in learning disability subtypes. The dimensions of predictive validity that are expected to emerge from such analyses can form the conceptual framework for testing subtype $\times$ treatment interactions in a more rigorous fashion than has heretofore been possible.

5. More emphasis on the developmental dimensions of learning disability subtypes would be a natural extension of what we now know about differences in these subtypes at different ages. More investigations of the sort carried out by Morris, Blashfield, and Satz (1987) and those described in Chapters 6, 13, and 14 of this book are to be expected. This type of cross-sectional and longitudinal tracking of learning disability subtypes is crucial for our understanding of the natural history of these subtypes as well as for our efforts to suggest and apply intervention techniques on a rational basis. In the same vein, knowing as much as we can about adults with various subtypes of learning disabilities should be of considerable benefit, both for science and for clinical practice.

6. The application of biopsychological technology in the study of learning disability subtype validity should grow by leaps and bounds. Event-related potential studies of carefully defined subtypes of learning-disabled children (e.g., Stelmack & Miles, 1990) should provide the sort of data needed to piece together the brain–behavior relationships that are of interest to neuropsychological investigators. Dividends flowing from such investigations for both theory and clinical practice should be substantial.

7. That learning disability subtypes appear to be replicable across cultures is an important validity dimension. Currently, systematic replications have been made in Canada, the United States, and The Netherlands. Recent work in Finland (Korhonen, 1988) suggests that such efforts can be extended to other Western cultures. The challenge for the future lies in the cross-validation of learning disability subtypes in other Western and non-Western cultures.

8. Investigation of the socioemotional dimensions of learning disabilities is growing in an exponential fashion. A synthesis of this work will soon appear (Rourke, Fuerst, & DeLuca, in preparation). There is every reason to believe that the psychosocial functioning of learning disability subtypes will be the subject of intensive inquiry over the next few years. One very encouraging aspect of this work is that validity studies have already been carried out with some success (see Chapter 9, this volume). With considerations regarding reliability now largely resolved and initial validity studies showing considerable promise, the way is open to answering significant questions relating to socioemotional adaptation of subtypes of learning-disabled children and adults.

9. Educational validation studies are absolutely essential if we are to further our understanding of the scientific and professional practice implications of the learning disability subtype enterprise. Hence, it is expected that those bold enough to try will pursue this avenue of investigation. We are very much in need of data in this area.

10. The concurrent, predictive, construct, and clinical validity of the NLD subtype is proceeding apace. Extensions of this work to the testing

of deductions derived from the NLD model will expand considerably over the next few years. The extensions of particular interest may very well be in the area of neurological disease and developmental disabilities such as fragile-X syndrome, Williams syndrome, Turner's syndrome, congenital hypothyroidism, autism, closed head injury, hydrocephalus, cerebral palsy, callosal agenesis, multiple sclerosis, AIDS, and the diseases resulting from some neurotoxins and teratogens. The white-matter hypothesis that forms the basis of the NLD neurodevelopmental model will probably come under intensive scientific scrutiny over the next decade.

11. Theory and model building will increase dramatically over the next decade. Circumspect, comprehensive evaluations of the applications of classification methodology (e.g., Morris & Fletcher, 1988) as well as comprehensive models of various learning disability subtypes (e.g., Rourke, 1989) are very much needed if we are to make scientific advances in this area.

Finale

We began this book with the specification of various forms of truth. This epistemological effort was followed by reports on a wide-ranging series of investigations designed to designate the content, concurrent, predictive, construct, and clinical validity of various subtyping efforts. We end with some truth and some additional questions. There is much more to learn, and, undoubtedly, some respecification of what we think we have already learned. Science is like that; the clinical imperatives of learning-disabled children and adults demand it. Let us continue.

References

Francis, D. J., Fletcher, J. M., & Rourke, B. P. (1988). Discriminant validity of lateral sensorimotor measures in children. *Journal of Clinical and Experimental Neuropsychology, 10*, 779–799.

Korhonen, T. (1988) External validity of subgroups of Finnish learning-disabled children. *Journal of Clinical and Experimental Neuropsychology, 10*, 56.

Morris, R., Blashfield, R., & Satz, P. (1986). Developmental classification of reading-disabled children. *Journal of Clinical and Experimental Neuropsychology, 8*, 371–392.

Morris, R. D., & Fletcher, J. M. (1988). Classification in neuropsychology: A theoretical framework and research paradigm. *Journal of Clinical and Experimental Neuropsychology, 10*, 640–658.

Rourke, B. P. (1983a). Outstanding issues in research on learning disabilities. In M. Rutter (Ed.), *Developmental neuropsychiatry* (pp. 564–574). New York: Guilford Press.

Rourke, B. P. (1983b). Reading and spelling disabilities: A developmental neuropsychological perspective. In U. Kirk (Ed.), *Neuropsychology of language, reading, and spelling* (pp. 209-234). New York: Academic Press.

Rourke, B. P. (1985). Overview of learning disability subtypes. In B. P. Rourke (Ed.), *Neuropsychology of learning disabilities: Essentials of subtype analysis* (pp. 3-14). New York: Guilford Press.

Rourke, B. P. (1989). *Nonverbal learning disabilities: The syndrome and the model.* New York: Guilford Press.

Rourke, B. P., Fuerst, D. R., & DeLuca, J. W. (in preparation). *Psychosocial funtioning of learning-disabled children.* New York: Guilford Press.

Stelmack, R. M., & Miles, J. (1990). Effect of picture priming on event-related potentials of normal and disabled readers during a word recognition memory task. *Journal of Clinical and Experimental Neuropsychology, 12.*

Index